Sports Medicine

Editor

BRIAN J. KRABAK

PHYSICAL MEDICINE AND REHABILITATION CLINICS OF NORTH AMERICA

www.pmr.theclinics.com

Consulting Editor
GREGORY T. CARTER

November 2014 • Volume 25 • Number 4

ELSEVIER

1600 John F. Kennedy Boulevard • Suite 1800 • Philadelphia, Pennsylvania, 19103-2899

http://www.theclinics.com

PHYSICAL MEDICINE AND REHABILITATION CLINICS OF NORTH AMERICA Volume 25, Number 4
November 2014 ISSN 1047-9651, ISBN 978-0-323-32385-7

Editor: Jennifer Flynn-Briggs
Developmental Editor: Don Mumford

Reprints. For copies of 100 or more of articles in this publication, please contact the Commercial Reprints Department, Elsevier Inc., 360 Park Avenue South, New York, NY 10010-1710. Tel.: 212-633-3874; Fax: 212-633-3820; E-mail: reprints@elsevier.com.

Physical Medicine and Rehabilitation Clinics of North America (ISSN 1047-9651) is published quarterly by Elsevier Inc., 360 Park Avenue South, New York, NY 10010-1710. Months of issue are February, May, August, and November. Business and Editorial Offices: 1600 John F. Kennedy Blvd., Suite 1800, Philadelphia, PA 19103-2899. Customer Service Office: 3251 Riverport Lane, Maryland Heights, MO 63043. Periodicals postage paid at New York, NY and additional mailing offices. Subscription price per year is $275.00 (US individuals), $486.00 (US institutions), $145.00 (US students), $335.00 (Canadian individuals), $640.00 (Canadian institutions), $210.00 (Canadian students), $415.00 (foreign individuals), $640.00 (foreign institutions), and $210.00 (foreign students). Foreign air speed delivery is included in all *Clinics* subscription prices. All prices are subject to change without notice. **POSTMASTER:** Send address changes to *Physical Medicine and Rehabilitation Clinics of North America*, Customer Service Office: Elsevier Health Sciences Division, Subscription Customer Service, 3251 Riverport Lane, Maryland Heights, MO 63043. **Customer Service: 1-800-654-2452 (US). From outside of the United States, call 314-447-8871. Fax: 314-447-8029. E-mail: JournalsCustomer Service-usa@elsevier.com (for print support); JournalsOnlineSupport-usa@elsevier.com (for online support).**

Physical Medicine and Rehabilitation Clinics of North America is indexed in *Excerpta Medica, MEDLINE/ PubMed (Index Medicus), Cinahl,* and *Cumulative Index to Nursing and Allied Health Literature.*

Contributors

CONSULTING EDITOR

GREGORY T. CARTER, MD, MS
Consulting Medical Editor, Medical Director, St Luke's Rehabilitation Institute, Spokane, Washington; University of Washington, School of Medicine, Seattle, Washington

EDITOR

BRIAN J. KRABAK, MD, MBA, FACSM
Clinical Associate Professor, Rehabilitation, Orthopedics and Sports Medicine, University of Washington and Seattle Children's Sports Medicine; Team Physician, University of Washington and Seattle University; Medical Director, 4 Deserts Ultramarathon and Seattle Rock N Roll Marathon, Seattle, Washington

AUTHORS

PETER J. AMBROSE, PharmD, FASHP
Professor, Department of Clinical Pharmacy, School of Pharmacy, University of California at San Francisco, San Francisco, California

BERDALE COLORADO, DO, MPH
Assistant Professor, Department of Orthopaedic Surgery, Washington University School of Medicine, St Louis, Missouri

LEAH G. CONCANNON, MD
Clinical Assistant Professor, Sports and Spine Division, Department of Rehabilitation Medicine, University of Washington, Seattle, Washington

ARTHUR JASON DE LUIGI, DO
Associate Professor; Director of Sports Medicine, Department of Rehabilitation Medicine, Georgetown University School of Medicine, Washington, DC

NICKOLAS G. GARBIS, MD
Instructor, Department of Orthopaedic Surgery and Rehabilitation, Loyola University, Maywood, Illinois

GARY A. GREEN, MD, Clinical Professor, Division of Sports Medicine, Pacific Palisades Medical Group, University of California, Los Angeles, Pacific Palisades, California

CAROLINE K. HATTON, PhD
Sports Antidoping Science Consultant, Culver City, California

JOHN HEIL, DA
Private Practice, Psychological Health Roanoke, Roanoke, Virginia

STANLEY A. HERRING, MD
Clinical Professor, Departments of Rehabilitation Medicine, Orthopaedics and Sports Medicine, and Neurological Surgery, University of Washington; Co-Medical Director, Sports Concussion Program, Zackery Lystedt Sports Concussion Endowed Professorship; Team Physician, Seattle Seahawks; Team Physician, Seattle Mariners, Seattle, Washington

DEVYANI HUNT, MD
Associate Professor, Department of Orthopaedic Surgery, Washington University School of Medicine, St Louis, Missouri

NANCY KADEL, MD
Orthopaedic Surgeon, Group Health Physicians, Seattle, Washington

MARLA S. KAUFMAN, MD
Clinical Associate Professor, Department of Rehabilitation, Orthopaedics and Sports Medicine, University of Washington, Seattle, Washington

DAVID J. KENNEDY, MD
Clinical Assistant Professor, Department of Orthopaedic Surgery, Stanford University, Redwood City, California

LEE KNEER, MD
Assistant Professor, Departments of Physical Medicine and Rehabilitation and Orthopaedics, Emory Orthopaedics and Spine Center, Atlanta, Georgia

BRIAN J. KRABAK, MD, MBA, FACSM
Clinical Associate Professor, Rehabilitation, Orthopedics and Sports Medicine, University of Washington and Seattle Children's Sports Medicine; Team Physician, University of Washington and Seattle University; Medical Director, 4 Deserts Ultramarathon and Seattle Rock N Roll Marathon, Seattle, Washington

GRANT LIPMAN, MD
Co-Director, Wilderness Medicine Fellowship; Clinical Associate Professor, Division of Emergency Medicine, Department of Surgery, Stanford University School of Medicine, Stanford, California

GERARD MALANGA, MD
Clinical Professor, Department of Physical Medicine & Rehabilitation, Rutgers University-New Jersey Medical School, Newark, New Jersey; Founder and Partner, New Jersey Regenerative Institute, Cedar Knolls, New Jersey

KEN MAUTNER, MD
Director, Primary Care Sports Medicine; Assistant Professor, Departments of Physical Medicine and Rehabilitation and Orthopaedics, Emory Orthopaedics and Spine Center, Atlanta, Georgia

EDWARD G. McFARLAND, MD
The Wayne H Lewis Professor of Orthopaedics and Shoulder Surgery; Co-Director, Division of Shoulder Surgery, Department of Orthopaedic Surgery, The Johns Hopkins University, Baltimore, Maryland

REINA NAKAMURRA, MD
Resident, Department of Physical Medicine & Rehabilitation, Rutgers University-New Jersey Medical School, Newark, New Jersey

STEPHEN PAULUS, MD
Clinical Instructor, Department of Orthopaedic Surgery, Stanford University, Redwood City, California

JUDITH R. PETERSON, MD
Private Practice, Yankton Medical Clinic, Yankton, South Dakota; Clinical Associate Professor, Department of Neurosciences, Sanford School of Medicine, University of South Dakota, Sioux Falls, South Dakota

LESLIE PODLOG, PhD
Department of Exercise and Sport Science, University of Utah, Salt Lake City, Utah

HEIDI PRATHER, DO
Professor, Department of Orthopaedic Surgery, Washington University School of Medicine, St Louis, Missouri

STEFANIE SCHULTE, PhD
Department of Exercise and Sport Science, University of Utah, Salt Lake City, Utah

BRANDEE WAITE, MD
Associate Director, Sports Medicine Fellowship; Associate Professor, Physical Medicine and Rehabilitation, University of California Davis Sports Medicine; Team Physician, University of California Davis, Sacramento, California

Contents

treatment of spinal injuries in adolescent athletes require a coordinated effort between the clinician, patients, parents/guardians, coaches, therapists, and athletic trainers. Treatment should not only help alleviate the current symptoms but also address flexibility and muscle imbalances to prevent future injuries by recognizing and addressing risk factors. Return to sport should be a gradual process once the pain has resolved and the athlete has regained full strength.

Heidi Prather, Berdale Colorado, and Devyani Hunt

Hip and groin pain is commonly experienced by athletes. The differential diagnosis should include both intra-articular and extra-articular sources for pain and dysfunction. A comprehensive history and physical examination can guide the evaluation of hip pain and the potential need for further diagnostics. Treatment of athletes with hip disorders includes education, addressing activities of daily living, pain-modulating medications or modalities, exercise and sports modification, and therapeutic exercise. Surgical techniques for prearthritic hip disorders are expanding and can offer appropriate patients a successful return to athletic endeavors when conservative measures are not effective.

Judith R. Peterson and Brian J. Krabak

Anterior cruciate ligament (ACL) injury is a common sports injury which can have severe negative consequences. Neuromuscular factors that increase risk, such as knee landing kinematics, may be ameliorated through training. Effective ACL injury prevention programs exist, although the ideal program is yet to be determined. It is recommended that athletes engaged in high-risk sports participate in an ACL injury prevention program to reduce the risk of sustaining this injury.

Nancy Kadel

The dancer's foot and ankle are subjected to high forces and unusual stresses in training and performance. Injuries are common in dancers, and the foot and ankle are particularly vulnerable. Ankle sprains, ankle impingement syndromes, flexor hallucis longus tendonitis, cuboid subluxation, stress fractures, midfoot injuries, heel pain, and first metatarsophalangeal joint problems including hallux valgus, hallux rigidus, and sesamoid injuries will be reviewed. This article will discuss these common foot and ankle problems in dancers and give typical clinical presentation and diagnostic and treatment recommendations.

Brian J. Krabak, Brandee Waite, and Grant Lipman

Participation in ultramarathon races and knowledge of these athletes continues to increase as the sport becomes more popular. Physicians and athletes need to better understand the impact of the unique aspects of ultramarathon races, such as race environment (temperature, humidity, and altitude), race distance, race stages, nutritional requirements and equipment, on athlete injuries and illness. Proper treatment of injuries and illnesses during an ultramarathon race is important for avoiding long-term medical issues. In this article, the evaluation and treatment of common musculoskeletal injuries and medical illnesses in ultramarathon runners are reviewed.

Pain and dysfunction related to tendinopathy are often refractory to traditional treatments and offer a unique challenge to physicians, because no gold standard treatment exists. Injectable biologics may represent a new modality in conjunction with a multifaceted treatment approach. Platelet-rich plasma (PRP) injections are not associated with the systemic or tendon degradation risks of corticosteroids or the inherent risks of surgery. Studies are promising but have not been replicated with high-powered evidence at the clinical level. Further evidence to expand understanding of the role of PRP in the treatment of tendinopathy is needed.

Traditional treatment of sports injuries includes use of the PRICE principle (Protection, Rest, Ice, Compression, Elevation), nonsteroidal anti-inflammatories, physical therapy modalities, and corticosteroid injections. Recent evidence has raised concerns over this traditional treatment approach regarding the use of anti-inflammatories and injectable corticosteroids. More recent treatments, known as regenerative medicine, include platelet-rich plasma and stem cell therapies. Evidence for their efficacy in a variety of sports injuries has emerged, ranging from tendinopathy and muscle tears to ligament and chondral injuries. This article reviews the literature regarding established treatments for sports injuries and these more innovative treatments.

To help clinicians understand the risks associated with performance-enhancing drugs, this overview covers prohibited lists of substances and methods, therapeutic use exemptions, the legitimate indications and adverse effects, including for megadose and polypharmacy doping of stimulants, anabolic steroids, erythropoiesis-stimulating agents, and growth hormone and ways in which physicians or patients risk committing anti-doping rule violations inadvertently.

This article discusses the principles and practices that guide psychological intervention with injury, and encourages a psychological approach to injury for clinicians. Part 1 reviews the research literature, and serves as a foundation for the review of clinical practices in part 2. Examination of the research literature highlights 4 areas: (1) psychological factors influencing rehabilitation, (2) social factors affecting rehabilitation, (3) performance concerns among returning athletes, and (4) tools/inventories for assessing psychological readiness to return. A synopsis of an injury intervention plan is provided, and the influence of pain and fear in the rehabilitation process is described.

PHYSICAL MEDICINE AND REHABILITATION CLINICS OF NORTH AMERICA

VISIT THE CLINICS ONLINE!
Access your subscription at:
www.theclinics.com

NOW AVAILABLE FOR YOUR iPhone and iPad

Foreword

Sports Medicine

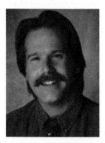

Gregory T. Carter, MD, MS
Consulting Editor

Sports medicine has always been a little bit difficult to define in my mind. A lot of medical specialties and ancillary health care providers have laid claim to the term. Sports medicine is truly a field that cannot be confined to a singular group. Much like our own parent field of physical medicine and rehabilitation, sports medicine involves health care professionals, researchers, and educators from a wide variety of disciplines, in an interdisciplinary fashion, to help prevent and treat injuries in athletes.

Given the importance and broad applicability of this topic, I wanted a really strong issue on sports medicine and I knew just the guy to ask to be guest editor: Dr Brian Krabak. Brian brings so much to the table here. First and foremost, he is a brilliant academic physician, specializing in sports medicine. However, he is also himself an elite athlete, having competed in more than 30 endurance events, including 24-hour and 36-hour adventure races. He not only "talks the talk" but he also "walks the walk" (granted he might be doing sprinting intervals while using the walking part to recover). I knew Brian would recruit the best of the best to be his authors, in a carefully selected list of important topics. Indeed, he came through in spades here.

Starting out this issue is a "Concussion Update" by Dr Stan Herring. Stan is medical director of Sports, Spine, and Orthopedic Health at University of Washington (UW) Medicine and co-medical director of the Sports Concussion Program, a partnership between UW Medicine and Seattle Children's Hospital. Dr Herring was a major contributor to the successful passage of the Zackery Lystedt Law[1] in Washington State and helped pass similar legislation in all fifty states and the District of Columbia.

---

[1] The key provisions of the Zackery Lystedt Law include immediate removal of an athlete from the game if concussion is suspected. Youth athletes who have been taken out of a game because of a suspected concussion are not allowed to return to play until after they are evaluated by a health care provider with specific training in the evaluation and management of concussions and receive a written clearance to return to play from that same health care provider.

Phys Med Rehabil Clin N Am 25 (2014) xiii–xv
http://dx.doi.org/10.1016/j.pmr.2014.10.001
1047-9651/14/$ – see front matter © 2014 Elsevier Inc. All rights reserved.

His excellent article brings us up-to-date in this critically important area of sports medicine.

Leading directly from this is an excellent overview entitled, "Treatment of Cervical Spine Injuries and Return to Play Decisions," provided by one of Dr Herring's former mentees, DJ Kennedy, MD. DJ is now faculty in the renowned sports medicine program at Stanford University. Cervical spine injuries are often seen with head injuries and the timely and appropriate management of these injuries is of critical importance. Dr Kennedy's article provides critical guidelines.

"Shoulder Pain in the Throwing Athlete" is provided by Edward McFarland, MD, the Wayne H. Lewis Professor of Orthopedics and Shoulder Surgery at Johns Hopkins School of Medicine. Dr McFarland is world renowned for his work in shoulder surgery and provides a fantastic treatise on the workup and management of shoulder pain in the athlete.

Back pain in the adolescent athlete is thoroughly covered and discussed by Dr Arthur Jason De Luigi, the Director of Sports Medicine at Med Star National Rehabilitation Hospital, and Program Director of the Med Star National Rehabilitation Hospital/Georgetown University Hospital Sports Medicine Fellowship. Dr De Luigi is internationally recognized as a leader in Adaptive Sports Medicine through his extensive experience with disabled athletes, holding positions as the Medical Director and Head Team Physician for the US Adaptive Alpine Ski Team.

An excellent summary of "Managing Hip Pain in the Athlete" is provided by Dr Heidi Prather, Associate Professor of Orthopedic Surgery and Chief of the Section in Physical Medicine and Rehabilitation at Washington University School of Medicine. Dr Prather is also faculty in the Center for Adolescent and Young Adult Hip Disorders at Washington University.

"Prevention of ACL Injuries in the Athlete" is very nicely covered by Dr Judith Peterson from the University of South Dakota. ACL injuries are common in athletes of all ages. As youth sports become increasingly competitive, ACL tears are occurring in athletes at younger ages. Sustaining the injury can mean surgery, months of rehab, thousands of dollars in medical bills, and a higher likelihood of knee problems later in life; so, prevention is critical.

Foot and Ankle Injuries in the Dancer are covered in a remarkable article by Nancy Kadel, MD, a dancer herself, who founded the Seattle Dance Medicine Free Clinic at Group Health. Dr Kadel's idea was to have a multidisciplinary clinic for evaluating common dance-related injuries available for dancers at no cost. Many working dancers are uninsured or underinsured so this guarantees access and allows Dr Kadel and her staff to educate the dancers about their bodies, proper rest, and recovery to their training.

Dr Krabak himself takes on the "Evaluation and Treatment of Injuries in the Ultra-Endurance Running Athlete." Brain is well suited for this topic because he cares for endurance athletes and has plenty of experience himself in the intense mental and physical preparation needed to take on the relentless challenges faced by ultra-endurance running athletes.

A superb overview of "Treatment of Tendonopathies with Platelet-rich Plasma" is provided by Dr Ken Mautner. Dr Mautner is a nationally recognized expert in diagnostic and interventional musculoskeletal ultrasound and regularly performs platelet-rich plasma injections for patients with chronic tendinopathy in his clinics at Emory University.

Regenerative medicine is an emerging branch of medicine focused on replacing, engineering, or regenerating human cells, tissues, or organs to restore or establish normal function. This topic is sublimely covered by Dr Gerry Malanga in his article entitled, "Role of Regenerative Medicine." Dr Malanga is the Director of PM&R Sports Medicine Fellowship at Atlantic Sports and Health Director and Pain Management at Overlook Hospital. He is the head team physician for New Jersey City University and is a consultant to the Rutgers University Athletic Department as well.

Following the rise and fall of Lance Armstrong, the role of drugs that athletes might use to gain an edge on the competition is a paramount topic today in sports medicine. Dr Caroline Hatton, former Associate Director of the University of California at Los Angeles Olympic Laboratory, has spent her career helping improve methods of testing athletes for performance-enhancing drugs. Her article on "Performance-enhancing Drugs: Understanding the Risks" is a first-rate overview of this critically important topic. In her spare time, she writes books for children and also about drugs in sports for readers of all ages.

Finally, another tremendous article entitled, "Psychosocial Factors Impact on Sports Rehabilitation," is provided by Dr Leslie Podlog, from the Department of Exercise and Sport Science at the University of Utah School of Medicine.

I want to give my sincerest thanks to Dr Krabak and to all of the extraordinary authors he recruited to bring together this timely and very useful issue of the *Physical Medicine and Rehabilitation Clinics of North America*. I suspect this issue will find its way out of physician offices and into locker rooms and onto training tables and even on to the fields of competition themselves.

Gregory T. Carter, MD, MS
St Luke's Rehabilitation Institute
711 South Cowley Street
Spokane, WA 99202, USA

E-mail address:
gtcarter@uw.edu

Preface

Sports Medicine

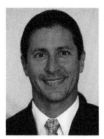

Brian J. Krabak, MD, MBA, FACSM
Editor

The field of sports medicine is living in a tale of two cities: the best of times and the worst of times. It's an exciting time, where the boundaries of athleticism and technology are being pushed. We have seen the evolution of extreme sports, including the X Games and long distance running races in extreme terrains for hundreds of miles. Athletes are sustaining a level of peak fitness at an older age, challenging our notion of athletic decline. Technological advances have now allowed us to better understand the pathophysiology of injury and recovery. We can now tap into an athlete's own cells and tissue to optimize growth factors and, potentially, stem cells, to promote healing and speed recovery.

At the same time, it's a time where athletes are willing to utilize anything in order to win. The pressure stems from astronomical salaries in excess of $100 million and egos enjoying fame. Athletes are now willing to fly anywhere in the world to try interventions that still need better randomized controlled studies to see if they truly work. Longitudinal studies are needed to understand the long-term implications of these interventions. Unfortunately, this sends the wrong message to youth athletes, who are more likely to notice the tweets, notoriety, and "money shots" on the Internet than the disability and dementia these athletes may experience later in life.

With this in mind, the current issue on "Sports Medicine" is a comprehensive, multidisciplinary state-of-the-art review focusing on the athlete as a whole in the world we live in. The articles explore the impact of excessive activity, new therapies, and performance enhancement interventions on the musculoskeletal, neurological, and psychological aspects of the athlete. Only by better understanding the balance of

Phys Med Rehabil Clin N Am 25 (2014) xvii–xviii
http://dx.doi.org/10.1016/j.pmr.2014.06.014
pmr.theclinics.com

these factors and potential risks will we be able to promote healthy athleticism for current and future athletes.

Brian J. Krabak, MD, MBA, FACSM
Rehabilitation, Orthopedics, and Sports Medicine
University of Washington
and Seattle Children's Sports Medicine
Seattle, WA 98195, USA

E-mail address:
bkrabak@uw.edu

Evaluation and Treatment of the Concussed Athlete - Update

Marla S. Kaufman, MD[a], Leah G. Concannon, MD[b],*,
Stanley A. Herring, MD[c]

KEYWORDS

- Concussion • Sports injuries • Neuropsychological testing
- Sport Concussion Assessment Tool

KEY POINTS

- Any athlete suspected of sustaining a concussion must be removed from play and evaluated by a health care professional. There is no same day return to play.
- Athletes with persistent symptoms for greater than 10 days should be managed in a multidisciplinary clinic.
- Current research does not allow us to determine a cause and effect relationship between a history of concussions and development of chronic traumatic encephalopathy (CTE).

INTRODUCTION

Each year in the United States there are an estimated 3.8 million concussions that occur as a result of sports and recreational injuries[1]; however, many more may go unreported because athletes may not recognize or report their symptoms, or there may be a lack of proper diagnosis. Motor vehicles remain the leading cause of concussions among individuals aged 15 to 24 years, with sports the second most common.[2] Although this topic has drawn massive media attention, solid data are certainly lacking in many aspects of the management of adolescent athletes with concussions.

The passage of the Zackery Lystedt Law in Washington State on May 14, 2009 marked the beginning of a new era in the management of concussions, especially in youth athletes. Although clinicians strive for patient management based on empirical

[a] Department of Rehabilitation, Orthopaedics and Sports Medicine, University of Washington, 325 Ninth Avenue, Box 359721, Seattle, WA 98104, USA; [b] Department of Rehabilitation Medicine, Sports and Spine Division, University of Washington, 325 Ninth Avenue, Box 359721, Seattle, WA 98104, USA; [c] Departments of Rehabilitation Medicine, Orthopaedics and Sports Medicine, and Neurological Surgery, University of Washington, 325 Ninth Avenue, Box 359721, Seattle, WA 98104, USA
* Corresponding author.
E-mail address: lgconcan@uw.edu

Phys Med Rehabil Clin N Am 25 (2014) 707–722
http://dx.doi.org/10.1016/j.pmr.2014.06.002
1047-9651/14/$ – see front matter © 2014 Elsevier Inc. All rights reserved.

data, in actuality clinical practices are based on a combination of scientific evidence, recommendations provided by the Fourth International Consensus Conference on Concussion most recently held in Zurich in 2012, and anecdotal evidence derived from direct experience in patient care. As such, the goal of this article is to provide an updated review of the management of youth sports concussions. However, this is certainly a moving target as much work is currently under way to provide a structure for more evidence-based care.

DEFINITION, DEMOGRAPHICS, EPIDEMIOLOGY, PATHOPHYSIOLOGY

A concussion is a mild traumatic brain injury (mTBI) that occurs as a result of a direct impact to the head or an impact to the body that causes transmission of forces to the head and brain. Although every patient with a concussion presents differently, common features of a concussion typically include:

- Rapid onset of symptoms that evolve within minutes to hours
- Short-lived neurologic impairment
- Functional, rather than structural, process
- Only 10% of patients present with loss of consciousness (LOC)[3]
- Spontaneous resolution of symptoms (85% within 7–10 days)[4]

The diagnosis of a concussion is based on the recognition of certain symptoms following an impact. These symptoms can be divided into 4 different categories: cognitive, somatic, affective, and sleep. The first 3 can be evaluated at the time of the initial injury, and the fourth category, sleep, should be included in subsequent evaluations **(Table 1)**.[5] Serial evaluations are imperative because of the dynamic nature of concussion presentation, with possible emergence of symptoms minutes to hours after concussion.

According to the National Federation of State High School Associations, more than 7.7 million high school students (more than 3.2 million girls and 4.4 million boys) participated in sports during the 2012-2103 school year, which accounts for more than 50% of all high school students.[6] In a recent study by Marar and colleagues,[2] concussions represented more than 10% of all reported injuries, which is greater than rates reported in previous studies.[7–9] Rates of concussion remain highest in football, followed by girls' soccer, boys' wrestling, and girls' basketball.[2] In all activities except for cheerleading, the rate of concussion is reported as higher in competition than in practice.[2]

Table 1
Selected signs and symptoms associated with concussion

Cognitive	Somatic	Affective	Sleep
Confusion	Headache	Emotional lability	Sleep pattern changes
Amnesia	Fatigue	Irritability	Drowsiness
Loss of consciousness	Disequilibrium	Depression	Awakening at night
Delayed verbal/motor responses	Dizziness	Anxiety	Difficulty initiating sleep
Feeling "in a fog"	Nausea		
Vacant stare	Vomiting		
Inability to focus	Blurry/double vision		
Disorientation	Photophobia		
Slurred/incoherent speech	Phonophobia		

Of note, for all gender-comparable sports, girls had a higher rate of concussion than their male counterparts.[2] In addition, several studies have suggested that female athletes report a higher number and greater severity of symptoms.[3] Several hypotheses for this exist, including differences in head-neck segment mass contributing to increased forces on the head, hormonal factors, or self-reporting practices.[3]

At present there is no way to accurately predict time to recovery after concussion. Impact seizures and brief LOC (<1 minute) have not been shown to predict prolonged recovery. However, there are several known risk factors for prolonged recovery (**Box 1**).[10–17]

PRESEASON PLANNING

A formal Emergency Action Plan (EAP) should be in place before the beginning of practice for any sport. This EAP should include specific management guidelines pertaining to concussions, with a preassigned multidisciplinary treatment team.[18] Preseason planning may include implementation of baseline assessment, particularly in high-risk sports. It may also include computerized neuropsychological (NP) testing, although, as discussed in a later section, this is not required.[3] The preparticipation examination also offers a prime opportunity to discuss the risk of concussions and the importance of reporting with the athlete, and to modify behavior if appropriate.[19] In addition, ongoing education of parents, coaches, and officials is necessary, as an EAP is only as effective as its implementation, and all involved parties need to be a part of the broader framework of concussion management and return to play (RTP) decision making.

ON-THE-FIELD MANAGEMENT

Any athlete suspected of having suffered a concussion should be removed from practice or play immediately.[18] In a collapsed or unconscious athlete, assessment must begin with the ABCs (airway, breathing, circulation) and determination of cervical spine status before dedicated neurologic testing. Initial disposition for emergency transport or sideline evaluation must be determined.[17]

On the sideline, injured athletes should be supervised at all times and continually reassessed to ensure there is no deterioration of mental status. In addition to a

---

Box 1
Selected risk factors for prolonged recovery after concussion

- Younger age
- Number, severity, and proximity of concussions
- Increased number of symptoms (≥4)
- Self-reported cognitive/memory issues
- Prolonged headache, fatigue, or fogginess
- Amnesia
- History of prior concussions
- Attention-deficit disorder/attention-deficit hyperactivity disorder
- History of chronic headaches and/or migraine disorder
- History of learning disability
- History of psychiatric illness (such as anxiety or depression)

more in-depth history and neurologic examination, the Sport Concussion Assessment Tool 3 (SCAT3) or NFL Sideline Concussion Assessment Tool can be used to evaluate a concussion. These tools may be even more valuable if baseline testing data have been obtained before the season. If the athlete is to be discharged home, detailed instructions and precautions should be reviewed with the athlete and the caregiver and follow-up care should be coordinated.[17]

There should be no same-day RTP for any athlete suspected of sustaining a concussion, at any level (youth, collegiate, professional), even if initial symptoms resolve quickly.[18] Concussions continue to evolve, and in some cases symptoms may not be fully present until several hours after the initial insult.[18] In addition, although the athlete may appear asymptomatic at the time of the impact, he or she may actually experience cognitive deficits that are not readily apparent on immediate sideline evaluation. The adage "when in doubt, sit them out" becomes even more paramount in these situations.

Younger athletes face additional risks related to head trauma and concussions. In comparison with their older counterparts, research has shown that younger athletes are more vulnerable to both concussions and potentially catastrophic outcomes of mismanagement.[20] Consensus statements and legislation that require immediate removal from play until a player has returned to baseline have been put in place, at least in part, to help eliminate the occurrence of second impact syndrome (SIS) and other catastrophic injuries. SIS is thought to occur when an athlete suffers a second head injury while still symptomatic from an earlier head injury, resulting in either death or severe disability. This problem seems to occur primarily in adolescents, and is thought to stem from a loss of cerebral autoregulation, leading to rapid cerebral vascular congestion, increased intracranial pressure, and brain herniation.[21] SIS usually progresses rapidly, and the athlete may walk off the field only to be comatose and in respiratory arrest several minutes later.[20] In its original description, there is no associated intracranial hemorrhage. More recent descriptions, however, do demonstrate cases of SIS with a concomitant thin subdural hematoma. The extent of the mass effect and midline shift in these cases is disproportional to the volume of the subdural hematoma, and is thought to be consistent with the loss of autoregulation that is a hallmark of SIS.[22]

CLINICAL MANAGEMENT

Beyond initial physical and relative cognitive rest, there is no effective treatment for curing a concussion. Excessive exertion, however, may delay recovery. In addition, as previously discussed, premature return to contact activity could result in catastrophic brain injury. Clinical management should be performed by a medical professional trained in the diagnosis and management of youth sports concussions. Initial identification is often performed by athletic trainers on the field, and a team approach is often necessary for comprehensive and proper management, especially for those with persisting symptoms. This multidisciplinary team includes physicians, athletic trainers, neuropsychologists, physical therapists, school counselors, and others.

The initial clinic visit should include a detailed history and physical examination (**Boxes 2** and **3**).

Unfortunately, there is no definitive test for diagnosing a concussion. In certain scenarios, however, imaging, laboratory testing, and/or NP testing may be used as part of the workup or management of the postconcussive athlete.

Imaging is not typically indicated for athletes who have sustained a sports-related concussion, especially those with an uncomplicated recovery pattern. Standard

---

Box 2
History at initial evaluation

Have you ever had:

☐ X-ray, MRI, or CT scan of your head or neck

☐ Neuropsychological testing (such as ImPACT)

Have you ever been diagnosed with:

☐ learning disability/dyslexia ☐ ADD/ADHD ☐ seizure disorder

☐ migraine headache ☐ anxiety, depression, or any psychiatric condition

Have you had any delay in your developmental milestones? (ie, walking, talking, etc) ☐ Yes ☐ No

Where do you go to school and what grade are you in? _____

What kind of grades do you normally receive? _____

Are you still able to attend school? Yes ☐ No ☐ N/A

What sports do you play? _____

What other medical problems do you have?

☐ diabetes ☐ thyroid disorder ☐ anemia ☐ asthma ☐ other _____

What surgeries have you had?_____ _____

What medications do you take on a regular basis? _____

Which medications have you been taking since this injury? _____

Do you have any allergies? _____

If you are currently experiencing headaches, please describe:

Location: ☐ front ☐ back ☐ right ☐ left ☐ behind eye ☐ other _____

Character: ☐ throbbing ☐ stabbing ☐ aching ☐ vise-like ☐ other _____

Worse with physical activity/exertion? ☐ Yes ☐ No

Worse with mental exertion? ☐ Yes ☐ No

Have you had an issue with headaches prior to this injury? ☐ Yes ☐ No

Abbreviations: ADD, Attention-deficit disorder; ADHD, attention-deficit hyperactivity disorder; CT, computed tomography; MRI, magnetic resonance imaging.

---

imaging, such as magnetic resonance imaging (MRI) or computed tomography (CT), is expected to be normal given the predominately functional, rather than structural, etiology.[3,18] In the acute setting such as the emergency department, imaging, typically CT, should be pursued if there is suspicion of a skull fracture or an intracranial bleed,[3] and should be considered in cases where there has been a prolonged LOC, focal neurologic deficits, or other concerning findings. In the postacute setting, brain MRI may be used in cases where focal neurologic deficit is identified on physical examination. In addition, MRI may be used if there is a prolonged course with persistent symptoms, or if underlying abnormality such as tumor, arteriovenous malformation, or Chiari malformation is considered. Other imaging modalities, such as positron emission tomography, single-photon emission CT, functional MRI, diffusion tensor imaging, and magnetic resonance spectroscopy have demonstrated findings of structural and physiologic changes and should currently be considered research tools, with hopes for future use in the clinical setting.[3,18]

Box 3
Neurologic/musculoskeletal examination

Cranial nerves:

Extraocular movements: intact ☐ Yes ☐ No

Nystagmus: ☐ Absent ☐ Present

PERRL: ☐ Yes ☐ No

Facial sensation V1 to V3: intact ☐ Yes ☐ No

Facial movements bilateral: intact ☐ Yes ☐ No

Hearing bilateral: intact ☐ Yes ☐ No

Tongue, uvula, palate midline: ☐ Yes ☐ No

Shoulder shrug bilateral: intact ☐ Yes ☐ No

Visual fields: intact ☐ Yes ☐ No

Strength/sensation/reflexes:

Manual muscle testing 5/5 bilateral upper and lower extremities: ☐ Yes ☐ No

Sensation: intact LT BUE/BLE: ☐ Yes ☐ No

Reflexes symmetric/intact BUE/BLE: ☐ Yes ☐ No

Hoffman's bilateral: ☐ Absent ☐ Present

Clonus: ☐ Absent ☐ Present

Babinski: ☐ Absent ☐ Present

Cervical spine:

Range of motion intact all planes: ☐ Yes ☐ No

Focal tenderness to palpation: ☐ No ☐ Yes

Spurling bilateral: ☐ Negative ☐ Positive

Explanation of any **abnormal** findings above: _____

Abbreviations: BLE, bilateral lower extremities; BUE, bilateral upper extremities; LT, left; PERRL, pupils equal, round, reactive to light.

NP testing can be a very useful adjunct with many aspects of management, including diagnosis, scholastic issues, and RTP timing. Full cognitive recovery should occur before RTP, although this may lag behind resolution of clinical symptoms. NP testing should not be solely relied on for RTP decisions, especially in the infrequent cases where cognitive function returns to baseline before full resolution of clinical symptoms. According to Zurich guidelines,[18] NP testing is not required; however, several investigators have proposed that baseline NP testing be obtained in all athletes participating in contact sports as part of their preparticipation assessment. In the realm of youth athletes, this is typically done in the form of easily accessible computerized testing. This testing may be very helpful in the case of subsequent concussions, in that it can be used to assist with the timing of RTP. Before an athlete becomes clinically asymptomatic, NP testing may be used to evaluate for deficits initially after injury, and may be useful in assisting with return to school issues and guidelines for teachers. Regardless of the form of testing, it is the opinion of the authors that all NP testing is best interpreted with the involvement of a well-trained neuropsychologist.

A study by Guskiewicz and Register-Mihalik[23] demonstrated significant disagreement between symptom severity total scores, computerized neurocognitive testing, and balance testing. Each of these measures may be sensitive to specific deficits that other tests are not able to capture, underscoring the importance of using multiple tools for each assessment. Regardless of the specific tools used, it is imperative that evaluation and management after concussion uses tools that evaluate multiple facets, including a symptoms checklist and measurement of symptom severity, cognitive function (including concentration, memory, delayed recall), and a thorough neurologic and musculoskeletal examination, including balance testing.

At present there are no specific biomarkers or laboratory data that can be used to diagnose or rule out a concussion. During the initial evaluation, checking laboratory data is not likely to be of use. In the setting of persistent postconcussion symptoms, however, it may be useful to rule out other confounding factors or potential causes that can cause similar symptoms, such as hypothyroid/hyperthyroid and anemia.

At present there is no pharmacologic therapy that can be used to cure a concussed athlete. Any medications should be used judiciously, especially in the acute setting (<24 hours), during which time any substance that may alter mental status should be avoided. During recovery, medications may be considered for symptomatic relief. However, attention should be directed to those with potential cognitive and neurologic side effects, as they may interfere with recognition of true symptoms. When considering timing of RTP, it is important to take into account that symptoms may be masked or underreported in the presence of certain medications. The management of headaches is discussed later in this article.

Many athletes report sleep disturbance after concussion, may have difficulty with sleep initiation and maintenance, and may report increased daytime somnolence. Medications should be avoided for several days after concussion, and good sleep hygiene should be encouraged. There is no evidence for the use of stimulants or sleep-promoting medications in the acute setting[3]; however, both medication and cognitive therapies may be considered for poor sleep associated with postconcussion syndrome (PCS).

Several medications that aim to modify underlying pathophysiology to decrease symptom duration have been investigated, such as drugs that inhibit arachidonic acid metabolism, calcium-channel antagonists, corticosteroids, thyrotropin-releasing hormone (TRH)/TRH analogues, free radical scavengers, antioxidants, and drugs that modify monoamine function.[24] In addition, treatment such as hyperbaric oxygen therapy has been considered. Caution should be exercised when trialing therapies with limited supportive data, as they certainly can have unwanted complications, such as possible psychiatric side effects with cholinergic antagonists.

Rest, both physical and cognitive, is the cornerstone of the treatment of concussions. Iatrogenic complications from mandated rest should be considered. Although physical rest should be encouraged during the initial period after concussion, there is some evidence that subthreshold activity may be safe and useful in treating the athlete with persistent symptoms. A preliminary study by Leddy and colleagues[25] in 2010 demonstrated that monitored and controlled subthreshold exercise improved PCS symptoms in a comparison with patients who did not exercise, without any adverse events reported.

In addition, it is the opinion of the authors that the term "relative mental rest" is preferable to the commonly used term "mental rest." Complete mental rest is not even a possibility, and youth athletes should be educated that thinking is not going to harm their brains. There is no concrete evidence that cognitive activity will either prolong symptoms or have any impact on the ultimate course of recovery[26]; however, it is true that cognitive stressors such as video games, loud or bright TV/movies, and prolonged computer usage may worsen symptoms during the acute recovery period. School and schoolwork should be a priority, and students should be encouraged to continue school as tolerated. Missing school can create many unintended consequences, such as anxiety from having to make up lost time and incomplete projects, and altered mood arising from limited social contact. In addition, patients with moderate and severe traumatic brain injury who are admitted to inpatient rehabilitation programs are required to perform 3 hours of therapy per day, with the intention to augment, rather than inhibit, their recovery.

The recent publication of the Child SCAT-3[27] reminds us that children experience concussions differently than older adolescents and adults. Young children may have difficulty reporting symptoms, and input from parents is often essential. Health care providers may need to work more closely with teachers and school officials for return-to-school issues, and return to learning should be emphasized before return to sport. A more conservative approach to RTP is also recommended, which may include a longer asymptomatic period before adding physical activity, and/or a longer period of time at each stage of the graduated RTP protocol.[18]

Children and adolescents may require accommodations for a successful return to school. For those with prolonged symptoms, this may take the form of a 504 plan or an Individualized Education Program. Informal adjustments and accommodations may include a shortened school day or scheduled breaks during the day, providing preprinted class notes, delaying graded work such as tests and projects until symptom improvement, and providing increased time for testing once it is reintroduced.[3,25]

RETURN TO PLAY

RTP should not begin until the athlete's concussion-related symptoms have resolved and he or she returns to preconcussion baseline. Although athletes should be asymptomatic in relation to the concussion, they may indicate either preexisting or unrelated symptoms on the checklist. Jinguji and colleagues[28] demonstrated that at baseline, 25% to 35% of athletes reported 1 to 3 symptoms. As noted previously, NP testing, if completed, should have returned to baseline before considering a return to contact activities.

An individualized, graded, monitored RTP protocol is suggested.[18] Many schools and teams require more than 1 contact practice before return to competition, and this should be considered in any RTP plan. Athletes should remain at baseline during and in between steps, and they should not proceed to the next step if symptoms recur. Each step should have a duration of at least 24 hours to evaluate for symptom recurrence, and the duration of each step may be longer in athletes with a longer duration of symptoms.

Example of RTP protocol
Step 1: Rest until symptoms have returned to baseline (physical and relative mental rest)
Step 2: Light aerobic exercise (walking, stationary bike, and so forth)
Step 3: Sport-specific exercise, including push-ups/sit-ups
Step 4: Noncontact training drills and light resistance training
Step 5: Full contact training
Step 6: Return to competition

The RTP process should be medically supervised at each step. Written, as opposed to verbal, instructions are preferable so as to ensure adequate communication with patients, families, and medical providers. In their clinic the authors provide written clearance before resumption of physical activity (step 2) and again for progression to contact activity (step 5). Medical clearance for RTP after a concussion is now the law in all 50 states and the District of Columbia.

HEADACHE

Headache is the most commonly reported symptom following a concussion, seen in 86% of athletes in a study by Guskiewicz and colleagues.[29] Concussion may also exacerbate a preexisting headache disorder.[30] Often the headache will resolve as the concussion resolves, but some athletes are left with persistent headache as the only symptom. The experience of pain, in and of itself, can cause impairment in concentration, mental processing, and reaction time.[31] This situation may complicate the assessment of athletes with ongoing persistent headache in determining whether symptoms are still attributable to the brain injury, or simply to the headache itself.

Posttraumatic headaches (PTH) occurring after a traumatic brain injury are classified as secondary headache types by the International Classification of Headache Disorders.[32] To fulfill these criteria, headaches must begin within 7 days from the date of injury and are classified into acute (lasting less than 3 months) or chronic (lasting greater than 3 months). Whiplash-associated headaches, which occur after an acceleration-deceleration injury and with associated neck pain,[31] can also occur after a concussion, and the two may coexist in the same patient.

In retrospective studies, the prevalence of PTH following traumatic brain injury ranges between 30% and 90%.[33] Headaches can present as either tension type or migraine, with or without aura. Medication rebound headache can also occur, particularly if the initial headache type is improperly managed with overuse of over-the-counter medication.[34] Athletes with migrainous features after concussion may suffer from greater cognitive impairment, and report higher postinjury symptom scores, than athletes with nonmigrainous headaches.[35]

A recent systematic review found that there is insufficient evidence to support treatment protocols for headaches following concussion, but some guidelines are offered[33]:

1. Clinical management should be guided by the type of headache present.
2. Migraine headaches may respond to abortive medication, and may require prophylactic medication if symptoms are frequent.
3. Headaches with a cervicogenic origin may respond to gentle mobilization with the addition of active physical therapy if needed.
4. Behavioral therapy can be helpful in chronic, severe headaches.

In patients with persisting PTH, prophylactic medications may include β-blockers, antidepressants, and antiepileptics, although caution should be used given the sedative side effects of antiepileptics, which may further reduce cognitive function. Nonsteroidal anti-inflammatories, acetaminophen, and triptans are often used for symptomatic treatment. Narcotics are not recommended, as they are commonly associated with medication overuse headache.[36] More aggressive options include occipital nerve blocks and Botox injections.[30]

In adolescent and young adult athletes, more aggressive care should be undertaken only with caution, and in a multidisciplinary setting, with expert management by a headache specialist. Medications should be prescribed only for prolonged, disabling headache, as they can mask unresolved concussive symptoms.[35] Unless otherwise specified by a treating headache specialist, athletes should be asymptomatic and off of all medications before RTP. This aspect makes RTP especially complicated with Botox, given that a single injection lasts for 3 months.[35,36]

PERSISTENT POSTCONCUSSION SYMPTOMS

Although most athletes recover from a concussion within a short time frame, at least 10% to 15% may have symptoms persisting past 10 days.[18] In these athletes, it is important to consider other coexisting abnormalities that may affect symptom reporting, such as preexisting headache disorders, depression, and anxiety.[3,37]

A small number of these individuals with persistent symptoms may go on to develop PCS, characterized by symptoms lasting longer than 3 months. The term PCS refers to the somatic, cognitive, emotional, motor, or sensory symptoms ascribed to a concussion or head injury, and generally includes headache, fatigue, and difficulties with attention.[38]

Persistent PCS is believed to be due to either the biological effects of the injury, psychological factors, or a combination of both.[39] Social factors may also play a role.[40] Reported symptoms for both depression and chronic pain can be similar, or even identical, to those of persistent PCS, which makes it challenging for the clinician to differentiate between the two. Even without suffering head trauma, 89% of general trauma patients reported symptoms consistent with PCS.[38] Healthy, noninjured young adults also demonstrate similar symptoms on self-report questionnaires, emphasizing that symptoms are nonspecific to individuals with a history of mTBI.[41]

Several factors have been evaluated to determine which individuals are at risk for PCS, including sex, age, and educational level. Perhaps more relevant, however, are the risk factors that may potentially be modified, or at least mitigated.

In a prospective study by Ponsford and colleagues[38] comparing trauma patients with mTBI patients and those without mTBI, premorbid psychiatric history and anxiety reported at 1 week postinjury strongly predicted continuing postconcussion symptoms at 3 months. At 3 months, individuals who had suffered an mTBI were no more likely than the trauma controls to report ongoing symptoms; however, individuals in either group who reported anxiety, posttraumatic stress disorder (PTSD), or other life stressors were more likely to report continued symptoms. In a different study, the presence of comorbid depression or PTSD was associated with postconcussion symptoms at 3 months, and depressive symptoms were found to persist despite cognitive recovery in patients with mTBI.[42] It is important for the treating physician to recognize how ongoing psychological complaints unrelated to the mTBI can influence management.

Negative illness perceptions and expectations may also be risk factors for PCS. Whittaker and colleagues[43] found that patients who early in their course consider that their symptoms will have serious negative consequences on their lives are more likely to experience PCS. Patients who interpret their symptoms as serious and enduring are also more likely to experience enduring symptoms.

Hou and colleagues[40] describe the risks for development of persistent symptoms in terms of:

1. Predisposing factors: premorbid vulnerability including anxiety or somatic complaints
2. Precipitating factors: the brain injury itself, which triggers initial symptoms
3. Perpetuating factors: cognitive, behavioral, and emotional reactions to the injury, which may contribute to ongoing symptoms

Patients who attribute preexisting, nonspecific somatic complaints to the injury are also at greater risk of developing PCS.

Early identification of those individuals at risk for developing PCS may allow for the implementation of counseling or behavioral strategies to help mitigate the risk.[37] It is also important to recognize that owing to the nonspecific nature of many of the symptoms, not all individuals reporting postconcussion symptoms are continuing to suffer from an ongoing biological effect stemming from the mTBI. Overdiagnosis of psychosocial effects as ongoing concussion symptoms may lead to unnecessary treatments and activity restrictions,[18] and can also hinder recovery.

CHRONIC NEUROLOGIC IMPAIRMENT

Individuals who have suffered a concussion are at increased risk of future concussions, and this risk increases in a dose-dependent manner.[11] An increasing number of previous concussions may also be correlated with increased symptom duration,[3,11] and has been linked with increased rates of self-reported depression in retired professional American football players.[44,45] There is conflicting evidence for chronic cognitive impairment following multiple concussions.[3] A study by Guskiewicz and colleagues[46] showed earlier onset of dementia, but without an increase in prevalence. A recent study with 50-year follow-up showed no increased rates of dementia, Parkinson disease, or amyotrophic lateral sclerosis in former high school football players when compared with controls.[47] Prospective, longitudinal studies are needed, and care should be taken not to generalize currently available data.

CHRONIC TRAUMATIC ENCEPHALOPATHY

Chronic traumatic encephalopathy (CTE) is a rare, progressive neurologic disorder that is postulated to result from repetitive brain trauma, with symptoms usually presenting years to decades after exposure.[48] Histopathologically, CTE is a distinct tauopathy, and currently can be diagnosed only at autopsy. Permanent PCS is not known to cause CTE, and indeed the two are distinct entities.[49]

In 1928, Martland[50] described punch drunk syndrome in boxers; however, current descriptions of CTE differ from early accounts. Whereas Martland's subjects often lived into old age, with dementia developing only later, more recent cases have a high rate of suicidality, often culminating in a violent end in middle age.[51]

The clinical symptoms of CTE can be broadly categorized into cognitive, mood and behavioral, and neurologic symptoms (**Table 2**).[48,52]

Much remains unknown about CTE, and future prospective longitudinal studies will be needed to answer unresolved questions. The current literature reports a correlation between prior brain trauma and the development of CTE, but cannot prove causality.[53] The true incidence and prevalence are unknown, but given the large number of athletes participating in contact sports, and the relatively small number who develop clinical symptoms and a pathologic diagnosis of CTE, the goal of future research will be to determine which of a multitude of risk factors contribute to its development.[3] At this point it is not even known what type, frequency, and amount of trauma is needed to develop CTE.[54] Risk factors may include comorbid medical or psychiatric illness,

Table 2			
Clinical symptoms associated with chronic traumatic encephalopathy			
Cognitive	**Mood**	**Behavioral**	**Neurologic**
Memory deficits	Apathy	Poor impulse control	Dysarthria
Attention deficits	Depression	Substance abuse	Parkinsonian features
Executive function deficits	Suicidality	Violence	Chronic traumatic encephalomyelopathy

drug and alcohol abuse, or genetic factors.[55] It is not yet known how head impacts at a younger age, or cumulative subconcussive forces, may affect the development of CTE. It is also not clear whether playing while symptomatic increases risk. Given the available knowledge, the authors recommend proper management of each concussive episode, with consideration of retirement from contact or collision sports in certain circumstances, although it is not yet clear if such will be enough to prevent the development of CTE. As with the other neurologic issues discussed herein, it is important not to generalize the available data regarding CTE.

PREVENTION

Helmets decrease the incidence of skull trauma; however, despite technological advancements that can in some cases reduce impact forces, no currently available helmet can prevent concussions.[3,17,18,56] Mouth guards can prevent dental trauma, but do not prevent concussion.[55,57] Similarly, protective headgear in sports such as rugby can decrease soft-tissue trauma, but has not been shown to reduce the risk of concussion.[17,58]

Rule changes, such as the elimination of spear tackling in American football, checking from behind in ice hockey, and upper limb to the head in soccer, have been shown to reduce injury.[3] Other options for improving safety include teaching proper tackling techniques and progression,[59] limiting the number of contact practices, and limiting contact before a certain age; the goal is to reduce concussions simply by reducing exposure. Overly aggressive behavior and behavior with the intent to harm should be discouraged by officials, while abiding by the rules of fair play should be promoted by coaches, parents, and teammates.

LEGISLATION

A concussion that is never brought to medical attention cannot be managed properly. Education of coaches, parents, and athletes about the signs and symptoms of a concussion can help to increase the identification of concussions, which can thereby improve management.[3] The Zackery Lystedt Law, the first robust youth sports concussion law, was passed in Washington State in 2009 to create more uniform management of concussion and to help forestall preventable brain injury.

The law has 3 basic tenets[60,61]:

- Inform and educate youth athletes, their parents and guardians, and require them to sign a concussion information form
- Removal of a youth athlete who appears to have suffered a concussion from play or practice at the time of the suspected concussion
- Require a youth athlete to be cleared by a licensed health care professional trained in the evaluation and management of concussions before returning to play or practice

The Zackery Lystedt Law, and those modeled after it, are living documents that can be modified as more information is learned about proper management of concussions.[62]

COUNSELING

When discussing the risks of concussions with athletes and families, it is important to differentiate between what is known and what is unknown, and what is based on evidence rather than consensus statement. This approach holds particularly true for long-term consequences, including CTE, and when discussing retirement from contact sports.

With all of these unknowns surrounding CTE, it is likely most prudent to allay unnecessary fear from sensationalized media reports and to provide families with access to information and guidance, while recognizing the limitations in the available literature to date.[18]

The indications for retirement from contact sports are sometimes vague and always based on expert opinion. An open discussion between all involved parties is necessary when making recommendations. It is clear that athletes with prolonged unresolved postconcussion symptoms, permanent neurologic signs or symptoms, NP testing that has not returned to baseline, or a report of decreased academic performance should not return to sports.[63] It is more challenging to make recommendations to the athlete who has fully recovered, but whose history puts him or her at potentially increased risk in the future. Cantu[64] suggests that retirement be considered in any athlete in whom symptoms have lasted for months. In addition, any athlete with more than 3 concussions who is experiencing increasing symptom duration, especially if longer than 3 months, and/or lowering of the concussion threshold, should also consider retirement. Given that the brain is still developing in youth and adolescent athletes, it may be prudent to be even more conservative in young athletes than in adults.[21]

SUMMARY

Although concussion management has made great strides in recent years, further research is needed to improve the safety of athletes. In the absence of a test to confirm diagnosis or resolution of a concussion, all athletes suspected of a concussion need to be removed from play, and prevented from returning to play on the same day. Mismanagement of concussion can have detrimental short-term and long-term consequences, many of which are preventable.

REFERENCES

1. Halstead ME, Walter KD. American Academy of Pediatrics. Clinical report - sport-related concussion in children and adolescents. Pediatrics 2010;126(3):597–615.
2. Marar M, McIlvain NM, Fields SK, et al. Epidemiology of concussions among United States high school athletes in 20 sports. Am J Sports Med 2012;40(4):747–55.
3. Harmon KG, Drezner JA, Gammons M, et al. American Medical Society for Sports Medicine position statement: concussion in sport. Br J Sports Med 2013;47(1): 15–26.
4. McCrory P, Johnston K, Meeuwisse W, et al. Summary and agreement statement of the 2nd International Conference on Concussion in Sport, Prague 2004. Br J Sports Med 2005;39:196–204.
5. SCAT3. Br J Sports Med 2013;47(5):259.
6. National Federation of State High School Associations participation data. Available at: http://www.nfhs.org/content.aspx?id=3282. Accessed November 2, 2013.
7. Powell JW, Barber-Foss KD. Traumatic brain injury in high school athletes. JAMA 1999;282(10):958–63.
8. Schulz MR, Marshall SW, Mueller FO, et al. Incidence and risk factors for concussion in high school athletes, North Carolina, 1996-1999. Am J Epidemiol 2004;160(10):937–44.
9. Gessell LM, Fields SK, Collins CL, et al. Concussions among United States high school and collegiate athletes. J Athl Train 2007;42(4):495–503.

10. Collins MW, Field M, Lovell MR, et al. Relationship between postconcussion headache and neuropsychological test performance in high school athletes. Am J Sports Med 2003;31(2):168–73.

11. Collins MW, Iverson GL, Lovell MR, et al. On-field predictors of neuropsychological and symptom deficit following sports-related concussion. Clin J Sport Med 2003;13(4):222–9.

12. Guskiewicz KM, McCrea M, Marshall SW, et al. Cumulative effects associated with recurrent concussion in collegiate football players: the NCAA Concussion Study. JAMA 2003;290(19):2549–55.

13. Asplund CA, McKeag DB, Olsen CH. Sport-related concussion: factors associated with prolonged return to play. Clin J Sport Med 2004;14(6):339–43.

14. Slobounov S, Slobounov E, Sebastianelli W, et al. Differential rate of recovery in athletes after first and second concussion episodes. Neurosurgery 2007;61(2):338–44.

15. Lau B, Lovell MR, Collins MW, et al. Neurocognitive and symptom predictors of recovery in high school athletes. Clin J Sport Med 2009;19(3):216–21.

16. Makdissi M, Darby D, Maruff P, et al. Natural history of concussion in sport: markers of severity and implications for management. Am J Sports Med 2010;38(3):464–71.

17. Castile L, Collins CL, McIlvain NM, et al. The epidemiology of new versus recurrent sports concussions among high school athletes, 2005-2010. Br J Sports Med 2012;46(8):603–10.

18. Herring SA, Cantu RC, Guskiewicz KM, et al. Concussion (mild traumatic brain injury) and the team physician: a consensus statement–2011 update. Med Sci Sports Exerc 2011;43(12):2412–22.

19. McCrory P, Meeuwisse WH, Aubry M, et al. Consensus statement on concussion in sport: the 4th International Conference on Concussion in Sport held in Zurich, November 2012. Br J Sports Med 2013;47(5):250–8.

20. Buzzini SR, Guskiewicz KM. Sport-related concussion in the young athlete. Curr Opin Pediatr 2006;18(4):376–82.

21. Cantu RC. Recurrent athletic head injury: risks and when to retire. Clin Sports Med 2003;22(3):593–603, x.

22. Cantu RC, Gean AD. Second-impact syndrome and a small subdural hematoma: an uncommon catastrophic result of repetitive head injury with a characteristic imaging appearance. J Neurotrauma 2010;27(9):1557–64.

23. Guskiewicz KM, Register-Mihalik JK. Postconcussive impairment differences across a multifaceted concussion assessment protocol. PM R 2011;3(10 Suppl 2):S445–51.

24. McCrory P. Should we treat concussion pharmacologically? The need for evidence based pharmacological treatment for the concussed athlete. Br J Sports Med 2002;36(1):3–5.

25. Leddy JJ, Kozlowski K, Donnelly JP, et al. A preliminary study of subsymptom threshold exercise training for refractory post-concussion syndrome. Clin J Sport Med 2010;20(1):21–7.

26. Halstead ME, McAvoy K, Devore CD, et al. Returning to learning following a concussion. Pediatrics 2013;132(5):948–57.

27. Child SCAT3. Br J Sports Med 2013;47(5):263.

28. Jinguji TM, Bompadre V, Harmon KG, et al. Sport Concussion Assessment Tool-2: baseline values for high school athletes. Br J Sports Med 2012;46(5):365–70.

29. Guskiewicz KM, Weaver NL, Padua DA, et al. Epidemiology of concussion in collegiate and high school football players. Am J Sports Med 2000;28(5):643–50.

30. Seifert TD. Sports concussion and associated post-traumatic headache. Headache 2013;53(5):726–36.
31. Register-Mihalik J, Guskiewicz KM, Mann JD, et al. The effects of headache on clinical measures of neurocognitive function. Clin J Sport Med 2007;17(4):282–8.
32. Headache Classification Committee of the International Headache Society. The international classification of headache disorders, 2nd edition. Cephalalgia 2004;24(Suppl 1):9–160.
33. Hoffman JM, Lucas S, Dikmen S, et al. Natural history of headache after traumatic brain injury. J Neurotrauma 2011;28(9):1719–25.
34. Watanabe TK, Bell KR, Walker WC, et al. Systematic review of interventions for post-traumatic headache. PM R 2012;4(2):129–40.
35. Mihalik JP, Stump JE, Collins MW, et al. Posttraumatic migraine characteristics in athletes following sports-related concussion. J Neurosurg 2005;102(5):850–5.
36. Conidi FX. Sports-related concussion: the role of the headache specialist. Headache 2012;52(Suppl 1):15–21.
37. Makdissi M, Cantu RC, Johnston KM, et al. The difficult concussion patient: what is the best approach to investigation and management of persistent (>10 days) postconcussive symptoms? Br J Sports Med 2013;47(5):308–13.
38. Ponsford J, Cameron P, Fitzgerald M, et al. Predictors of postconcussive symptoms 3 months after mild traumatic brain injury. Neuropsychology 2012;26(3):304–13.
39. Iverson GL. Misdiagnosis of the persistent postconcussion syndrome in patients with depression. Arch Clin Neuropsychol 2006;21(4):303–10.
40. Hou R, Moss-Morris R, Peveler R, et al. When a minor head injury results in enduring symptoms: a prospective investigation of risk factors for postconcussional syndrome after mild traumatic brain injury. J Neurol Neurosurg Psychiatry 2012;83(2):217–23.
41. Ettenhofer ML, Barry DM. A comparison of long-term postconcussive symptoms between university students with and without a history of mild traumatic brain injury or orthopedic injury. J Int Neuropsychol Soc 2012;18(3):451–60.
42. McCauley SR, Boake C, Levin HS, et al. Postconcussional disorder following mild to moderate traumatic brain injury: anxiety, depression, and social support as risk factors and comorbidities. J Clin Exp Neuropsychol 2001;23(6):792–808.
43. Whittaker R, Kemp S, House A. Illness perceptions and outcome in mild head injury: a longitudinal study. J Neurol Neurosurg Psychiatry 2007;78(6):644–6.
44. Guskiewicz KM, Marshall SW, Bailes J, et al. Recurrent concussion and risk of depression in retired professional football players. Med Sci Sports Exerc 2007;39(6):903–9.
45. Kerr ZY, Marshall SW, Harding HP Jr, et al. Nine-year risk of depression diagnosis increases with increasing self-reported concussions in retired professional football players. Am J Sports Med 2012;40(10):2206–12.
46. Guskiewicz KM, Marshall SW, Bailes J, et al. Association between recurrent concussion and late-life cognitive impairment in retired professional football players. Neurosurgery 2005;57(4):719–26.
47. Savica R, Parisi JE, Wold LE, et al. High school football and risk of neurodegeneration: a community-based study. Mayo Clin Proc 2012;87:335–40.
48. McKee AC, Stein TD, Nowinski CJ, et al. The spectrum of disease in chronic traumatic encephalopathy. Brain 2013;136(Pt 1):43–64.
49. Baugh CM, Stamm JM, Riley DO, et al. Chronic traumatic encephalopathy: neurodegeneration following repetitive concussive and subconcussive brain trauma. Brain Imaging Behav 2012;6(2):244–54.

50. Martland HS. Punch drunk. JAMA 1928;91(15):1103–7.

51. Omalu BI, Bailes J, Hammers JL, et al. Chronic traumatic encephalopathy, suicides and parasuicides in professional American athletes: the role of the forensic pathologist. Am J Forensic Med Pathol 2010;31(2):130–2.

52. Gavett BE, Stern RA, McKee AC. Chronic traumatic encephalopathy: a potential late effect of sport-related concussive and subconcussive head trauma. Clin Sports Med 2011;30(1):179–88, xi.

53. McCrory P, Meeuwisse WH, Kutcher JS, et al. What is the evidence for chronic concussion-related changes in retired athletes: behavioural, pathological and clinical outcomes? Br J Sports Med 2013;47(5):327–30.

54. McCrory P. Sports concussion and the risk of chronic neurological impairment. Clin J Sport Med 2011;21(1):6–12.

55. Concannon LG, Kaufman MS, Herring SA. Counseling athletes on the risk of chronic traumatic encephalopathy. SportsHealth, in press.

56. Benson BW, Hamilton GM, Meeuwisse WH, et al. Is protective equipment useful in preventing concussion? A systematic review of the literature. Br J Sports Med 2009;43(Suppl 1):i56–67.

57. Knapik JJ, Marshall SW, Lee RB, et al. Mouthguards in sport activities: history, physical properties and injury prevention effectiveness. Sports Med 2007; 37(2):117–44.

58. McIntosh AS, McCrory P, Finch CF, et al. Does padded headgear prevent head injury in rugby union football? Med Sci Sports Exerc 2009;41(2):306–13.

59. Available at: http://usafootball.com/health-safety/how-to-tackle. Accessed February 12, 2014.

60. Available at: http://www.nflevolution.com/article/Concussion-Legislation-by-State? ref=767. Accessed January 5, 2014.

61. Certification of Enrollment, Engrossed House Bill 1824, Chapter 475, Laws of 2009, 61st Legislature, 2009 Regular Session, Youth Sports—Head Injury Policies, effective date: 07/26/09, State of Washington. Available at: http://ssl.csg.org/ dockets/2011cycle/31B/31Bbills/0531b01bwayouthsportsheadinjurypolicies.pdf. Accessed September 29, 2013.

62. Adler RH, Herring SA. Changing the culture of concussion: education meets legislation. PM R 2011;3(10 Suppl 2):S468–70.

63. Sedney CL, Orphanos J, Bailes JE. When to consider retiring an athlete after sports-related concussion. Clin Sports Med 2011;30(1):189–200, xi.

64. Cantu RC. When to disqualify an athlete after a concussion. Curr Sports Med Rep 2009;8(1):6–7.

Return to Play Considerations for Cervical Spine Injuries in Athletes

Stephen Paulus, MD, David J. Kennedy, MD*

KEYWORDS

- Return to play • Cervical fractures • Stingers • Cervical stenosis
- Cervical cord neuropraxia • Disc herniation

KEY POINTS

- Describe typical mechanisms of injury for common cervical vertebral fractures.
- Understand the contribution of electrodiagnostic medicine to return to play considerations in stingers.
- Describe controversies in both screening for cervical stenosis in the athletic population and management of athletes with cervical injuries and identified stenosis.
- Know relative and absolute contraindications for return to play following cervical disc herniation.

INTRODUCTION

Cervical spine injuries are significant concerns in the athletic population, and they can occur with a variety of mechanisms and severities. Although catastrophic sports-related cervical spine injuries are relatively rare, they have been reported in multiple contact and noncontact sports, including American football,[1] rugby,[2] wrestling,[3] hockey,[4] recreational diving,[5] horseback riding,[6] skiing, and snowboarding.[7] Sports injuries were the fourth most common cause of spinal cord injury (SCI) in the United States between 2005 and 2010, after motor vehicle accidents, violence, and falls, and are the second most common cause of SCI in the first 30 years of life.[8]

Noncatastrophic injuries of the cervical spine occur with even greater frequency. These less grave injuries are typically amendable to functional rehabilitation and return-to-play (RTP) for the affected athlete. Although some cervical spine injuries have clearer guidelines, RTP decisions for many cervical injuries remain controversial. Authors have proposed criteria to guide RTP decision-making in cervical spine

Department of Orthopaedic Surgery, Stanford University, 450 Broadway Street, Redwood City, CA 94063, USA
* Corresponding author.
E-mail address: djkenned@stanford.edu

Phys Med Rehabil Clin N Am 25 (2014) 723–733
http://dx.doi.org/10.1016/j.pmr.2014.06.005
1047-9651/14/$ – see front matter © 2014 Elsevier Inc. All rights reserved.

fractures,[9–12] stingers,[13–15] cervical stenosis and cervical cord neuropraxia (CCN),[12,14,16] and herniated nucleus pulposis.[17–19] However, the relative infrequency of these injuries has limited the ability to perform randomized clinical trials, elucidate their epidemiology and risk factors, or produce validated outcomes measurements. Much of the current RTP guidelines are based on retrospective case series and expert opinion pieces.

The general principles that guide RTP decision-making, namely being free of pain with full range of motion (ROM) and normal or near-normal strength, are not unique to injuries in the cervical spine. However, because of the presence of adjacent neuro-vascular systems, team physicians, trainers, and parents must proceed with care in deciding when an athlete may return to the field. This article attempts to aggregate both the current published literature and the clinical experience of field leaders in the recommendations that follow.

CERVICAL FRACTURES

Cervical spine fractures may occur by a variety of mechanisms in the athletic popula-tion. They vary greatly in severity depending on the location of fracture, extent of involvement of adjacent neurovascular structures, and time required for bone healing. In the 2012 assessment of spine injuries in National Football League (NFL) players from 2000 to 2010, the spectrum of cervical fractures occurred with the lowest frequency, 1.8% of all cervical injuries, but carried the longest mean number of days lost at 119.7 days.[20] Tator and colleagues[21] described 188 cervical fractures and/or disloca-tions in competitive ice hockey players between 1966 and 1993, 130 of which occurred without neurologic involvement.

Spinous process fractures are not uncommon forms of isolated cervical vertebral fracture and typically have a benign clinical course. They most commonly occur in the lower levels of the cervical spine and were described with 4 postulated injury mechanisms by Meyer and colleagues.[22] The first mechanism involves avulsion of the spinous process by forceful co-contraction of trapezius, rhomboid minor, and/or serratus posterior muscles, the pattern of which is often referred to as "clay shoveler's fracture (**Fig. 1**)."[23] Other injury mechanisms include hyperflexion-hyperextension whiplash injuries that have been observed in football, hockey, and gymnastics,[11] as well as sharp direct blows to the spinous process, and avulsion injury associated with fracture/dislocation of the rest of the cervical spine.

Jefferson[24] described fractures of the C1 vertebrae following traumatic falls and direct cranial impact, with force transmission to the lateral masses from axial loading of head impact and continued torso momentum, with resultant fractures of the anterior and/or posterior vertebral arches (**Fig. 2**). In the athletic population, inappropriate tackling technique with cervical flexion has been implicated in Jefferson C1 burst frac-tures in football and rugby players,[25] as well as heads-first form checking into the boards in hockey players.[26]

Compression fractures in the cervical spine are significantly less common than those in the thoracolumbar spine. Such injuries may happen sporadically in the athletic population, postulated as a result of hyperflexion forces in contact sports. The severity of the compression fracture may vary from mild deformation of superior or inferior endplate to significant anterior wedging of the vertebral body. Simple cervical compression fractures are typically benign in clinical course when properly identified, because they retain structural integrity of the anterior and posterior longitudinal liga-ments as well as the posterior vertebral body. However, the mechanism of contact hyperflexion with higher magnitude forces may also result in more severe cervical

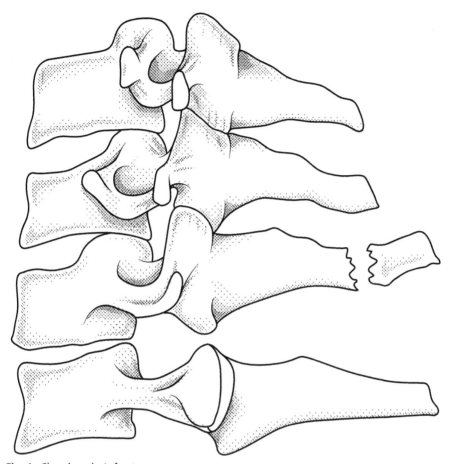

Fig. 1. Clay shoveler's fracture.

fractures with posterior element involvement, often referred to as chance fractures; therefore, the clinician should proceed with caution when evaluating what appears to be an isolated cervical compression fracture (**Fig. 3**).[27]

A combination of cervical axial loading with flexion or distraction may result in more catastrophic cervical spine fractures with failure of 2 spinal columns and resultant involvement of the spinal cord. Classically, posterior element collapse is followed by anteroinferior fragmentation of the vertebral body, known as a teardrop fracture (**Fig. 4**). However, there are multiple possible patterns of ligamentous and bony injury with 2-column instability, such as burst fractures with retropulsion involvement of the spinal canal and facet dislocation/distractions. In such cases, the degree of neurovascular involvement and resultant functional limitations will dictate treatment options and RTP decision-making.[9,14,28]

Because of the necessity for completion of bone healing in simple cervical fractures without neurovascular compromise, no such injured athlete should return to full competition before a minimum of 8 to 10 weeks. Most fractures, including those only involving the spinous process, will require at least semi-rigid cervical collar immobilization until pain free. Once pain-free, the collar can be discontinued and a gradual

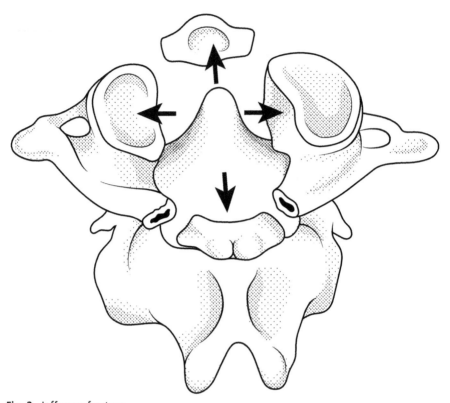

Fig. 2. Jefferson fracture.

resumption of ROM activities and subsequent cervical rehabilitation program that progresses to sports-specific activities can be engaged. Once pain-free, it is also recommended to obtain dynamic (flexion/extension) lateral radiographs of the cervical spine to assess cervical stability. The necessity of dynamic imaging may be illustrated by the

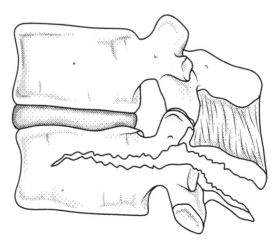

Fig. 3. Chance fracture.

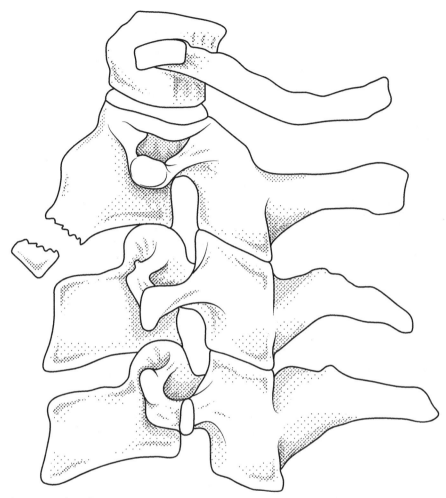

Fig. 4. Teardrop fracture.

Mazur and Stauffer[29] discovery that 6 of 27 patients with isolated compression fractures of the cervical spine exhibited instability on follow-up radiographs.

Permanent avoidance of return to contact sports following some cervical fractures may be prudent when limitations from the initial injury persist or risk of additional injury is significantly increased. Such cases include atlanto-occipital and/or atlanto-axial fusion or instability, dynamic subaxial instability defined as greater than 3.5 mm translation or greater than 11° of angulation, multilevel fusions, and/or significantly limited cervical ROM. Diagnosis of spear tackler's spine, which is the reversal of cervical lordosis and evidence of prior vertebral injury in a football player who has been confirmed to use a head first, or "spearing," tackling technique is also an absolute contraindication to resumption of contact sports participation. Relative contraindications of RTP following cervical fracture include healed fractures of the C1-C2 complex such as type 1 or type 2 odontoid fracture and nondisplaced Jefferson fracture, minimally displaced compression fractures, and 1-level to 2-level posterior fusions.

STINGERS

Cervical "Stingers" or "burners" are one of the most common sports-related injuries to the cervical spine and have perhaps the most well-delineated body of literature for their epidemiology, pathophysiology, and RTP decision-making. They are the most common complaint for which college football players are referred to emergency departments and orthopedic clinics for cervical spine evaluation.[30] The prevalence of stingers in college football players has been estimated between 15% and 65% over their collegiate seasons,[30,31] with recurrent injuries reported in up to 87% of players.[32] In an electrodiagnostic assessment of 185 upper extremity nerve injuries in athletes, 40 (21.6%) were diagnosed with stingers, 30 of which occurred in football players and 10 of which occurred in wrestlers.[33] Stingers may well be underreported in cases with only transient or mild symptoms.

Stingers represent transient peripheral nervous system injuries typically caused by either concussion or tensile/stretch overload to the brachial plexus or its supplying nerve roots. They typically present as radiating upper extremity pain and paresthesias in a dermatomal distribution with myotomal muscle weakness following a tackle or blow to the neck. Electromyographic evidence of axonal damage has been localized in different cases to the levels of the roots, trunks, divisions, cords, and branches of the plexus[34,35]; however, they most commonly affect the C5 nerve root. Strength evaluation for athletes with these injuries must include C5 innervated muscles, such as the deltoids and biceps. Stingers are exclusively unilateral, and when similar symptoms occur bilaterally, the physician should immediately consider and evaluate for SCI. Pain symptoms in stinger injuries often resolve over the course of hours, but may persist for up to several days or longer. Myotomal weakness may persist after resolution of pain, and physicians may consider electrodiagnostic testing if it lasts for greater than 2 weeks, to determine the extent of axonal involvement.[36]

An athlete who sustains a first stinger may return to play once symptoms of pain and weakness have resolved, and full ROM of the neck and shoulder are assessed. In many transient cases, this could occur as early as minutes after sustaining the injury, but if symptoms persist, the player should be withheld from competition until they resolve. If the athlete sustains a second stinger during the same season, it is proposed that he or she should be withheld from the remainder of that game but may return the following game only if all symptoms have completely resolved.[37] A third stinger, regardless of symptom duration, necessitates radiological evaluation of the cervical spine to assess for neuroforaminal or uncovertebral stenosis that may predispose the player to repeat injuries, or disc herniation with atypical radicular presentation. Prolonged persistence of pain and/or weakness of any stinger requires electrodiagnostic testing to guide RTP decision-making. Although a normal electromyography is not required for the athlete to return to play, absence of ongoing acute denervation (spontaneous potentials) with evidence of reinnervation (polyphasicity with appropriate recruitment) should be established before the athlete is returned to competition (**Table 1**).[36]

CERVICAL STENOSIS, TRANSIENT QUADRIPARESIS, AND CERVICAL CORD NEUROPRAXIA

Transient quadriparesis, also referred to as cervical cord neuropraxia (CCN), is a rare injury in the athletic population in which the player experiences temporary typically bilateral sensory and/or motor deficits following a fall or contact injury. The degree of sensorimotor impairment is highly variable, ranging from mild tingling and dysesthesias to complete numbness and paralysis of all 4 extremities. Torg and colleagues[38]

Table 1 Return to play following cervical stinger	
Injury	**RTP Recommendation**
First stinger	RTP after pain-free full ROM with normal strength
Second stinger	Withhold from remainder of the game; RTP after pain-free full ROM with normal strength
Third stinger	Withhold from remainder of game; perform advanced cervical spine imaging; RTP after pain-free full ROM with normal strength
Any stinger, persistent pain/weakness	Withhold from athletic activity; electrodiagnostic evaluation to guide RTP decision-making

described a classification system with 3 grades based on symptom duration. Grade I is defined by symptoms less than 15 minutes; grade II has symptoms between 15 minutes to 24 hours, and grade III patients experience symptoms for greater than 24 hours. They also described upper limb, lower limb, quad-variants, and hemi-variants. In some mild cases with rapid recovery, bilateral symptoms are the primary means by which to distinguish an episode of CCN from a cervical stinger.

Transient quadriparesis has been more frequently observed in high-velocity sports, such as football, rugby, and hockey, but has also been described in other contact sports, including wrestling, boxing, and basketball.[39] It was described in 24 of 39,377 (0.06%) collegiate football players in a 1984 assessment,[40] with 56% recurrence in affected athletes who returned to play.[38] The pathophysiology of these episodes is thought to be caused by hyperextension of the neck with axial loading, which narrows the anteroposterior diameter of the cervical canal and compresses the cervical cord between the posterior-inferior vertebral body and the superior lamina of the level below.[41] Most cases of CCN are retrospectively found to occur in the context of significant functional cervical stenosis.

There is considerable controversy over the best manner in which to characterize and screen for cervical stenosis in athletes, and the degree to which each is prognostic for risk and recovery. Canal measurements may be affected by positioning, target distance during imaging, posture and body habitus, and axial canal characteristics. Herzog and colleagues[42] illustrated that broad shoulder habitus in athletes increases variability in lateral radiographs by 6% to 11% versus the general population, and Pavlov and colleagues[43] attempted to describe a ratio of canal diameter to vertebral body diameter on lateral imaging. They defined a ratio of less than 0.8 as significant for cervical stenosis. However, Herzog observed that more than 40% of professional American football players could be labeled as stenotic because of congenitally large vertebral bodies. This and the results of other studies have similarly depicted the excessively high sensitivity in the setting of a low positive predictive value for the 0.8 Torg ratio.[44] Castro and colleagues[31] attempted to redefine stenosis as a Torg ratio of 0.7 or less, which increases the screening radiograph's positive predictive value but still does not take into account the functional disparities of cord thickness, disc protrusions, mitigating effect of cerebral spinal fluid, or posterior element variability. Although advanced imaging techniques such as computed tomography myelograms, plain film myelography, and magnetic resonance imaging (MRI) better capture these variables, their higher costs limit their utility for screening use in asymptomatic athletes.

Any episode of transient quadriparesis, even with symptom resolution, necessitates plain radiograph and MRI screening for functional stenosis and neural compression. In the absence of cord signal changes or cervical canal stenosis, the player may return to competition when he or she is asymptomatic with full ROM of the neck.

As there is controversy over screening methods for cervical stenosis in the athletic population, so too is there considerable variability among expert opinions for when an athlete may return to play after an episode of transient quadriparesis in the context of identifiable stenosis. Torg and Ramsey-Emrhein[45] consider one episode of CCN with a ratio of 0.8 or less to be a relative contraindication to RTP, with the case-by-case decision contingent on severity and length of initial episode symptoms, severity of stenosis, and sport in question. An episode of CCN with MRI evidence of cord edema should be considered an absolute contraindication to return to contact sports. Cantu[46] thinks that documented cervical stenosis alone should be a contraindication to collision sports and describes a case of permanent quadriplegia in a stenotic patient after a single episode of CCN without any other radiologic abnormality. Identification of significant congenital cervical stenosis on imaging modalities without prior injury, while not routinely done, can lead to a discussion with athlete, parents, and physicians as to the best interest of the player, increased risk for neurologic injury in comparison to other athletes, and sport of choice. Cantu proposes that a second episode of transient quadriparesis is a contraindication to contact sports, even in the absence of cervical stenosis or cord injury, but does not limit participation in noncontact sports (**Table 2**).

INTERVERTEBRAL DISC HERNIATION

Cervical disc herniation occurs with lower frequency than in the lumbar spine, and typically in athletes older than collegiate age. Although contact sports may increase the risk for cervical herniations, noncontact sports may be protective against disc herniation by improved dynamic muscular support for the spine that reduces injurious forces on the intervertebral discs.[17] Cervical disc herniation with radiculopathy was observed in 19 of 185 referrals (10.3%) for electrodiagnostic evaluation of upper extremity nerve injuries in 180 athletes: 6 cases occurred in football players, 2 in wrestlers, 5 in weight lifters, and 6 in all other sports.[33] Disc herniation accounted for 57 of 987 (5.8%) of cervical injuries to NFL players from 2000 to 2010, with 84.8 mean days of lost play per episode.[20]

As with the nonathlete population, symptoms of neck and upper extremity pain, numbness, and/or weakness may significantly vary from patient to patient and is not expected to correlate directly with degree of herniation seen on imaging. However, the extent to which the symptoms of disc herniation and radiculopathy prove functionally limiting may be higher in the athletic population, given the increased physical requirements of their chosen profession or hobby.

Table 2		
Return to play following cervical cord neuropraxia		
Injury	**Advanced Imaging Findings and Symptoms**	**RTP Recommendation**
First CCN	Myelomalacia	Absolute contraindication
	Cervical stenosis and/or prolonged symptoms in contact sports	Relative contraindication
	Unremarkable MRI, pain-free full ROM with normal strength	No contraindication
Second CCN		Absolute contraindication to contact sports

Traditional conservative management techniques for cervical disc herniation should be practiced in the athletic population, including relative rest, nonsteroidal anti-inflammatory medications, dynamic cervical ROM, and strengthening exercises as part of a comprehensive cervical rehabilitation regimen with progression to sport-specific exercises. Epidural injections may be pursued in cases refractory to conservative management techniques, and surgery is indicated for failure of conservative care, in cases of unrelenting or severe neurologic compromise, or for cervical myelopathy.

RTP after cervical disc herniation and associated radiculopathy is a more challenging decision for practitioners and athletes than with cases of simple cervical sprain/strain or bony fracture. Conventional principles of attaining pain-free full ROM with full strength are a reasonable guide for the treatment of most patients; however, residual upper extremity pain and numbness may persist despite appropriate conservative, interventional, and surgical management. In high-level professional athletes, some residual discomfort and/or subtle muscle weakness may be a relative, rather than absolute, contraindication to returning to sports participation when the spectrum of proper management techniques fail. Single-level or 2-level cervical fusions are also relative contraindications. Multilevel fusions, cervical myelopathy, and cases with significant residual muscle weakness and/or pain remain absolute contraindications to return to contact sports, given the risk for permanent neurologic damage or worsened injury.

SUMMARY

Although catastrophic injuries to the cervical spine can occur during the course of athletic play, most neck injuries are of benign clinical course and do not completely prevent the athlete's RTP. Any injury to the cervical spine must be evaluated with caution to assess its severity, and with a low threshold for imaging given of the presence of adjacent neurovascular structures. Much of RTP decision-making is based on expert opinions and extrapolated general guidelines of pain relief without weakness or limitation of ROM, and this article attempted to summarize the current literature to date. Standardized guidelines do not exist to direct the decision-making process in athletes who have sustained a cervical spine injury, because the relative infrequency of each category of injury limits the ability to perform randomized clinical trials and validate outcomes measurements. Although these are stark limitations to establishing definitive treatment parameters at this point, they clearly demonstrate the areas where future research is needed to elucidate treatment decisions.

REFERENCES

1. Rihn JA, Anderson DT, Lamb K, et al. Cervical spine injuries in American football. Sports Med 2009;39(9):697–708.
2. Shelly MJ, Butler JS, Timlin M, et al. Spinal injuries in Irish rugby: a ten-year review. J Bone Joint Surg Br 2006;88(6):771–5. http://dx.doi.org/10.1302/0301-620X.88B6.17388.
3. Boden BP, Lin W, Young M, et al. Catastrophic injuries in wrestlers. Am J Sports Med 2002;30(6):791–5.
4. Tator CH, Provvidenza C, Cassidy JD. Spinal injuries in Canadian ice hockey: an update to 2005. Clin J Sport Med 2009;19(6):451–6. http://dx.doi.org/10.1097/JSM.0b013e3181bd0db6.
5. Tator CH, Edmonds VE, New ML. Diving: a frequent and potentially preventable cause of spinal cord injury. Can Med Assoc J 1981;124(10):1323–4.

6. Hamilton MG, Tranmer BI. Nervous system injuries in horseback-riding accidents. J Trauma 1993;34(2):227–32.

7. Tarazi F, Dvorak MF, Wing PC. Spinal injuries in skiers and snowboarders. Am J Sports Med 1999;27(2):177–80.

8. DeVivo MJ, Go BK, Jackson AB. Overview of the national spinal cord injury statistical center database. J Spinal Cord Med 2002;25(4):335–8.

9. Bailes JE, Hadley MN, Quigley MR, et al. Management of athletic injuries of the cervical spine and spinal cord. Neurosurgery 1991;29(4):491–7.

10. Zmurko MG, Tannoury TY, Tannouty CA, et al. Cervical sprains, disc herniations, minor fractures, and other cervical injuries in the athlete. Clin Sports Med 2003; 22(3):513–21. http://dx.doi.org/10.1016/S0278-5919(03)00003-6.

11. Marks MR, Bell GR, Boumphrey FR. Cervical spine injuries and their neurologic implications. Clin Sports Med 1990;9(2):263–78.

12. Torg JS, Ramsey-Emrhein JA. Management guidelines for participation in collision activities with congenital, developmental, or postinjury lesions involving the cervical spine. Clin J Sport Med 1997;7(4):273–91.

13. Shannon B, Klimkiewicz JJ. Cervical burners in the athlete. Clin Sports Med 2002; 21(1):29–35. http://dx.doi.org/10.1016/S0278-5919(03)00055-3.

14. Cantu RC, Bailes JE, Wilberger JE. Guidelines for return to contact or collision sport after a cervical spine injury. Clin Sports Med 1998;17(1):137–46.

15. Standaert CJ, Herring SA. Expert opinion and controversies in musculoskeletal and sports medicine: stingers. Arch Phys Med Rehabil 2009;90(3):402–6. http://dx.doi.org/10.1016/j.apmr.2008.09.569.

16. Page S, Guy JA. Neurapraxia, "stingers," and spinal stenosis in athletes. South Med J 2004;97(8):766–9.

17. Mundt DJ, Kelsey JL, Golden AL, et al. An epidemiologic study of sports and weight lifting as possible risk factors for herniated lumbar and cervical discs. The Northeast Collaborative Group on low back pain. Am J Sports Med 1993; 21(6):854–60.

18. Eck JC, Riley LH 3rd. Return to play after lumbar spine conditions and surgeries. Clin Sports Med 2004;23(3):367–79. http://dx.doi.org/10.1016/j.csm.2004.03. 002, viii.

19. Watkins RG 4th, Williams LA, Watkins RG 3rd. Microscopic lumbar discectomy results for 60 cases in professional and Olympic athletes. Spine J 2003;3(2): 100–5.

20. Mall NA, Buchowski J, Zebala L, et al. Spine and axial skeleton injuries in the National Football League. Am J Sports Med 2012;40(8):1755–61. http://dx.doi. org/10.1177/0363546512448355.

21. Tator CH, Carson JD, Edmonds VE. Spinal injuries in ice hockey. Clin Sports Med 1998;17(1):183–94.

22. Meyer PG, Hartman JT, Leo JS. Sentinel spinous process fractures. Surg Neurol 1982;18(3):174–8.

23. Nuber GW, Schafer MF. Clay shovelers' injuries a report of two injuries sustained from football. Am J Sports Med 1987;15(2):182–3.

24. Jefferson G. Fracture of the atlas vertebra: report of four cases, and a review of those previously recorded. Br J Surg 1920;7:407–22.

25. Torg JS, Vegso JJ, O'Neill MJ, et al. The epidemiologic, pathologic, biomechanical, and cinematographic analysis of football-induced cervical spine trauma. Am J Sports Med 1990;18(1):50–7.

26. Torg J. Athletic injuries to the head, neck, and face. 2nd edition. St Louis (MO): Mosby-Year Book Inc; 1991.

27. Laporte C, Laville C, Lazennec JY, et al. Severe hyperflexion sprains of the lower cervical spine in adults. Clin Orthop 1999;363:126–34.
28. Morganti C. Recommendations for return to sports following cervical spine injuries. Sports Med 2003;33(8):563–73.
29. Mazur JM, Stauffer ES. Unrecognized spinal instability associated with seemingly "simple" cervical compression fractures. Spine 1983;8(7):687–92.
30. Meyer SA, Schulte KR, Callaghan JJ, et al. Cervical spinal stenosis and stingers in collegiate football players. Am J Sports Med 1994;22(2):158–66.
31. Castro FP Jr, Ricciardi J, Brunet ME, et al. Stingers, the Torg ratio, and the cervical spine. Am J Sports Med 1997;25(5):603–8.
32. Levitz CL, Reilly PJ, Torg JS. The pathomechanics of chronic, recurrent cervical nerve root neurapraxia. The chronic burner syndrome. Am J Sports Med 1997; 25(1):73–6.
33. Krivickas LS, Wilbourn AJ. Peripheral nerve injuries in athletes: a case series of over 200 injuries. Semin Neurol 2000;20(2):225–32. http://dx.doi.org/10. 1055/s-2000-9832.
34. Wilbourn A, Hershman E, Bergfeld J. Brachial plexopathies in athletes, the EMG findings. Muscle Nerve 1986;(9):254.
35. Poindexter DP, Johnson EW. Football shoulder and neck injury: a study of the G findings. Arch Phys Med Rehabil 1984;65(10):601–2.
36. Weinstein SM. Assessment and rehabilitation of the athlete with a "stinger": a model for the management of noncatastrophic athletic cervical spine injury. Clin Sports Med 1998;17(1):127–35.
37. Kepler CK, Vaccaro AR. Injuries and abnormalities of the cervical spine and return to play criteria. Clin Sports Med 2012;31(3):499–508. http://dx.doi.org/10. 1016/j.csm.2012.03.005.
38. Torg JS, Corcoran TA, Thibault LE, et al. Cervical cord neurapraxia: classification, pathomechanics, morbidity, and management guidelines. J Neurosurg 1997; 87(6):843–50. http://dx.doi.org/10.3171/jns.1997.87.6.0843.
39. Torg JS, Pavlov H, Genuario SE, et al. Neurapraxia of the cervical spinal cord with transient quadriplegia. J Bone Joint Surg Am 1986;68(9):1354–70.
40. Torg JS, Naranja RJ Jr, Pavlov H, et al. The relationship of developmental narrowing of the cervical spinal canal to reversible and irreversible injury of the cervical spinal cord in football players. J Bone Joint Surg Am 1996;78(9):1308–14.
41. Torg JS, Thibault L, Sennett B, et al. The Nicolas Andry Award. The pathomechanics and pathophysiology of cervical spinal cord injury. Clin Orthop 1995;(321):259–69.
42. Herzog RJ, Wiens JJ, Dillingham MF, et al. Normal cervical spine morphometry and cervical spinal stenosis in asymptomatic professional football players. Plain film radiography, multiplanar computed tomography, and magnetic resonance imaging. Spine 1991;16(Suppl 6):S178–86.
43. Pavlov H, Torg JS, Robie B, et al. Cervical spinal stenosis: determination with vertebral body ratio method. Radiology 1987;164(3):771–5. http://dx.doi.org/10. 1148/radiology.164.3.3615879.
44. Cantu RC. Sports medicine aspects of cervical spinal stenosis. Exerc Sport Sci Rev 1995;23:399–409.
45. Torg JS, Ramsey-Emrhein JA. Suggested management guidelines for participation in collision activities with congenital, developmental, or postinjury lesions involving the cervical spine. Med Sci Sports Exerc 1997;29(Suppl 7):S256–72.
46. Cantu RC. Stingers, transient quadriplegia, and cervical spinal stenosis: return to play criteria. Med Sci Sports Exerc 1997;29(Suppl 7):S233–5.

Understanding and Evaluating Shoulder Pain in the Throwing Athlete

Nickolas G. Garbis, MD[a], Edward G. McFarland, MD[b],*

KEYWORDS

- Throwing athletes • Biomechanics • Throwing motion • Rehabilitation
- Surgical management • Overhead athlete

KEY POINTS

- Evaluation of the throwing athlete requires the ability to perform a thorough physical examination of the shoulder.
- The most common adaptive changes seen in the shoulder of overhead athletes include loss of shoulder rotation, a protracted position of the scapula, and relative weakness of external rotation.
- The most common arthroscopic findings in throwing athletes are superior labrum anterior posterior tears (SLAP lesions) and partial-thickness tears of the rotator cuff.
- Despite increased knowledge about the throwing shoulder, the cause of what generates pain is poorly understood.
- The major indication for surgical intervention is failure of nonoperative treatment.

INTRODUCTION

Shoulder pain in the throwing athlete can often be a challenge to manage, for a variety of reasons: (1) the pain typically occurs without trauma, and the mechanism is typically some obscure overuse; (2) a variety of conditions can contribute to the pain, but the cause remains unknown, (3) the treatment of pain in the throwing shoulder remains one of the most challenging tasks of the sports medicine physician; and (4) the amount

There was no external source of funding for this article. All authors, their immediate family members, and any research foundation with which they are affiliated did not receive any financial payments or other benefits from any commercial entity related to the subject of this article.

[a] Department of Orthopaedic Surgery and Rehabilitation, Loyola University, 2160 South 1st Avenue, Maywood, IL 60153, USA; [b] Division of Shoulder Surgery, Department of Orthopaedic Surgery, The Johns Hopkins University, 601 North Caroline Street, Baltimore, MD 21287, USA
* Corresponding author. c/o Elaine P. Henze, BJ, ELS, Medical Editor and Director, Editorial Services, Department of Orthopaedic Surgery, The Johns Hopkins University/Johns Hopkins Bayview Medical Center, 4940 Eastern Avenue, #A665, Baltimore, MD 21224-2780.
E-mail address: ehenze1@jhmi.edu

of stress placed on the shoulder of the throwing athlete is high, and the results of treatment are not as predictable as the patient, family, trainer, coach, and doctor would like to think.

Most of the current literature on the throwing athlete focuses on the baseball pitcher, but much of the information can be applied to players of other sports that require rapid acceleration and deceleration of the upper extremity, such as tennis, softball, javelin, handball, water polo, and so forth. The primary scope of this article is to focus on understanding and evaluating shoulder pain in the throwing athlete. Specifically, we review (1) the biomechanical reasons that the throwing motion is so deleterious to the shoulder, (2) the historical and physical examination findings that help in the assessment, (3) the role of imaging in the evaluation of the shoulder of the throwing athlete, and (4) the treatment of these injuries. Although knowledge about these injuries continues to evolve, the results of treatment have come under increasing scrutiny with regard to returning athletes to participation in their sports.

THROWING BIOMECHANICS

The overhead throwing motion used in baseball generates a large amount of stress on one of the most vulnerable joints in the body. Injuries occur not just from the magnitude of the force but also from the number of repetitions involved. The internal rotation of the humerus during a pitch has been measured as high as 7000° per second.[1] Elite pitchers repeat this high-stress cycle with nearly every throw. After ball release, the cycle must be reversed, and the forward inertia of the arm and body must be slowed to a stop.

The throwing motion is complex and involves using the lower extremities, the core muscles, and the upper extremity to generate the forces necessary to accelerate the ball. There is increasing appreciation that the forces transferred to the arm, which allow it to reach these velocities, are generated in large part by a coordinated transfer of torque from the legs to the trunk and to the distal parts of the extremity. This coordinated torque transfer is commonly referred to as the kinetic chain.[2,3]

An overhead thrower must be able to have extreme shoulder range of motion (ROM) to assist with acceleration, yet have enough stability in the bony and soft tissues to prevent injury from the high forces generated in the pitching motion. Any disruption in this balance can lead to excess stress on 1 or multiple anatomic structures involved in the kinetic chain. Wilk and colleagues[4] refer to these conflicting demands as the thrower's paradox. The phases of throwing have been well documented in the literature (**Fig. 1**).[5–9] At the transition between late cocking and acceleration, external rotation of the shoulder in relationship to the torso has been reported to reach 165°, whereas normal external rotation in most nonathletes is approximately 90°.[10]

In addition to the high angular velocities mentioned earlier, the magnitude of force across the shoulder during a baseball pitch can be high. An analysis of 40 professional pitchers calculated a 947 N (108% of body weight) distraction force across the shoulder joint.[11] A similar study in collegiate pitchers calculated an average of 81% of body weight distraction force during fastballs.[12] This difference is likely the result of differences in average pitch speed: professional pitchers, 143 km/h (89 mph); college pitchers, 125.5 km/h (78 mph).[13,14] To counteract these high distraction forces, the deltoid and rotator cuff have been estimated to produce nearly 1090 N of compressive force, 400 N of posterior shear, and 97 N-m of horizontal abduction torque during the deceleration phase.[10] It is postulated that these high forces place stress on the rotator cuff and the supporting structures of the shoulder, especially the superior labrum

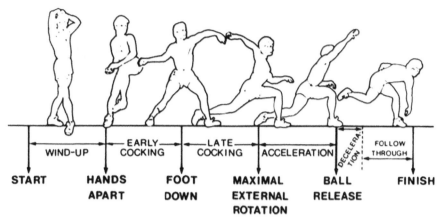

Fig. 1. The phases of the baseball pitch are the windup, early cocking, late cocking, acceleration, deceleration, and follow-through. The forces on the shoulder vary according to which part of the baseball pitch is evaluated. (*From* DiGiovine NM, Jobe FW, Pink M, et al. An electromyographic analysis of the upper extremity in pitching. J Shoulder Elbow Surg 1992;1(1):16; with permission.)

where the biceps tendon attaches. One theory is that this high distraction force creates shear forces in the rotator cuff tendons, causing them to begin to tear.[10]

ANATOMIC ADAPTATIONS

Several anatomic adaptations occur in the shoulder of overhead throwers in response to these high forces. Major changes such as increased musculature in the throwing arm, forward drooping of the shoulder (protracted scapula), and slight asymmetry of the shoulder were first described in tennis players,[15] but they have been noted in athletes who perform overhead sports of any kind. In baseball, they have become common, and seem to be more prevalent in the dominant extremity when overhead throwing is started at a young age.[16] However, it is controversial if these changes are adaptive or maladaptive: some suggest these changes are normal adaptations, whereas others think they can result in injury if not corrected.

Osseous Adaptations in the Humerus

It has been believed that humeral torque in youth baseball pitchers contributes to deformation of the proximal epiphyseal cartilage. This deformation, in combination with repetitive stresses of throwing, has been implicated in the development of proximal humeral retrotorsion or epiphysiolysis (Little League shoulder) (**Fig. 2**).[17] Statistically significant side-to-side differences of humeral retrotorsion have been measured via ultrasonography in adolescent pitchers.[16] This difference in humeral retrotorsion has also been found in college[18,19] and professional[20] baseball pitchers. The increased stress on the throwing arm has also been implicated in side-to-side bone mineral density differences in overhead athletes.[21,22]

Altered proximal humeral anatomy is also believed to contribute to the change of position in the throwing shoulder's total arc of motion (maximum external rotation to maximum internal rotation with the arm in 90° of abduction). The total arc of motion in most nonathletic individuals ranges from 160° to 180°.[4,19] In throwing athletes, this arc is shifted posteriorly, allowing more external rotation and decreased internal

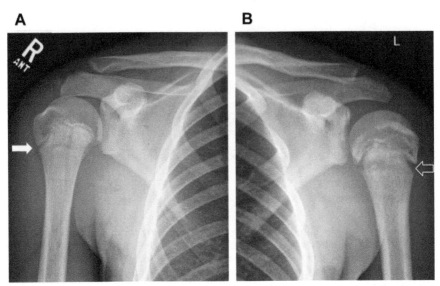

Fig. 2. The high forces on the proximal humeral growth plate can result in widening of the growth plate and pain. Anteroposterior radiographs show (*A*) the normal proximal shoulder growth plate (*closed arrow*) and (*B*) a wide growth plate (*open arrow*) in the throwing arm of an adolescent baseball pitcher. The presence of the wide growth plate and pain is known as Little League shoulder.

rotation.[23] This difference in the total arc of motion has been shown in asymptomatic throwing athletes at multiple levels, but it is unknown if it is a normal adaptation or if it is maladaptive.[18–20,23–25]

Capsulolabral Adaptations

The anterior inferior glenohumeral ligament is an important restraint of external rotation with the arm in the throwing position. Adaptations secondary to repetitive stress can lead to lengthening of the capsule and allow increased external rotation.[26–28] However, the role that this increased external rotation plays in the development of shoulder injuries is not known. Biomechanical studies have shown that the stress of throwing can transmit substantial forces to the biceps attachment at the superior glenoid,[27,29] and this stress has been postulated as a cause of labral tears in the superior aspect of the shoulder.

Muscular Adaptations

In baseball, muscular adaptations about the shoulder girdle secondary to repetitive throwing and conditioning are more prevalent in pitchers than in position players.[30] Hypertrophy of the muscles can be a normal response to increases in physiologic load, and pitchers can develop loss of external rotation strength. Although the reason for this development is unknown, it has been postulated that the throwing motion may create tension in the infraspinatus branch of the suprascapular nerve, resulting in infraspinatus weakness.[31] Baseball players often have weaker external to internal rotation in their dominant arms compared with their nondominant arms, as measured by isokinetic strength devices.[32] Nevertheless, their dominant arms often have stronger adduction and internal rotation than the opposite extremities.[30,32,33]

DIAGNOSTIC APPROACH

A painful throwing shoulder can often be confusing and frustrating for the examiner. There are 3 general areas that can contribute to this confusion: anatomy, diagnostic test results, and presenting symptoms. First, there are 4 joints or articulations that comprise the shoulder girdle: the acromioclavicular, sternoclavicular, scapulothoracic, and glenohumeral joints. Dysfunction in any of these structures can affect performance and cause pain. Furthermore, many of the affected structures are deep in the shoulder and difficult to palpate, making it challenging to localize the symptoms. Second, although multiple examination maneuvers are available, they are of varying degrees of helpfulness in determining the source of pain.[34,35] Indirect examination maneuvers can often be inaccurate and misleading. In addition, multiple tests for specific diagnoses can be positive,[36,37] because of the difficulty in examining just 1 structure at a time. Third, pain patterns in the shoulder are not specific.[38] For example, an athlete can present with anterior shoulder pain that can result from causes such as rotator cuff tendinosis or partial or complete rotator cuff tears, biceps tendinosis, shoulder instability, frozen shoulder, superior labrum anterior and posterior (SLAP) lesions, or cervical radiculopathy. The other challenge in the examination of the throwing athlete is that although the most common lesions are partial rotator cuff tears or superior labrum tears, there can occasionally be a "zebra", or uncommon, cause (eg, vascular occlusions, neurologic lesions, and thoracic outlet syndrome[39]) with a presentation similar to that of the more common conditions. Also, stress fractures of the humerus, glenoid, or scapula, although rare, can present with symptoms similar to those of other more common shoulder conditions and should be considered in the differential diagnosis.[40,41]

However, a systematic approach, and some experience, can help the clinician become more familiar with which constellation of findings in these athletes is not normal.

Initial Evaluation

As with any complete evaluation, a thorough history of the thrower's complaints must be the first step. Who was the first person who noticed an issue? Was it the athlete complaining of pain, or was it a coach, trainer, or family member who noticed? Often, the first complaint is a loss of velocity on the pitches or loss of control of the pitches. Occasionally, there is no decrease in performance because some throwers play through the pain. Was there an acute traumatic event or was it insidious in nature? The clinician should also ask if there has been any change in throwing technique or change in mechanics, such as from a change that the players try to initiate or a change that the coaches try to initiate. Irritation of the shoulder occurs commonly when players try a new pitch or if they try to get the shoulder into throwing shape too rapidly, and the development of pain after this typically is a reversible overuse and not supportive of a pathologic lesion. What were the elements of the recent use during sport (eg, pitch counts, frequency of games, and innings per season)? Especially in younger athletes, it is also important to determine if they participate in other sports, concurrently or during different seasons. The examiner must also determine when the throwing athlete has symptoms. For example, does the pain occur when the ball is released or is it more during the late cocking phase? Is the pain located in the front of the shoulder, back, or scapula, and is there any referral down the arm? Pain at night or at rest can be a reason for more concern. Does the thrower have any history of, or does the thrower currently have, instability or a feeling that the shoulder is sliding part of the way out of the socket? When a ball is thrown, is there any popping, catching, clicking, or locking? If there is, is it associated with pain? The examiner must also ask about neurovascular symptoms, including paresthesias, weakness, coldness, swelling of the extremity, and any color changes compared with the opposite side.

In addition to all the pain-specific questions, the clinician should enquire about the history of attempted treatments and any medications used, including performance-enhancing supplements. Often, players take a variety of over-the-counter antiinflammatory agents, and it is important to establish the doses because those too large or too small can have different effects. Any history of injections, rehabilitation protocols, or treatments can be helpful in the evaluation because the success or failure of such treatments can help determine the severity of the injury. Another point to establish is what the thrower's aspirations and goals are at that time. Is the thrower in high school? Planning on playing in college? Close to the postseason? Typically, 6 to 9 months of recovery are required after surgical procedures around the shoulder, which can affect the decision-making process.

Physical Examination

The shoulder examination varies by individual examiner, and the following is our preferred order for evaluating throwing athletes.[42]

- First, inspect the entire shoulder girdle. The clinician must be able to see both shoulders and the upper back. Men must remove their shirts; women should use a sports bra or an examination gown that leaves the shoulders bare (**Fig. 3**). Any deformity or asymmetry in the shoulder girdle should be noted. Special attention should be paid to atrophy in the periscapular musculature. If the injury is traumatic, the examiner should look for swelling or ecchymosis.

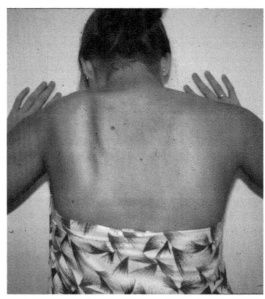

Fig. 3. When examining the shoulders, it is imperative that the patient's bilateral shoulders are completely visible. Men should not wear a shirt or t-shirt. Women should wear a sports bra or a gown that exposes the shoulders. This photograph shows a patient whose winging was missed because her shoulders were not adequately exposed initially.

- Second, evaluate shoulder ROM. It is important to inspect active ROM of both shoulders from in front of and behind the patient. The clinician can evaluate for scapular dyskinesis or asymmetry of scapular motion by viewing the patient from behind as the arm is elevated. ROM in multiple planes should be assessed:
  - External rotation with the arm at the side
  - External rotation at 90° of abduction
  - Active internal rotation up the back and with the arm at 90° of abduction
  - Passive evaluation if there is any side-to-side difference or restriction
  Motion that is restricted actively and passively may point to true shoulder stiffness, whereas restricted active motion alone can be the result of pain or weakness.
- Third, compare rotator cuff and other periscapular muscle strength of the affected side with that of the contralateral side.
- Fourth, perform distal neurovascular and cervical spine examinations.
- Fifth, palpate the bony prominences and soft tissue of the shoulder to determine points of tenderness or crepitus. This procedure is performed before special examinations or provocative maneuvers that might cause the patient discomfort.

IMAGING

When evaluating a painful shoulder in an overhead athlete, it is recommended that conventional radiographs be obtained as the initial imaging study. Conventional radiographs are especially helpful in adolescent athletes, who have open growth plates. In this population, the condition known as Little League shoulder shows widening of the growth plate of the proximal humerus compared with the other extremity (**Fig. 2**). The recommended radiograph series is an anteroposterior view with the shoulder in internal rotation, an anteroposterior view with the arm in external rotation (also called a Grashey view or true anteroposterior view of the shoulder), and an axillary view. A scapular Y view offers little important information and is no longer recommended.

If the conventional radiographs are normal and further evaluation is considered important, then, the next best imaging study is magnetic resonance arthrography with gadolinium. Studies have shown that this imaging study has better sensitivity and specificity for labrum lesion and partial tears of the rotator cuff than magnetic resonance imaging without arthrography.[43,44] The presence of lesions does not necessarily mean a surgical procedure is necessary; SLAP tears or partial rotator cuff tears are often detected in asymptomatic shoulders.

Ultrasonography can be a good screening test for rotator cuff conditions,[45] but it may not be as useful for detecting superior labrum disease.[46] Although ultrasonography is helpful at delineating biceps disease, isolated biceps tendon issues beyond the confines of the joint (ie, in the bicipital groove) are unusual in throwing athletes.

COMMON CONDITIONS
Glenohumeral Internal Rotation Deficit

Description
Posterior capsular tightness is believed to be a contributor to internal derangements of the shoulder in the throwing shoulder.[47] The large distraction force during follow-through has been implicated in the development of posterior capsular contractures.[11] When the posterior capsule is contracted, there may be a tendency to shift the head superiorly and posteriorly.[27] Internal and external rotation is typically measured with the patient supine. The examiner stabilizes the scapula to prevent scapulothoracic motion, bilateral glenohumeral motion alone is measured (**Fig. 4**) with a hand-held goniometer, and the measurements are compared. Typically, the throwing shoulder

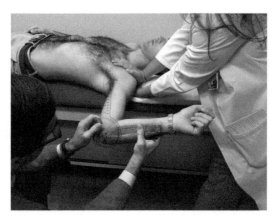

Fig. 4. When measuring glenohumeral motion, it is important to stabilize the scapula to prevent motion of the shoulder blade on the thorax. This goal can be accomplished with the patient supine and 1 examiner stabilizing the scapula while the other examiner measures the rotations.

has greater external rotation and less internal rotation than the nonthrowing shoulder. Although there is some controversy about the degree of loss of internal rotation that defines glenohumeral internal rotation deficit (GIRD), the most commonly quoted criterion is more than 20° of loss of internal rotation, or less than 10% of the total ROM, of the contralateral arm.[48]

The mainstay of treatment of GIRD is initial posterior capsular stretches, known as sleeper stretches (**Fig. 5**), which alone have been reported to provide a more than 90% success rate for symptomatic players with GIRD.[49] If the nonoperative management fails, the athlete may need referral to a surgeon for selective capsular release. However, to our knowledge, the success of a surgical approach to this problem has not been reported, and this treatment remains controversial.

Examination

The technique described earlier should be used. Typically, the athletic trainer or the physical therapist makes these measurements, but it is best if the individual who

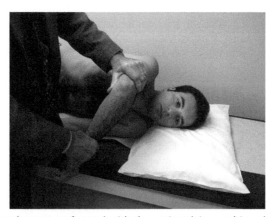

Fig. 5. Sleeper stretches are performed with the patient lying on his or her unaffected side while the therapist or trainer internally rotates the affected arm.

makes the first measurements also makes each subsequent measurement to minimize interobserver error. The accuracy of measuring shoulder ROM with goniometers has an intraobserver reliability of 87% to 99% but a lower interobserver reliability rate (horizontal abduction, adduction, extension, and internal rotation: 26% to 55%; flexion, abduction, and external rotation: 84% to 90%).[50] However, these measurements are likely accurate only to within 5°, even with a goniometer.[51,52] Throwing athletes should have screening for GIRD before the start of the season and be reevaluated if they develop any pain or issues throughout the course of the season.

SLAP Lesions

Description
The amount of literature addressing SLAP lesions in the overhead throwing athlete is substantial. This lesion, in which the biceps attachments to the bone (superior glenoid tubercle) and to the superior labrum are disrupted, is one of the most common in overhead athletes. The athlete often reports a loss of throwing velocity and pain in the shoulder. The attachment of the biceps tendon is primarily to the bone of the superior glenoid tubercle just above the glenoid rim. The remaining portion of the biceps tendon splays out anteriorly and posteriorly and is continuous with the superior labrum, which is attached to the glenoid along its periphery (**Fig. 6**). The definition of what is a SLAP lesion may vary from surgeon to surgeon, but there is some evidence that experienced surgeons can agree on whether a SLAP lesion is or is not present.[53]

Pathophysiology
There is controversy about the cause of superior labrum lesions seen in overhead athletes. The superior labrum and biceps anchor are subjected to a high compressive

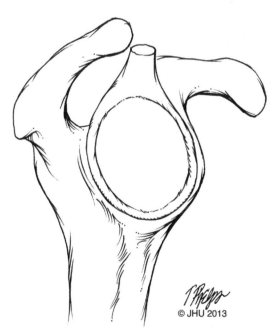

Fig. 6. The biceps tendon attachment to the superior labrum anteriorly and posteriorly at the superior end of the glenoid. (*Courtesy of* The Johns Hopkins University, Baltimore, MD, 2013; with permission.)

force when the arm is in maximum abduction and external rotation during the throwing motion,[54] and some clinicians think that the labrum is physiologically impinged between the humeral head and the glenoid at this point of the throwing motion, which has been called internal impingement.[55] However, the highest distraction forces on the biceps tendon and superior labrum occur at ball release and follow-through. It is not known which of these forces creates SLAP lesions, but they are common in the throwing shoulder.

Examination

The literature describes multiple examination maneuvers for the diagnosis of SLAP lesions, but the clinical usefulness of these tests remains controversial. Many of the tests were derived with the concept that the labrum functioned similarly to a meniscus in a knee. Some tests describe a positive result with a click during the examination maneuver, but clicks have been described in 5% of patients with and without SLAP lesions.[56] Despite this finding, 1 study suggested that the presence of a click or a pop increased the accuracy of the examination maneuvers for labral tears, but that study did not restrict the labrum tears to SLAP lesions only.[57]

The active compression (O'Brien) test is one of the more commonly used tests for evaluating SLAP lesions.[58] Although it is a popular test, studies have shown that its sensitivity and specificity for SLAP lesions are modest at best and cannot be relied on to make the diagnosis.[59,60] The test is performed with the patient standing and in 90° of forward elevation with the arm adducted 10° across the body (**Fig. 7**). For part 1 of the test, the elbow is in a position of maximal extension and the thumb should point down. The examiner applies a downward inferior force, and the patient is asked to resist this force. If the patient has pain with this maneuver, the location of the pain for a SLAP lesion should be deep in the shoulder. Care should be taken to ascertain the location of the pain, because this test is positive for multiple conditions, especially in patients with acromioclavicular joint disease. For part 2 of the test, the patient has the arm in the same position but the palm is turned up and the maneuver is repeated.

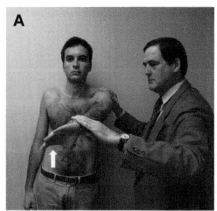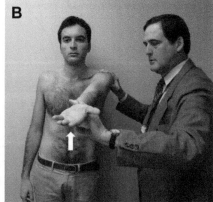

Fig. 7. The active compression test is performed with the patient standing, with the arm elevated 90° and adducted 10°. The arm is held with the thumb down, and the patient resists (*arrow*) a downward force by the examiner (*A*). This maneuver should create pain deep in the shoulder. The test is then repeated with the arm in the same position but with the arm rotated and the thumb up (*B*) as the patient resists (*arrow*) the downward pressure by the examiner. It is a positive test if the patient reports that the pain was less in this position than with the thumb down.

The production of pain in the palm-up position than in the thumb-down position is a positive test for a SLAP lesion. The presence of a painful click with the thumb down but not with the palm up is also considered a positive test. This test has been extensively studied and has been shown not to be highly accurate for SLAP tears.[61,62]

Another test, which is also controversial, is the dynamic shear test.[63,64] This test is performed with the examiner behind a standing patient and the patient's arm in abduction and external rotation (**Fig. 8**). The examiner elevates the arm between 70° and 120° while pushing the humeral head anteriorly. A positive test is achieved when the patient reports pain in the posterior and superior shoulder in this ROM. One study suggested that a slightly modified version of this test had a likelihood ratio of 30 and was an excellent test for making the diagnosis of SLAP lesions.[63] However, another study found that it was not effective in making that diagnosis.[61] This test should be used with caution in patients who might have shoulder instability, because it could potentially dislocate the shoulder.

Several studies have shown that no single physical examination maneuver is sensitive and specific for SLAP lesions.[65–67] Multiple examination techniques may increase diagnostic accuracy in the office. As mentioned earlier in the section on imaging, MR arthrography can be helpful in identifying labral disease. The most reliable way to diagnose a SLAP lesion is with a diagnostic arthroscopy,[65] but this procedure should be reserved for patients who have undergone appropriate rehabilitation unsuccessfully and continue to be symptomatic.

Prognosis

The best treatment of SLAP lesions remains unknown. Nonoperative treatment with rest, frequent icing, nonsteroidal antiinflammatory drugs, and addressing GIRD or scapular imbalances are accepted treatments. When nonoperative treatment fails, the consensus is that operative intervention should be considered. Failure of nonoperative treatment can be defined as the inability to return to the previous level of play and a strong suspicion that the SLAP tear is responsible for the athlete's symptoms.[68,69] Although initial reports with repair of the most common SLAP lesions (type II) found that up to 87% of athletes with repair of a type II SLAP lesion return to play,[54,70] more recent studies have not proved those results to be accurate.[71,72] A recent meta-analysis concluded that the results of type II SLAP repair in the subset

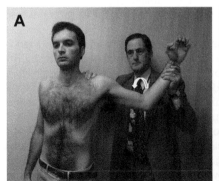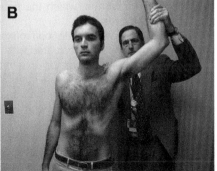

Fig. 8. The dynamic shear test is performed with the patient standing and the arm abducted and externally rotated. While placing an anteriorly directed force on the humerus (A, arrow), the examiner raises the arm from 70° to 120° (B). The test is positive if the patient reports posterior shoulder pain or a click, or both.

of overhead athletes are inconclusive and different from those for nonoverhead athletes.[73]

Rotator Cuff Lesions

Description

Rotator cuff disease, a frequent occurrence in the symptomatic throwing athlete, includes painful rotator cuff tendinosis, a partial rotator cuff tear, and (less commonly) a full-thickness rotator cuff tear.[74] Night pain can also be a common finding when the shoulder is inflamed, and when severe, the pain may refer down to the elbow or hand. A common site of rotator cuff disease in the throwing athlete is the posterior half of the supraspinatus and anterosuperior half of the infraspinatus.[75] In the case of a partial-thickness tear, rest, rehabilitation, and consideration of a shoulder injection can be helpful. Although a discussion of biologics such as platelet-rich plasma is beyond the scope of this article, they can be considered in lieu of corticosteroids in the presence of tendinosis or tears. More high-quality studies are needed to determine its efficacy.[76,77] If nonoperative treatment of partial tears fails, operative repair is an option; it may have a success rate as high as an 89% return-to-play rate in college and professional throwers.[78] However, operative intervention for full-thickness rotator cuff tears in throwing athletes does not have as good a prognosis. Mazoue and Andrews[74] reported that only 1 of 12 (8%) professional baseball players who had repair of a full-thickness rotator cuff tear were able to return to the same level of competition.

Examination

Testing for the rotator cuff can be categorized into strength testing and impingement testing. The supraspinatus muscle is most effectively tested by what is called the Jobe test.[79] It is performed with the patient's arm elevated to 90° of abduction in the scapular plane (**Fig. 9**). The examiner then provides an inferiorly directed force against patient resistance. The initial report by Jobe and Moynes[79] suggested that the best position for testing was with the thumb down, but it can often be painful for patients. Subsequent study has shown that the Jobe test can be performed with the thumb up or in a neutral position.[80–82]

The infraspinatus is tested with the patient standing and the elbows at the side. The elbows are bent 90°, and the forearms are held slightly adducted from neutral to minimize supraspinatus and deltoid contribution.[81] The examiner applies an internal rotation force to the forearms, which the patient attempts to resist. Pain or weakness indicates a positive test.

The integrity of the third rotator cuff muscle, the subscapularis muscle, and its tendinous attachment should be evaluated with a variety of physical examination tests. The subscapularis is not likely to be torn in a throwing athlete, but there is the possibility of a lesser tuberosity avulsion fracture in the adolescent throwing athlete.[83] The subscapularis muscle and its attachment can be difficult to test with strength testing alone. Testing internal rotation strength with the patient's arms at the side is confounded with contributions from the pectoralis major and latissimus dorsi.[84] The lift-off test has been shown by electromyogram and clinical study to be the most accurate and valid examination for the subscapularis (**Fig. 10**).[85,86] The hand is placed into a position of internal rotation up the back and allowed to rest on the patient's lumbar spine. The patient is then asked to lift the hand off the back. An inability to lift the hand is considered a positive test. It is a relatively accurate examination for full-thickness tears but has limited usefulness for a patient with a partial-thickness tear.[87] Two other tests for subscapularis are the belly press and the bear-hug test. The belly press is

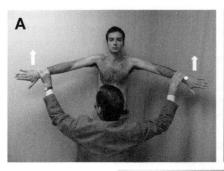
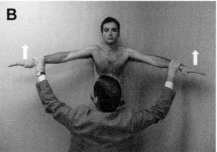
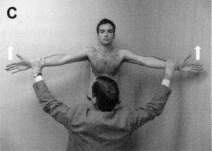

Fig. 9. Resisted abduction with the arms elevated 90° and adducted 30° in the plane of the scapula has been known as the Jobe test. A positive test is pain or weakness when the examiner pushes down on the arm while the patient resists the force (*arrows*). This test can be painful if performed with thumb down (*A*) and is just as accurate with the thumb in neutral (*B*) or external rotation (*C*).

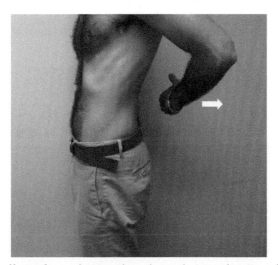

Fig. 10. The lift-off test for evaluating the subscapularis tendon is performed with the patient standing and with the arm internally rotated up the back. A positive test is achieved if the patient cannot lift the hand off the back (*arrow*).

performed with the patient standing with the palm flat on the abdomen. The elbow is brought forward, internally rotating the shoulder, and the patient is asked to press their hand against the abdomen. In a positive test, the wrist flexes and the elbow moves posteriorly (**Fig. 11**).[87] The bear-hug test is performed by having the patient place the hand of the affected extremity on the nonaffected shoulder. The patient is asked to keep the hand on the shoulder while the examiner attempts to externally rotate the arm. A positive test is failure of the patient to maintain this hand position. To our knowledge, only 1 study has evaluated this test; it showed a sensitivity and specificity of 60% and 90%, respectively.[88]

Several clinical tests have been described for evaluation of rotator cuff pathology, including the Kennedy-Hawkins sign,[35] the painful arc,[89] the Neer impingement sign,[90,91] and the Whipple test.[92]

The Kennedy-Hawkins sign is performed with the patient standing or sitting and the examiner to the side of the patient. The arm is elevated in the plane of the scapula until resistance is met and then the arm is internally rotated. A positive result is when this test produces pain, typically into the deltoid anteriorly or laterally. Although this test has some usefulness for making the diagnosis of rotator cuff tendinitis, it can be positive in many shoulder conditions, which limits its clinical usefulness.[93]

The painful arc is a test in which the patient is asked to elevate the arm to full elevation in abduction and with the arm in the plane of the scapula. The test is considered positive if there is pain between 70° and 120° of elevation.[94] This test has been found to be helpful in making the diagnosis of full-thickness rotator cuff tears in patients older than 65 years, but its usefulness in overhead throwers who are substantially younger has not been shown.[93]

The Neer impingement sign can be performed with the patient standing or seated.[91] The examiner stabilizes the scapula and passively moves the arm into forward flexion. If the patient's anterior shoulder or deltoid pain is reproduced near full flexion, the test is considered positive. The Neer impingement sign can be positive in a variety of shoulder conditions, including partial tears, and is not specific for rotator cuff disease.[93]

The Whipple test was evaluated clinically by Savoie and colleagues[92] in 2001. It is performed by having the patient stand with the arm in 90° of forward flexion and adducted with the ipsilateral hand in line with the contralateral shoulder (**Fig. 12**).

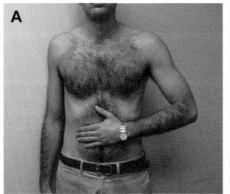 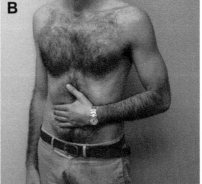

Fig. 11. The belly press test for the subscapularis tendon is performed by having the patient place a hand on the abdomen and bring the elbow forward (*A*). A positive test is achieved when the wrist flexes and the elbow falls backward with this maneuver (*B*).

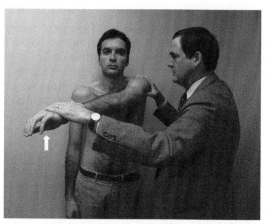

Fig. 12. The Whipple test is performed by placing the patient's flexed arm opposite the other shoulder. The examiner pushes down, and the patient resists the downward force (*arrow*). The test is positive if the patient has weakness and cannot hold the arm in this position to resistance. A positive test for weakness means that there is a rotator cuff tear.

The examiner applies an inferiorly directed force against patient resistance. It is a positive test if there is pain or weakness in the deltoid or anterior shoulder. One study found that this test is not helpful for making the diagnosis of labrum tears or partial rotator cuff tears, and it is most often positive in patients with massive rotator cuff tears.[95]

In general, the examination maneuvers for the rotator cuff are better at detecting full-thickness tears as opposed to partial-thickness tears or tendinosis.[42] These tests are also less useful in detecting full-thickness tears in patients younger than 60 years. The examiner should be cautious with these impingement-type maneuvers because the throwing athlete with stiffness, a SLAP lesion, or chondral lesion may also have reproduction of their symptoms.

Scapular Dyskinesis

Description
There have been multiple observations of scapular asymmetry and bilateral differences in scapulothoracic motion. Priest and Nagel[15] first described this phenomenon in 1976 and termed it tennis shoulder. Their observation was that the dominant arm was positioned lower, its shoulder blade was held in more protraction, and its musculature was better developed. Other investigators have also described scapular abnormalities that are associated with the symptomatic overhead throwing athlete.[2,3,96,97] The theory is that a tight posterior shoulder capsule can be a contributing factor to inferior positioning and protraction during throwing.[3,8] This abnormal positioning of the scapula can alter the mechanics of the throw and is postulated to decrease the clearance for the rotator cuff under the acromial arch. Athletes may complain of pain and impingement-type symptoms from late cocking all the way to follow-through.[98] Burkhart and colleagues[2] described the SICK (scapular malposition, inferior medial border prominence, coracoid pain and malposition, and dyskinesis of scapular movement) scapula syndrome as part of this constellation of findings. Although these findings are associated with the painful shoulder, it is not fully known if they are a cause or a result of pain or other conditions in the throwing shoulder.

Examination

The scapulae should be observed at rest, with the examiner behind the patient. The position of both scapulae on the thorax should be noted. Active forward flexion of the arms can show winging; it is not necessary for the patient to perform a push-up off the wall. The examiner can also ask the patient to abduct the arms 4 or 5 times and observe for any asymmetry. There are different opinions in the literature on whether scapular malpositioning is a primary or a secondary problem. Regardless of whether these findings are a result of pain or are inherently pathologic, a rehabilitation program emphasizing coordination of the periscapular musculature has been found to be helpful.[2]

Instability and Laxity

Description

One of the prevalent theories about the cause of pain in the shoulder of the overhead athlete is that the shoulder has increased ligamentous laxity, which has been interpreted as a form of shoulder instability. Rowe and Zarins[99] postulated that shoulder pain in the throwing athlete was secondary to anterior instability and occult subluxations. Jobe and colleagues[100] and Kvitne and Jobe[101] proposed that the rotator cuff symptoms seen in overhead throwing athletes were secondary to increased capsular laxity, which they interpreted as a form of anterior instability. These investigators recommended capsular shift or tightening to solve this problem and initially reported good results returning throwing athletes back to their sport. Since that time, a high degree of laxity in the shoulders of throwing athletes has become accepted as essentially a normal finding.[23,102] Normal laxity of the shoulder should not be interpreted as pathologic unless it causes symptoms of shoulder subluxation. Pain alone on examination has been found not to be a reliable sign to determine if a shoulder was unstable or not. However, this theory of instability of the shoulder remains unsettled and continues to be debated.[103]

Examination

An examiner can test a thrower's shoulder with laxity maneuvers and instability maneuvers. Shoulder laxity can be measured with anterior and posterior drawer tests and the load and shift tests.[35,100] Instability tests include the relocation test, apprehension test, and surprise maneuver.[103–105] The anterior and posterior drawer tests are performed with the patient supine, whereas the load and shift tests are performed with the patient sitting. For the drawer tests, the patient's arm is elevated by the examiner to 70° or 80° where the ligaments are the most loose. The glenohumeral joint is then loaded by the examiner with an axially directed force from the elbow. The examiner's other hand is then used to translate the humeral head anteriorly and posteriorly, using the glenoid rim as a reference. The modified Hawkins scale, which is based on what the examiner feels when trying to translate the humeral head over the rim of the socket (ie, the glenoid), can be used to classify the degree of translation (grade I: to rim; grade II: over rim; grade III: over rim and locks out).[102]

Laxity testing can be helpful, but there is wide variability even in asymptomatic athletes. More than half of asymptomatic high-school athletes can have translation posteriorly over the glenoid rim.[102] In 1 study of college athletes, 21% could be translated anteriorly and 54% could be translated posteriorly over the glenoid rim.[106] The usefulness of laxity testing is often to have the patient confirm if the sensation that is produced is the same as that experienced when the shoulder slides out of the socket.

The tests for instability are not to be confused with the tests described earlier that measure only the amount of ligamentous looseness. Instability tests are designed to reproduce symptoms typically seen in patients whose shoulders have frank dislocations or subluxations documented on examination or with radiologic confirmation. The anterior apprehension test,[99] which is a test for the presence of anterior shoulder dislocations, can be performed with the patient supine, standing, or seated. The arm is gradually brought to abduction, external rotation, and horizontal extension. A positive test is achieved when the patient relates a feeling of apprehension that the shoulder will come out of the socket. Pain alone without apprehension of instability is not a reliable indicator of anterior instability. The relocation test[101] is a highly accurate test for anterior instability. It is performed with the patient supine. The patient's arm is placed in abduction and external rotation until the patient feels apprehensive that the shoulder will dislocate. The examiner then stabilizes the humeral head with a posteriorly directed force; this maneuver stabilizes the shoulder and should take away the presence of apprehension. If the patient has pain with the arm in abduction and external rotation but no apprehension, then the test is less useful for anterior instability. There is controversy over what it means if the patient has pain with a relocation maneuver that is relieved by stabilizing the humeral head. It has been suggested that the relocation test for pain can be helpful in detecting SLAP lesions, but the examiner should be aware that a positive relocation test for pain is not diagnostic for any 1 condition.[54]

Impingement

Description

There is an evolution to the use of the term impingement as it relates to the shoulder. Historically, impingement has referred to a concept promoted by Neer[94] that suggests that rotator cuff disease, including tears of the rotator cuff, is the result of the rotator cuff impinging on the acromion when the arm is elevated above 90°. It has become increasingly appreciated that rotator cuff disease is, rather, the result of a combination of intrinsic and extrinsic factors. The intrinsic factors are the normal aging changes of the tendons, characterized by cell apoptosis and collagen disorganization, which lead to tendon degeneration and tears. The extrinsic factors are believed to be the rotator cuff tendons impinging or making contact with other structures around the shoulder. The structure most commonly believed to impinge on the rotator cuff has been the acromion. However, 1 study has shown that with the arm in a throwing position of abduction and external rotation, the rotator cuff makes contact with the top of the glenoid.[107] This type of contact has been called internal impingement.[108] It has been described as a normal arthroscopic finding by Walch and colleagues[108] and confirmed by another study,[109] in which 80% of shoulders undergoing arthroscopic surgery showed internal impingement regardless of the diagnosis. Another difficulty with this concept is that this contact has also been confirmed via magnetic resonance imaging in asymptomatic throwers.[55] Therefore, it is unknown when this phenomenon is physiologic and when it is pathologic.

Contact of the rotator cuff with the superior glenoid has also been shown when the arm is in flexion, and contact of the rotator cuff to the coracoid has been shown in some cases with the arm in adduction and internal rotation.[110,111] Although it is postulated that these types of contact may cause the rotator cuff to tear, there is no consensus on the causative pathophysiologic process.

Treatment

The presence of a partial rotator cuff tear in overhead athletes has been frequently documented.[112–116] The process may include some intrinsic components that have proved difficult to treat. As a result, the treatment of any type of what is believed to be impingement has been directed toward removing part of the acromion, but doing so has not proved to provide predictable pain relief.[117] Some clinicians are suggesting that it should no longer be called impingement but rather rotator cuff disease, to emphasize that the condition is multifactorial.[118] The mainstay of treatment of partial rotator cuff tears in athletes is nonsurgical interventions. The results of surgical debridement of the partial tears or even of repair of the partial tear have not been uniformly successful.[117]

NEUROVASCULAR INJURIES

Although neurovascular injuries in overhead athletes are rare, they can be devastating if not detected. As a result, when an athlete complains of numbness, tingling, and temperature differences in the throwing arm, he or she should be examined for neurovascular injuries.

Thoracic Outlet Syndrome

Description
Compression of the neurovascular structures as they exit the thoracic cavity into the upper extremity can cause neurologic or vascular symptoms. This constellation of symptoms can occur as the brachial plexus and the subclavian artery pass between the anterior and middle scalene muscles, above the first rib, below the clavicle, and more distally under the pectoralis minor and the coracoid.[119,120] Muscular development and scapular malpositioning can be potential contributors to thoracic outlet compression in the throwing athlete.[121]

Diagnosis and treatment
Symptoms can involve numbness of the small finger from compression of the lower trunk of the brachial plexus.[122] Multiple provocative tests have been described, including the Roos, Wright, and Adson tests.[119,123,124] Nonoperative treatment, including physical therapy, nonsteroidal antiinflammatory drugs, and a period of rest can be successful.[120,125,126]

Effort Thrombosis

Description
When the arm is in a position of abduction and external rotation, the humeral head can cause compression of the axillary vein. This condition is known as effort thrombosis or Paget-Schroetter syndrome.[127]

Diagnosis and treatment
Symptoms can include, pain, swelling, and discoloration of the upper extremity. Venography is the gold standard for diagnosis, but Doppler ultrasonography may also be helpful.[128] It can be difficult to make the diagnosis because of the intermittent nature of the symptoms. Thrombolytic therapy or surgical decompression has been shown to be effective.[128–130]

Quadrilateral Space Syndrome

Description
Quadrilateral space syndrome is compression of the posterior humeral circumflex artery or axillary nerve as is it passes to the posterior shoulder.[131]

Diagnosis and treatment
Symptoms can include posterior shoulder pain, but this finding is not specific. Tenderness to palpation over the quadrilateral space may be believed to aid in diagnosis, but

this finding, too, is not consistent.[132] There can also be weakness of the deltoid or deltoid atrophy in rare cases. Definitive diagnosis can be difficult because it requires electromyography, and the diagnosis of this entity must be made with an element of high clinical suspicion.[131,133,134] Treatment initially should be nonoperative, including rest and nonsteroidal antiinflammatory medications. If these modalities are not successful, then operative decompression of the quadrilateral space and axillary nerve can be performed.[131]

Nerve Palsies

Description
Nerve injuries in the throwing athlete can include suprascapular nerve and long thoracic lesions. These injuries can happen with or without the presence of a space-occupying lesion. The exact cause of suprascapular nerve injury is not known.[135,136] There is up to a 20% incidence of suprascapular nerve insufficiency with infraspinatus atrophy in professional volleyball players.[137]

Diagnosis and treatment
Surprisingly, this condition is entirely asymptomatic in most volleyball players. The athlete with symptoms from infraspinatus insufficiency can present with pain, weakness, and symptoms of tendinitis. The throwing athlete can develop winging of the scapula for a variety of different reasons. It can be secondary to an alteration of rhythm because of pain, as described by Kibler.[3] It is important to distinguish between winging of the scapula and scapular dyskinesis, because the former is the result of nerve injury, whereas the latter is a learned behavior secondary to pain. Winging is most often the result of a lesion of the long thoracic nerve, and electromyography can be helpful in confirming the diagnosis.[138–140] Magnetic resonance imaging can rule out a space-occupying lesion. The mainstay of treatment is rest, therapy, and antiinflammatory medication.

TREATMENT

Although the entire scope of treatment is not the focus of this article, most shoulder problems in throwing athletes should be initially addressed with nonoperative interventions. Generally, surgery in the throwing athlete should be a last resort, especially when the onset of pain is insidious and when the suspected lesions are partial rotator cuff tears or SLAP injuries. Injuries from trauma, such as an acute dislocation or acute full-thickness rotator cuff tear, might require early operative intervention before trying a therapy program.

The major goals when a thrower has shoulder pain are to relieve the symptoms and to return the shoulder to baseline performance. Rest from throwing may be helpful, but it should not be prolonged or the shoulder deconditions and recovery takes even longer. If possible, light toss should be performed to maintain some muscle strength and coordination. In baseball players who are not pitchers, typically the only thing that aggravates the shoulder is throwing a ball, so they are allowed to perform all other activities that do not hurt, including batting, running, or lifting weights. Patients with stress lesions such as Little League shoulder should also avoid throwing for approximately 3 months. A study by Carson and Gasser[141] found that most players with this entity can return to throwing within 12 weeks. In addition, youth pitchers should have their pitch counts monitored. The 2006 USA Baseball Guidelines and the 2010 Little League Baseball Regulations suggest that pitch counts be performed,[142] but there is little research to support absolute numbers. Adolescent players at risk are those who throw mostly fastballs and play on traveling teams. Overuse injuries in adolescent pitchers can lead to more serious mechanical injuries; implementing these pitch counts should reduce overuse injuries and decrease fatigue.[142,143]

The judicious use of nonsteroidal antiinflammatories can be helpful for patients in whom the symptoms are severe and keep them from participating in their sport. The usual precautions with the use of nonsteroidal antiinflammatory medications exist, and athletes should be queried about renal disease, liver disease, peptic ulcer disease, and aspirin sensitivity.

Cryotherapy can also be useful, especially in the early stages of irritation of the throwing shoulder. Although the use of cryotherapy is empirical only, we recommend that the athlete should ice the shoulder daily and after any athletic activity.[144,145]

Rehabilitation of the throwing athlete is focused on developing each part of the kinetic chain and restoring each unit of the chain to normal and synchronous function. Any muscular imbalance can be detrimental to the overall throwing motion, and efforts should be made to work agonist and antagonist muscle groups.[146,147] Most often, athletes are started on a phased program of nonoperative rehabilitation.[4]

The use of oral steroids in the form of dose packs or as injections remains controversial in overhead throwers. There are no known deleterious effects of a single cortisone dose pack or of a single cortisone shot into the subacromial space. However, to identify which diseases are being treated, these modalities should be used when the patient has been thoroughly evaluated and only with his or her informed consent. We do not recommend using these modalities for adolescents or to mask symptoms that might lead to more problems if the player is allowed to participate.

SUMMARY

Evaluation of the shoulder in the overhead and throwing athlete can be challenging. The cause of shoulder pain is often unclear, and the physical diagnosis may not be specific. The shoulder of the overhead throwing athlete can have a wide variety of conditions, such as partial rotator cuff tears, SLAP lesions, and ROM restrictions. A thorough examination can be helpful in obtaining a diagnosis. Conventional radiographs should be obtained first, supplemented as necessary by magnetic resonance arthrography. The mainstay of treatment should be nonoperative interventions. If nonoperative treatment fails, diagnostic arthroscopy, with potential repair or debridement of pathologic structures, can be attempted.

REFERENCES

1. Fleisig GS, Dillman CJ, Andrews JR. Biomechanics of the shoulder during throwing. In: Andrews JR, Wilk KE, editors. The athlete's shoulder. New York: Churchill Livingstone; 1994. p. 355–68.
2. Burkhart SS, Morgan CD, Kibler WB. The disabled throwing shoulder: spectrum of pathology. Part III: the SICK scapula, scapular dyskinesis, the kinetic chain, and rehabilitation. Arthroscopy 2003;19:641–61.
3. Kibler WB. The role of the scapula in athletic shoulder function. Am J Sports Med 1998;26:325–37.
4. Wilk KE, Meister K, Andrews JR. Current concepts in the rehabilitation of the overhead throwing athlete. Am J Sports Med 2002;30:136–51.
5. Gowan ID, Jobe FW, Tibone JE, et al. A comparative electromyographic analysis of the shoulder during pitching. Professional versus amateur pitchers. Am J Sports Med 1987;15:586–90.

6. Jobe FW, Moynes DR, Tibone JE, et al. An EMG analysis of the shoulder in pitching. A second report. Am J Sports Med 1984;12:218–20.
7. Kelly BT, Backus SI, Warren RF, et al. Electromyographic analysis and phase definition of the overhead football throw. Am J Sports Med 2002;30:837–44.
8. Meister K. Injuries to the shoulder in the throwing athlete. Part one: biomechanics/pathophysiology/classification of injury. Am J Sports Med 2000;28: 265–75.
9. Pappas AM, Zawacki RM, Sullivan TJ. Biomechanics of baseball pitching. A preliminary report. Am J Sports Med 1985;13:216–22.
10. Fleisig GS, Andrews JR, Dillman CJ, et al. Kinetics of baseball pitching with implications about injury mechanisms. Am J Sports Med 1995;23:233–9.
11. Werner SL, Gill TJ, Murray TA, et al. Relationships between throwing mechanics and shoulder distraction in professional baseball pitchers. Am J Sports Med 2001;29:354–8.
12. Werner SL, Guido JA Jr, Stewart GW, et al. Relationships between throwing mechanics and shoulder distraction in collegiate baseball pitchers. J Shoulder Elbow Surg 2007;16:37–42.
13. Feltner M, Dapena J. Dynamics of the shoulder and elbow joints of the throwing arm during a baseball pitch. Int J Sport Biomech 1986;2:235–59.
14. Fleisig GS, Barrentine SW, Zheng N, et al. Kinematic and kinetic comparison of baseball pitching among various levels of development. J Biomech 1999;32: 1371–5.
15. Priest JD, Nagel DA. Tennis shoulder. Am J Sports Med 1976;4:28–42.
16. Whiteley R, Ginn K, Nicholson L, et al. Indirect ultrasound measurement of humeral torsion in adolescent baseball players and non-athletic adults: reliability and significance. J Sci Med Sport 2006;9:310–8.
17. Sabick MB, Kim YK, Torry MR, et al. Biomechanics of the shoulder in youth baseball pitchers: implications for the development of proximal humeral epiphysiolysis and humeral retrotorsion. Am J Sports Med 2005;33:1716–22.
18. Osbahr DC, Cannon DL, Speer KP. Retroversion of the humerus in the throwing shoulder of college baseball pitchers. Am J Sports Med 2002;30:347–53.
19. Reagan KM, Meister K, Horodyski MB, et al. Humeral retroversion and its relationship to glenohumeral rotation in the shoulder of college baseball players. Am J Sports Med 2002;30:354–60.
20. Crockett HC, Gross LB, Wilk KE, et al. Osseous adaptation and range of motion at the glenohumeral joint in professional baseball pitchers. Am J Sports Med 2002;30:20–6.
21. Calbet JAL, Diaz Herrera P, Rodriguez LP. High bone mineral density in male elite professional volleyball players. Osteoporos Int 1999;10:468–74.
22. McClanahan BS, Harmon-Clayton K, Ward KD, et al. Side-to-side comparisons of bone mineral density in upper and lower limbs of collegiate athletes. J Strength Cond Res 2002;16:586–90.
23. Bigliani LU, Codd TP, Connor PM, et al. Shoulder motion and laxity in the professional baseball player. Am J Sports Med 1997;25:609–13.
24. Brown LP, Niehues SL, Harrah A, et al. Upper extremity range of motion and isokinetic strength of the internal and external shoulder rotators in major league baseball players. Am J Sports Med 1988;16:577–85.
25. King JW, Brelsford HJ, Tullos HS. Analysis of the pitching arm of the professional baseball pitcher. Clin Orthop Relat Res 1969;67:116–23.
26. Fitzpatrick MJ, Tibone JE, Grossman M, et al. Development of cadaveric models of a thrower's shoulder. J Shoulder Elbow Surg 2005;14:49S–57S.

27. Grossman MG, Tibone JE, McGarry MH, et al. A cadaveric model of the throwing shoulder: a possible etiology of superior labrum anterior-to-posterior lesions. J Bone Joint Surg Am 2005;87:824–31.
28. Kuhn JE, Bey MJ, Huston LJ, et al. Ligamentous restraints to external rotation of the humerus in the late-cocking phase of throwing. A cadaveric biomechanical investigation. Am J Sports Med 2000;28:200–5.
29. Kuhn JE, Lindholm SR, Huston LJ, et al. Failure of the biceps superior labral complex: a cadaveric biomechanical investigation comparing the late cocking and early deceleration positions of throwing. Arthroscopy 2003;19:373–9.
30. Newsham KR, Keith CS, Saunders JE, et al. Isokinetic profile of baseball pitchers' internal/external rotation 180, 300, 450 degrees.s-1. Med Sci Sports Exerc 1998;30:1489–95.
31. Ferretti A, Cerullo G, Russo G. Suprascapular neuropathy in volleyball players. J Bone Joint Surg Am 1987;69:260–3.
32. Noffal GJ. Isokinetic eccentric-to-concentric strength ratios of the shoulder rotator muscles in throwers and nonthrowers. Am J Sports Med 2003;31:537–41.
33. Magnusson SP, Gleim GW, Nicholas JA. Shoulder weakness in professional baseball pitchers. Med Sci Sports Exerc 1994;26:5–9.
34. McFarland EG. Preface. In: Kim TK, Park HB, El Rassi G, et al, editors. Examination of the shoulder: the complete guide. New York: Thieme; 2006. p. ix–xii.
35. Silliman JF, Hawkins RJ. Classification and physical diagnosis of instability of the shoulder. Clin Orthop Relat Res 1993;291:7–19.
36. Hegedus EJ, Goode A, Campbell S, et al. Physical examination tests of the shoulder: a systematic review with meta-analysis of individual tests. Br J Sports Med 2008;42:80–92.
37. McFarland EG, Selhi HS, Keyurapan E. Clinical evaluation of impingement: what to do and what works. J Bone Joint Surg Am 2006;88:432–41.
38. Itoi E, Minagawa H, Yamamoto N, et al. Are pain location and physical examinations useful in locating a tear site of the rotator cuff? Am J Sports Med 2006;34:256–64.
39. Ryu RKN, Dunbar WHV, Kuhn JE, et al. Comprehensive evaluation and treatment of the shoulder in the throwing athlete. Arthroscopy 2002;18:70–89.
40. Herickhoff PK, Keyurapan E, Fayad LM, et al. Scapular stress fracture in a professional baseball player: a case report and review of the literature. Am J Sports Med 2007;35:1193–6.
41. McFarland EG, Ireland ML. Rehabilitation programs and prevention strategies in adolescent throwing athletes. Instr Course Lect 2003;52:37–42.
42. McFarland EG, Tanaka MJ, Papp DF. Examination of the shoulder in the overhead and throwing athlete. Clin Sports Med 2008;27:553–78.
43. Flannigan B, Kursunoglu-Brahme S, Snyder S, et al. MR arthrography of the shoulder: comparison with conventional MR imaging. AJR Am J Roentgenol 1990;155:829–32.
44. Magee T, Williams D, Mani N. Shoulder MR arthrography: which patient group benefits most? AJR Am J Roentgenol 2004;183:969–74.
45. Teefey SA, Rubin DA, Middleton WD, et al. Detection and quantification of rotator cuff tears. Comparison of ultrasonographic, magnetic resonance imaging, and arthroscopic findings in seventy-one consecutive cases. J Bone Joint Surg Am 2004;86:708–16.
46. Taljanovic MS, Carlson KL, Kuhn JE, et al. Sonography of the glenoid labrum: a cadaveric study with arthroscopic correlation. AJR Am J Roentgenol 2000;174:1717–22.

47. Burkhart SS, Morgan CD, Kibler WB. Shoulder injuries in overhead athletes. The "dead arm" revisited. Clin Sports Med 2000;19:125–58.
48. Freehill MT, Ebel BG, Archer KR, et al. Glenohumeral range of motion in major league pitchers: changes over the playing season. Sports Health 2011;3: 97–104.
49. Burkhart SS, Morgan CD, Kibler WB. The disabled throwing shoulder: spectrum of pathology. Part I: pathoanatomy and biomechanics. Arthroscopy 2003;19: 404–20.
50. Riddle DL, Rothstein JM, Lamb RL. Goniometric reliability in a clinical setting. Shoulder measurements. Phys Ther 1987;67:668–73.
51. Awan R, Smith J, Boon AJ. Measuring shoulder internal rotation range of motion: a comparison of 3 techniques. Arch Phys Med Rehabil 2002;83:1229–34.
52. Boon AJ, Smith J. Manual scapular stabilization: its effect on shoulder rotational range of motion. Arch Phys Med Rehabil 2000;81:978–83.
53. Jia X, Yokota A, McCarty EC, et al. Reproducibility and reliability of the Snyder classification of superior labral anterior posterior lesions among shoulder surgeons. Am J Sports Med 2011;39:986–91.
54. Morgan CD, Burkhart SS, Palmeri M, et al. Type II SLAP lesions: three subtypes and their relationships to superior instability and rotator cuff tears. Arthroscopy 1998;14:553–65.
55. Halbrecht JL, Tirman P, Atkin D. Internal impingement of the shoulder: comparison of findings between the throwing and nonthrowing shoulders of college baseball players. Arthroscopy 1999;15:253–8.
56. McFarland EG, Kim TK, Savino RM. Clinical assessment of three common tests for superior labral anterior-posterior lesions. Am J Sports Med 2002;30: 810–5.
57. Walsworth MK, Doukas WC, Murphy KP, et al. Reliability and diagnostic accuracy of history and physical examination for diagnosing glenoid labral tears. Am J Sports Med 2008;36:162–8.
58. O'Brien SJ, Pagnani MJ, Fealy S, et al. The active compression test: a new and effective test for diagnosing labral tears and acromioclavicular joint abnormality. Am J Sports Med 1998;26:610–3.
59. Guanche CA, Jones DC. Clinical testing for tears of the glenoid labrum. Arthroscopy 2003;19:517–23.
60. Stetson WB, Templin K. The crank test, the O'Brien test, and routine magnetic resonance imaging scans in the diagnosis of labral tears. Am J Sports Med 2002;30:806–9.
61. Cook C, Beaty S, Kissenberth MJ, et al. Diagnostic accuracy of five orthopedic clinical tests for diagnosis of superior labrum anterior posterior (SLAP) lesions. J Shoulder Elbow Surg 2012;21:13–22.
62. Green RA, Taylor NF, Mirkovic M, et al. An evaluation of the anatomic basis of the O'Brien active compression test for superior labral anterior and posterior (SLAP) lesions. J Shoulder Elbow Surg 2008;17:165–71.
63. Kibler WB, Sciascia AD, Hester P, et al. Clinical utility of traditional and new tests in the diagnosis of biceps tendon injuries and superior labrum anterior and posterior lesions in the shoulder. Am J Sports Med 2009;37:1840–7.
64. O'Driscoll SW. Regarding "diagnostic accuracy of five orthopedic clinical tests for diagnosis of superior labrum anterior posterior (SLAP) lesions". J Shoulder Elbow Surg 2012;21:e23–4.
65. Jones GL, Galluch DB. Clinical assessment of superior glenoid labral lesions: a systematic review. Clin Orthop Relat Res 2007;455:45–51.

66. Kim TK, Queale WS, Cosgarea AJ, et al. Clinical features of the different types of SLAP lesions. An analysis of one hundred and thirty-nine cases. J Bone Joint Surg Am 2003;85:66–71.

67. Parentis MA, Glousman RE, Mohr KS, et al. An evaluation of the provocative tests for superior labral anterior posterior lesions. Am J Sports Med 2006;34: 265–8.

68. Edwards SL, Lee JA, Bell JE, et al. Nonoperative treatment of superior labrum anterior posterior tears: improvements in pain, function, and quality of life. Am J Sports Med 2010;38:1456–61.

69. Knesek M, Skendzel JG, Dines JS, et al. Diagnosis and management of superior labral anterior posterior tears in throwing athletes. Am J Sports Med 2013;41: 444–60.

70. Burkhart SS, Morgan C. SLAP lesions in the overhead athlete. Orthop Clin North Am 2001;32:431–41.

71. Neuman BJ, Boisvert CB, Reiter B, et al. Results of arthroscopic repair of type II superior labral anterior posterior lesions in overhead athletes: assessment of return to preinjury playing level and satisfaction. Am J Sports Med 2011;39: 1883–8.

72. Park HB, Lin SK, Yokota A, et al. Return to play for rotator cuff injuries and superior labrum anterior posterior (SLAP) lesions. Clin Sports Med 2004;23: 321–34.

73. Sayde WM, Cohen SB, Ciccotti MG, et al. Return to play after type II superior labral anterior-posterior lesion repairs in athletes: a systematic review. Clin Orthop Relat Res 2012;470:1595–600.

74. Mazoue CG, Andrews JR. Repair of full-thickness rotator cuff tears in professional baseball players. Am J Sports Med 2006;34:182–9.

75. Andrews JR, Gidumal RH. Shoulder arthroscopy in the throwing athlete: perspectives and prognosis. Clin Sports Med 1987;6:565–71.

76. Mautner K, Colberg RE, Malanga G, et al. Outcomes after ultrasound-guided platelet-rich plasma injections for chronic tendinopathy: a multicenter, retrospective review. PM R 2013;5:169–75.

77. Redler LH, Thompson SA, Hsu SH, et al. Platelet-rich plasma therapy: a systematic literature review and evidence for clinical use. Phys Sportsmed 2011;39: 42–51.

78. Conway JE. Arthroscopic repair of partial-thickness rotator cuff tears and SLAP lesions in professional baseball players. Orthop Clin North Am 2001;32:443–56.

79. Jobe FW, Moynes DR. Delineation of diagnostic criteria and a rehabilitation program for rotator cuff injuries. Am J Sports Med 1982;10:336–9.

80. Itoi E, Kido T, Sano A, et al. Which is more useful, the "full can test" or the "empty can test," in detecting the torn supraspinatus tendon? Am J Sports Med 1999; 27:65–8.

81. Kelly BT, Kadrmas WR, Speer KP. The manual muscle examination for rotator cuff strength. An electromyographic investigation. Am J Sports Med 1996;24: 581–8.

82. Malanga GA, Jenp YN, Growney ES, et al. EMG analysis of shoulder positioning in testing and strengthening the supraspinatus. Med Sci Sports Exerc 1996;28: 661–4.

83. Tarkin IS, Morganti CM, Zillmer DA, et al. Rotator cuff tears in adolescent athletes. Am J Sports Med 2005;33:596–601.

84. Chang YW, Hughes RE, Su FC, et al. Prediction of muscle force involved in shoulder internal rotation. J Shoulder Elbow Surg 2000;9:188–95.

85. Gerber C, Hersche O, Farron A. Isolated rupture of the subscapularis tendon. Results of operative repair. J Bone Joint Surg Am 1996;78:1015–23.
86. Greis PE, Kuhn JE, Schultheis J, et al. Validation of the lift-off test and analysis of subscapularis activity during maximal internal rotation. Am J Sports Med 1996; 24:589–93.
87. Gerber C, Krushell RJ. Isolated rupture of the tendon of the subscapularis muscle. Clinical features in 16 cases. J Bone Joint Surg Br 1991;73:389–94.
88. Barth JRH, Burkhart SS, De Beer JF. The bear-hug test: a new and sensitive test for diagnosing a subscapularis tear. Arthroscopy 2006;22:1076–84.
89. Kessel L, Watson M. The painful arc syndrome. Clinical classification as a guide to management. J Bone Joint Surg Br 1977;59:166–72.
90. Hawkins RJ, Kennedy JC. Impingement syndrome in athletes. Am J Sports Med 1980;8:151–7 [discussion: 157–8].
91. Neer CS II. Impingement lesions. Clin Orthop Relat Res 1983;173:70–7.
92. Savoie FH III, Field LD, Atchinson S. Anterior superior instability with rotator cuff tearing: SLAC lesion. Orthop Clin North Am 2001;32:457–61.
93. Park HB, Yokota A, Gill HS, et al. Diagnostic accuracy of clinical tests for the different degrees of subacromial impingement syndrome. J Bone Joint Surg Am 2005;87:1446–55.
94. Neer CS II. Anterior acromioplasty for the chronic impingement syndrome in the shoulder: a preliminary report. J Bone Joint Surg Am 1972;54:41–50.
95. Jia X, Petersen SA, Khosravi AH, et al. Examination of the shoulder: the past, the present, and the future. J Bone Joint Surg Am 2009;91:10–8.
96. Kibler WB. Biomechanical analysis of the shoulder during tennis activities. Clin Sports Med 1995;14:79–85.
97. Kibler WB, McMullen J. Scapular dyskinesis and its relation to shoulder pain. J Am Acad Orthop Surg 2003;11:142–51.
98. Fleisig GS, Barrentine SW, Escamilla RF, et al. Biomechanics of overhand throwing with implications for injuries. Sports Med 1996;21:421–37.
99. Rowe CR, Zarins B. Recurrent transient subluxation of the shoulder. J Bone Joint Surg Am 1981;63:863–72.
100. Jobe FW, Giangarra CE, Kvitne RS, et al. Anterior capsulolabral reconstruction of the shoulder in athletes in overhand sports. Am J Sports Med 1991;19: 428–34.
101. Kvitne RS, Jobe FW. The diagnosis and treatment of anterior instability in the throwing athlete. Clin Orthop Relat Res 1993;291:107–23.
102. McFarland EG, Campbell G, McDowell J. Posterior shoulder laxity in asymptomatic athletes. Am J Sports Med 1996;24:468–71.
103. Farber AJ, Castillo RC, Clough M, et al. Clinical assessment of three common tests for traumatic anterior shoulder instability. J Bone Joint Surg Am 2006;88: 1467–74.
104. Lo IKY, Nonweiler B, Woolfrey M, et al. An evaluation of the apprehension, relocation, and surprise tests for anterior shoulder instability. Am J Sports Med 2004;32:301–7.
105. Speer KP, Hannafin JA, Altchek DW, et al. An evaluation of the shoulder relocation test. Am J Sports Med 1994;22:177–83.
106. Lintner SA, Levy A, Kenter K, et al. Glenohumeral translation in the asymptomatic athlete's shoulder and its relationship to other clinically measurable anthropometric variables. Am J Sports Med 1996;24:716–20.
107. Walch G, Liotard JP, Boileau P, et al. Postero-superior glenoid impingement. Another impingement of the shoulder. J Radiol 1993;74:47–50.

108. Walch G, Boileau P, Noel E, et al. Impingement of the deep surface of the supraspinatus tendon on the posterosuperior glenoid rim: an arthroscopic study. J Shoulder Elbow Surg 1992;1:238–45.

109. McFarland EG, Hsu CY, Neira C, et al. Internal impingement of the shoulder: a clinical and arthroscopic analysis. J Shoulder Elbow Surg 1999;8:458–60.

110. Burns WC II, Whipple TL. Anatomic relationships in the shoulder impingement syndrome. Clin Orthop Relat Res 1993;294:96–102.

111. Kim TK, McFarland EG. Internal impingement of the shoulder in flexion. Clin Orthop Relat Res 2004;421:112–9.

112. Blevins FT. Rotator cuff pathology in athletes. Sports Med 1997;24:205–20.

113. Brockmeier SF, Dodson CC, Gamradt SC, et al. Arthroscopic intratendinous repair of the delaminated partial-thickness rotator cuff tear in overhead athletes. Arthroscopy 2008;24:961–5.

114. McConville OR, Iannotti JP. Partial-thickness tears of the rotator cuff: evaluation and management. J Am Acad Orthop Surg 1999;7:32–43.

115. Payne LZ, Altchek DW, Craig EV, et al. Arthroscopic treatment of partial rotator cuff tears in young athletes. A preliminary report. Am J Sports Med 1997;25:299–305.

116. Reynolds SB, Dugas JR, Cain EL, et al. Debridement of small partial-thickness rotator cuff tears in elite overhead throwers. Clin Orthop Relat Res 2008;466:614–21.

117. Roye RP, Grana WA, Yates CK. Arthroscopic subacromial decompression: two-to seven-year follow-up. Arthroscopy 1995;11:301–6.

118. McFarland EG, Maffulli N, Del Buono A, et al. Impingement is not impingement: the case for calling it "Rotator Cuff Disease". Muscles Ligaments Tendons J 2013;3:196–200.

119. Roos DB. Congenital anomalies associated with thoracic outlet syndrome. Anatomy, symptoms, diagnosis, and treatment. Am J Surg 1976;132:771–8.

120. Sanders RJ, Hammond SL. Management of cervical ribs and anomalous first ribs causing neurogenic thoracic outlet syndrome. J Vasc Surg 2002;36:51–6.

121. Esposito MD, Arrington JA, Blackshear MN, et al. Thoracic outlet syndrome in a throwing athlete diagnosed with MRI and MRA. J Magn Reson Imaging 1997;7:598–9.

122. Leffert RD, Perlmutter GS. Thoracic outlet syndrome. Results of 282 transaxillary first rib resections. Clin Orthop Relat Res 1999;368:66–79.

123. Adson AW. Surgical treatment for symptoms produced by cervical ribs and the scalenus anticus muscle. Surg Gynecol Obstet 1947;85:687–700.

124. Wright IS. The neurovascular syndrome produced by hyperabduction of the arms. The immediate changes produced in 150 normal controls, and the effects on some persons of prolonged hyperabduction of the arms, as in sleeping, and in certain occupations. Am Heart J 1945;29:1–19.

125. Leffert RD. Thoracic outlet syndrome. J Am Acad Orthop Surg 1994;2:317–25.

126. McGough EC, Pearce MB, Byrne JP. Management of thoracic outlet syndrome. J Thorac Cardiovasc Surg 1979;77:169–74.

127. Hughes ESR. Venous obstruction in the upper extremity (Paget-Schroetter's syndrome): a review of 320 cases. Surg Gynecol Obstet 1949;88:89–127.

128. Machleder HI. Evaluation of a new treatment strategy for Paget-Schroetter syndrome: spontaneous thrombosis of the axillary-subclavian vein. J Vasc Surg 1993;17:305–15 [discussion: 316–7].

129. AbuRahma AF, Sadler D, Stuart P, et al. Conventional versus thrombolytic therapy in spontaneous (effort) axillary-subclavian vein thrombosis. Am J Surg 1991;161:459–65.

130. Sheeran SR, Hallisey MJ, Murphy TP, et al. Local thrombolytic therapy as part of a multidisciplinary approach to acute axillosubclavian vein thrombosis (Paget-Schroetter syndrome). J Vasc Interv Radiol 1997;8:253–60.

131. Cahill BR, Palmer RE. Quadrilateral space syndrome. J Hand Surg Am 1983;8: 65–9.

132. Okino S, Miyaji H, Matoba M. The quadrilateral space syndrome. Neuroradiology 1995;37:311–2.

133. McClelland D, Paxinos A. The anatomy of the quadrilateral space with reference to quadrilateral space syndrome. J Shoulder Elbow Surg 2008;17:162–4.

134. Mochizuki T, Isoda H, Masui T, et al. Occlusion of the posterior humeral circumflex artery: detection with MR angiography in healthy volunteers and in a patient with quadrilateral space syndrome. AJR Am J Roentgenol 1994;163:625–7.

135. Bateman JE. Nerve injuries about the shoulder in sports. J Bone Joint Surg Am 1967;49:785–92.

136. Ferretti A, De Carli A, Fontana M. Injury of the suprascapular nerve at the spino-glenoid notch. The natural history of infraspinatus atrophy in volleyball players. Am J Sports Med 1998;26:759–63.

137. Sandow MJ, Ilic J. Suprascapular nerve rotator cuff compression syndrome in volleyball players. J Shoulder Elbow Surg 1998;7:516–21.

138. Gozna ER, Harris WR. Traumatic winging of the scapula. J Bone Joint Surg Am 1979;61:1230–3.

139. Kuhn JE, Plancher KD, Hawkins RJ. Scapular winging. J Am Acad Orthop Surg 1995;3:319–25.

140. Schultz JS, Leonard JA Jr. Long thoracic neuropathy from athletic activity. Arch Phys Med Rehabil 1992;73:87–90.

141. Carson WG Jr, Gasser SI. Little Leaguer's shoulder: a report of 23 cases. Am J Sports Med 1998;26:575–80.

142. American Sports Medicine Institute. Position statement for youth baseball pitchers. Available at: http://www.asmi.org/research.php?page=research&section=positionStatement. Accessed December 27, 2013.

143. Lyman S, Fleisig GS, Andrews JR, et al. Effect of pitch type, pitch count, and pitching mechanics on risk of elbow and shoulder pain in youth baseball pitchers. Am J Sports Med 2002;30:463–8.

144. Osbahr DC, Cawley PW, Speer KP. The effect of continuous cryotherapy on glenohumeral joint and subacromial space temperatures in the postoperative shoulder. Arthroscopy 2002;18:748–54.

145. Singh H, Osbahr DC, Holovacs TF, et al. The efficacy of continuous cryotherapy on the postoperative shoulder: a prospective, randomized investigation. J Shoulder Elbow Surg 2001;10:522–5.

146. Kibler WB, Livingston B. Closed-chain rehabilitation for upper and lower extremities. J Am Acad Orthop Surg 2001;9:412–21.

147. McMullen J, Uhl TL. A kinetic chain approach for shoulder rehabilitation. J Athl Train 2000;35:329–37.

Low Back Pain in the Adolescent Athlete

Arthur Jason De Luigi, DO

KEYWORDS

- Low back pain • Adolescents • Athletes • Spinal injuries

KEY POINTS

- Low back pain is frequently encountered in adolescent athletes.
- The adolescent athlete is at risk for significant structural injuries as well as nonmechanical problems.
- Adolescent athletes who present with low back pain are more likely to have structural injuries and therefore should be investigated fully.
- Any athlete with severe, persisting, or activity-limiting symptoms needs to be evaluated thoroughly.
- It is imperative to complete a comprehensive evaluation of back pain, and a cause such as muscle strain should be a diagnosis of exclusion.

INTRODUCTION

Low back pain is a common problem among adolescent athletes. It is estimated to occur in 10% to 15% of young athletes,[1,2] but the prevalence may be higher in certain sports.[1,3–7] Back pain has been reported as high as 27% in football and between 50% and 86% in gymnastics.[4–6] Although adolescent athletes are undergoing their pubescent changes into adulthood, they cannot be treated like young adults. Therefore, the approach to the treatment of adolescent athletes with low back pain can be difficult and requires thorough understanding of spinal development.

The demographics of adolescents with low back pain varies from that of adulthood, Although there are many conditions that occur in both adolescence and adulthood, there are certain spinal disease/injury processes that are unique to the growing adolescent spine.[8–11] One of the key factors to consider in the adolescent athlete is the ongoing growth and development of the adolescent spine. The growing spine introduces variables into the assessment and management of injuries to the spine that do not exist in the mature and developed spine of the adult population. For example, injuries of the pars interarticularis are more common in the adolescent spine, occurring

Department of Rehabilitation Medicine, Georgetown University School of Medicine, 3800 Reservoir Road, Washington, DC 20007, USA
E-mail address: Arthur.J.Deluigi@Medstar.net

Phys Med Rehabil Clin N Am 25 (2014) 763–788
http://dx.doi.org/10.1016/j.pmr.2014.06.004
1047-9651/14/$ – see front matter © 2014 Elsevier Inc. All rights reserved.

in up to 47% of young athletes,[9] whereas disk-related problems are uncommon in children; only 11% of children have disk-related disease, compared with 48% of adults.[9] Idiopathic pain is also less common in young athletes. Physicians who attribute low back pain in young athletes to simple back strains, without investigations, run the risk of delaying the diagnosis and appropriate treatment of more serious injuries, such as spondylolysis or spondylolisthesis.[8,11] Therefore, it is imperative that the clinician is aware the development of the spine and subsequent variances in injury patterns and frequencies when evaluating the adolescent athlete.

In addition to the structural considerations of the spine, the clinician should also be aware of potential physiologic, psychological, social, and cultural issues that may exist and affect the approach to diagnosis and management of adolescent spine disorders. To treat these athletes appropriately, clinicians need to develop a relationship with the athlete's parents/guardians, coaches, and other potential athletic support staff to facilitate compliance with the activity modifications and treatment necessary to provide optimal rehabilitation to the injured spine. The coordination of care with the athlete's support team facilitates the athlete's recovery, training, and performance.[12]

GROWTH AND DEVELOPMENT OF THE SPINE

There are distinct structural differences of the spine in adolescents from the adult spine, which affect the nature of injury. Compared with the adult spine, the relatively greater hydrophilic nature of the nucleus pulposus of the spine of a child allows for more effective force absorption and central distribution of force transfer to the adjacent vertebrae.[12] However, the composition of the nucleus pulposus begins to change as early as 7 or 8 years old, resulting in a more peripheral force distribution of the disk.[13] There are 3 primary ossification centers of the vertebrae: one in the vertebral body and 2 in the vertebral arch. The 2 ossifications in the center of the vertebral arch typically fuse by 2 to 6 years, and spinal bifida occulta results, caused by failure of fusion of these primary centers.[14,15] Pars interarticularis defects/fractures are more common in the adolescent spine, occurring in up to 47% of young athletes, and are postulated to be caused by incomplete bony maturation present in the neural arch.[9] Biomechanical studies have indicated that the bony strength of the vertebrae, particularly the neural arch, can increase into the fourth or fifth decade of life.[16]

The physes associated with the vertebral end plates facilitate the growth of the vertebral body. Hyaline cartilage adjacent to the nucleus pulposus and physeal cartilage adjacent to the vertebral body comprise the vertebral end plate. A ring apophysis and an end-plate physis comprise the physeal cartilage. The growth of the vertebral body is facilitated by the ring apophysis, which surrounds the periphery of the vertebral body and begins to ossify at 7 or 8 years old,[12] whereas vertical growth of the vertebral body is caused by end-plate physis, which begins to fuse with the vertebral body at about age 14 to 15 years, with final closure occurring around age 21 to 25 years.[12-14]

In addition to understanding the structural aspects of the growing adolescent spine, the clinician needs to be familiar with the variances of pubescent spinal development to assist in the diagnosis and management of spinal injuries. Schmorl nodes occur more frequently in children and adolescents compared with adults. Schmorl nodes are vertebral end-plate herniations of disk material, which are postulated to result from a combination of more central distribution of force via the nucleus pulposus combined with a relatively weak vertebral end plate.[12-15] The adolescent athlete is also at increased risk for apophyseal ring fractures during the ongoing physeal development until ossification.[12]

Another significant variation in injury patterns related to spinal development is disk-related disease in comparing the growing adolescent with mature adults, with the incidence at 11% in children compared with 48% in adults.[9] The proposed pathophysiologic basis for this significant age-related variance is the relative strength of the intervertebral disk compared with that of the adjacent bone in adolescents compared with those in adults.[12–15]

There is a significant variance in individual adolescents in the onset of puberty and the subsequent rate of growth and maturation. The variance between adolescents results in significant differences in size, strength, and skeletal maturity among children of the same chronologic age. Children between 6 and 10 years of age grow about 5 to 8 cm per year and gain about 2 to 3 kg per year.[17] During adolescence, the growth rate increases, leading first to increases in height followed by increases in weight. On average, girls enter adolescent growth spurt and reach their maximal growth velocity about 2 years before boys. Weight gain occurs during the maximal growth in height, with girls gaining about 7 kg in fat-free mass, whereas boys gain about twice this amount.[17]

DEMOGRAPHICS

Although low back pain commonly occurs in the adolescent population, adolescent athletes who participate in specific sports such as football or gymnastics may be at a more substantial risk of pain and structural injury than others at the same chronologic age.[4–6] The overall lifetime prevalence of low back pain by the midteenage years has been found to be 50% or greater in general population studies, with 1-year prevalence rates of 17% to 50%.[12,18–23] In several studies,[12,18–20,22,23] an increase in the prevalence of low back pain with age throughout childhood has been reported, with some of these studies also reporting higher rates of spinal injuries in girls than boys. A definitive connection has yet to be established between physical activity and low back pain, because the previous studies have had a significant variance in their results.[12,20,23–26] In an attempt to provide more objective evidence with the use of an accelerometer to assess activity levels in children and adolescents, Wedderkopp and colleagues[26] did not find any association between physical activity and low back pain. However, several studies[27] have identified an association in adolescents with low back pain between depression and other emotional problems. Another significant risk factor showing a strong correlation was that the development of low back pain during adolescence increased the likelihood for the development of low back pain as an adult in a large-scale twin study.[28]

There is a significant variance in the incidence and the specific spinal pathologic injury in adolescent athletes depending on the specific sport and also the position in a given sport.[12] Contact sports such as football and rugby have a significantly higher incidence of acute injuries from high-energy impacts.[6] In comparison, there is a greater incidence of overuse injuries with sports requiring repetitive flexion, extension, and torsion, such as gymnastics, figure skating, and rowing.[4,5,29] A significantly higher rate of low back pain in a group of female gymnasts and figure skaters and male hockey and soccer players compared with nonathletes has been noted (45% vs 18% over 3 years).[30] However, low back pain spans most sports in the adolescent population and was found to be a significant problem in golfers, rowers, and rugby players.[31–33]

Gymnasts in particular have shown a significantly high incidence of spinal injury (between 50% and 86%) in several studies.[4,5] These findings are limited not only to female gymnasts, because another study of male gymnasts showed that 79% of the male gymnasts had low back pain compared with 38% of their controls.[34] In another study assessing wrestlers, gymnasts, and soccer and tennis players, 65% of these athletes had a history of low back pain, with male gymnasts having the highest frequency, at 85%.[35]

RADIOLOGIC FINDINGS

There have been numerous studies regarding the incidence of radiologic findings in adolescent athletes. The results of these studies have shown that there are high rates of structural abnormalities on imaging studies of adolescent athletes in specific sports. As noted earlier, there was an increased incidence of low back pain symptoms in adolescent athletes who participate in gymnastics, and this trend also continues in the radiologic evaluation of their spines.[12] In a study on the incidence of findings of back pain in male gymnasts, magnetic resonance imaging (MRI) showed statistically significant differences in spinal diseases in gymnasts compared with controls, with findings of thoracolumbar disk degeneration (75% compared with 31%), Schmorl nodes (71% compared with 44%), and injuries to the ring apophysis (17% compared with 0%).[34] These findings were also shown in another study by Goldstein and colleagues,[36] who reported higher rates of various structural abnormalities on MRI studies of elite gymnasts compared with elite swimmers. Another study by Bennett and colleagues[37] performed MRI of the spine of elite female gymnasts, showing apophyseal injuries in almost half and disk degeneration in more than 60%.

Radiographic findings of spinal disease are not limited to adolescent gymnasts. Structural abnormalities on plain radiographs were shown in greater than 60% of the high-school and collegiate football players and in 74% of the rugby players assessed in 2 separate studies by Iwamoto and colleagues.[35,38] Several studies[39–42] have also shown higher rates of spondylolysis in high-level adolescent athletes participating in a variety of sports compared with nonathlete adolescents in the general population. Despite high levels of structural abnormalities on plain films and high rates of reported low back pain for young athletes competing in several sports, longer term follow-up studies[43–45] on many of these athletes did not show any significant increased risk for ongoing low back pain into adulthood compared with the general population.

CONSIDERATIONS IN THE EVALUATION OF LOW BACK PAIN IN THE ADOLESCENT ATHLETE

Injuries to the low back may be caused by an acute traumatic event; however, they are more frequently secondary to overuse injuries caused by chronic repetitive microtrauma.[29] It is imperative to complete a thorough assessment of all adolescent athletes who report symptoms of low back pain to evaluate for the presence of spinal disease. As noted earlier, because of the ongoing growth and development of the adolescent spine, the incidence of specific spinal diseases in adolescent athletes varies from adults. The clinician should also be cognizant of potential nonmechanical causes of low back pain, such as neoplasms, infection, developmental disorders, and systemic inflammatory rheumatisms.[12,28,45–48] One must formulate a strong differential diagnosis and subsequently through the evaluation process develop a rational diagnostic strategy based on a thorough history, review of systems, and physical examination. The clinician should always inquire about any potential red flag symptoms, such as unexplained weight loss, pain at night, pain with recumbency, progressive neurologic deficits, and any loss of bowel or bladder function. In addition, one should inquire about any additional symptoms during a review of symptoms, which may show a systemic process, such as a rheumatic disorder.

RISK FACTORS

As the adolescent athlete undergoes pubescent changes leading to periods of rapid growth, the muscles and ligaments are unable to maintain the pace of the rate of bone growth. This discrepancy places the adolescent athlete at greater risk of injury, as a result of muscle imbalance and a decrease in flexibility.[1,29,49] The skeletally immature spine of adolescent athletes is also vulnerable to injury of the growth cartilage and secondary ossifications centers, because these areas are the weakest link of force transfer and are susceptible to compression, distraction, and torsion injury.[1,7,29]

The vertebral bodies and intervertebral disks comprise the anterior column of the lumbar spine. Epiphyseal growth plates are located at both ends of the vertebral bodies and have overlying cartilaginous growth plates and ring apophyses, which attach to the outer annulus fibrosus. Repetitive flexion may lead to intervertebral disk herniation through the ring apophysis, a secondary ossification center, and injury to the ring apophysis can result in avulsion fractures.[28]

The facet joints, spinous process, and pars interarticularis make up the posterior column of the lumbar spine. Ossification of the posterior column of the spine progresses from anterior to posterior and may be congenitally incomplete in the area of the superior portion of the pars interarticularis of the lower lumbar vertebrae, particularly at the L5 level, predisposing to spondylolytic stress fractures.[1,11] The presence of spina bifida occulta at the lumbosacral junction seems to be an additional risk factor for spondylolysis. Traction from the dorsolumbar fascia and lordotic impingement may affect the growth cartilage of the facet joint and spinous process apophysis of the posterior arch.[1]

Because of the considerable variance in the timing and tempo of growth among children, smaller, less mature athletes may be at higher risk for injury from contact from larger athletes, particularly in contact sports.[11,49]

Several potential risk factors for spinal injury or low back pain in athletes have been identified. These factors include previous low back or lower extremity injuries, incomplete rehabilitation of previous injuries, decreased endurance, lower extremity muscle imbalance, high number of hours of participation per week, and the occurrence of stressful life events. Additional proximate causal factors associated with sports-related injury may include the individual mechanics and skill level associated with sports performance, training patterns, and equipment or facility problems.[47,50]

Training volume and intensity can also cause injuries, particularly when young athletes participate in a sport for longer periods, such as at tournaments and sports camps.[11] However, it is difficult to determine the appropriate amount of training for adolescent athletes, because of the variance in toleration of similar volumes of training. Overuse injuries present more often in athletes experiencing rapid growth,[1,11] suggesting that the volume and intensity of training that an athlete's body can tolerate vary as the athletes grow and mature.[11]

Poor technique, abdominal muscle weakness, hip flexor/hamstring/thoracolumbar fascia tightness, increased femoral anteversion, genu recurvatum, and increased thoracic kyphosis serve as additional risk factors for low back pain. These factors add additional stress to the posterior elements of the spine as a result of increased lumbar lordosis.[1,11]

PREVENTION

Although injuries are a part of sport, there are ways to reduce the risk of injury in young athletes. Recognizing risk factors is a key component to reducing injury.[11] Before the start of a sport season, a preparticipation evaluation may identify certain risk factors, such as previous injuries that have not been fully rehabilitated or muscle weaknesses or inflexibility. These areas can then be addressed before the start of the season. In addition, athletes should start general strength and fitness conditioning several weeks before the start of the season.[49] Increases in the frequency and intensity of training should be gradual, to allow for safe adaptation to the demands of the sport.

During periods of growth, young athletes are prone to loss of flexibility and muscle imbalances, which can predispose them to injury.[11,49] Because of this concern, young athletes should reduce the amount of training and the volume of repetitive motions during growth spurts. Certain sports require maneuvers that place a lot of stress on the posterior spine, such as layback spins in figure skating and walkovers in gymnastics. Athletes may need to limit the number of repetitions of these maneuvers, particularly if pain is associated with these maneuvers. Core strengthening exercises and stretches for tight hamstrings and hip flexors may help reduce the risk of low back pain.[11,49]

Proper technique should be emphasized in all athletes. It is important to correct posture to limit the amount of lordosis of the lumbar spine, which can help prevent injuries to the lumbar spine. In sports requiring lifting, such as pairs skating and dance, proper lifting techniques must be used to prevent back injuries.[11]

In team sports, there can be large discrepancies in the sizes and relative strengths of participants on any given team. Attempts should be made to match athletes in size and strength to prevent injuries from contact with larger, stronger participants.[11,49]

Another important aspect of prevention is recognizing that back pain is not part of the sport. Increasing complaints of pain, particularly if it is interfering with activity, should be taken seriously and addressed early to avoid significant injury.[11]

HISTORY AND PHYSICAL EXAMINATION

A comprehensive history is an essential initial step in the evaluation of adolescent athletes with low back pain. The mode of onset, location, quality, severity, and progression over time of the individual's symptoms provide useful insight into potential causes. Symptoms that remain mild for an extended period before presentation may be suggestive of less significant structural injuries or more indolent underlying processes, whereas more severe, acute, or progressive symptoms may suggest a more substantial structural injury or a rapidly progressive process, such as infection. In addition, the provider should inquire about back pain eliciting any neurologic symptoms and aggravating factors.[12]

The nature of an athlete's specific sport and the position played may also predispose that individual to particular problems as well as the volume of training and level of competition. The timing of injury or pain in relation to the competitive season or training cycle may be relevant for both diagnosis and treatment.[8,11] It is also important to inquire if there have been any recent increases in the training volume or intensity of the athlete. Thorough review of the dietary history, previous injuries, and the menstrual history of female athletes is also of importance.[11]

Primary importance should be placed on the potential of red flag symptoms, such as fever, malaise, unexplained weight loss, pain at night, morning stiffness, bowel or bladder incontinence, and progressive neurologic weakness. Pain at night is often believed to be suggestive of an infectious or neoplastic process.[12,51] Fever, lethargy, weight loss, rashes, headaches, and similar symptoms raise concern for significant systemic processes, including infection and malignancy.[12,48,51] Morning stiffness or additional joint symptoms may suggest a diffuse inflammatory process. A past history or family history of HLA-B27-associated conditions, such as psoriatic arthritis, ankylosing spondylitis, reactive (Reiter) arthritis, or inflammatory bowel disease, may help in determining systemic causes of low back pain.[29]

Isolated axial low back pain without lower extremity symptoms should be viewed differently from a presentation that includes leg pain or neurologic dysfunction, such as numbness, tingling, weakness, or changes in the bowel or bladder. Radicular symptoms such as radiation of pain down the leg and motor or sensory changes suggest the presence of nerve root or cord involvement.[12] Bilateral leg pain suggests bilateral foraminal involvement and should expand the clinician's differential diagnosis. At this point, one should consider and make specific assessment to help differentiate between a significant spondylolisthesis, central canal stenosis, disk herniation in the setting of a congenitally small spinal canal, or a cord process.[12] The presence of lower extremity symptoms does not always mean that they are of spinal origin, and the clinician should also assess for other concomitant nonspinal diseases such as stress fractures, compartment syndrome, or other musculotendinous injuries. The location of the back pain can also significantly affect the differential diagnosis. Thoracic or thoracolumbar pain may be associated with diskogenic processes or Scheuermann kyphosis. Low lumbar pain has many potential causes, including disk disease, central or foraminal stenosis, spondyloarthropathies, and myofascial pain. Pain in the sacral or gluteal region may be more associated with conditions such as sacroiliitis or a sacral stress fracture; however, one still must assess for referred pain from the lumbar facets or nerve root involvement.[12]

After the completion of a thorough history of present illness, the clinician should perform a comprehensive physical examination. The physical examination should be structured to identify significant and specific conditions that were formulated on the differential diagnosis. The result of a thorough history and physical examination should develop a strategic plan of further diagnostic and treatment options.[12]

The physical examination should always be thorough, including inspection of any structural imbalances or asymmetries, lumbar range of motion, lumbosacral and pelvic motion, palpation of the spine, lumbar paraspinals, sacroiliac (SI)/pelvic muscles and joints, and a neurologic examination. It is important to assess lower extremity alignment and function, balance, and spine-specific provocative maneuvers. Gait assessment should be performed to assess for abnormalities such as antalgia, ataxia, or Trendelenberg gait.[12]

The examiner should observe the athlete's spine by having the patient wear a gown open to the back. When observing the athlete from behind it is important in the spine, shoulders, and pelvis to identify that the bony and soft tissue structures on both sides of the midline are symmetric. Visual inspection of the spine should evaluate for the presence of any abnormalities such as hemangiomas, café-au-lait spots, hairy patches, or skin dimples that may indicate spinal disease.[49,52] Inspection should also identify any abnormal curvatures of the spine, such as scoliosis, excessive kyphosis, or lordosis.

Range of motion of the spine should be assessed in flexion, extension, rotation, and lateral flexion (bending). Adolescent athletes should be able to complete forward flexion of the spine and come close to touching their toes without knee flexion. Caution must be used to identify limitation of this motion because of tight hamstrings. Pain with flexion is suggestive of injury to the anterior spinal elements or lumbar muscle strain/spasms. The posterior elements of the spine can be assessed with hyperextension and facet loading (hyperextension with rotation).

Palpation for tenderness of the spine, lumbar paraspinals, and the SI joint is an integral part of the spinal assessment. Myofascial trigger points are taut, palpable bands in the lumbar paraspinal and gluteal muscles, which elicit or trigger the athlete's pain. Tenderness of the SI joint has a positive predictive value for SI disorder.[53]

Special tests include tests for the SI iliac joints, facet joints, and neural tension signs. These tests include FABER (flexion-abduction-external rotation), Gaenslen sign, Gillet test, seated slump test, straight leg raise, Lasègue maneuver, Bragard sign, Lazarević sign, and facet loading.[11,54]

Additional assessment should be completed to assess the hip to rule out hip disease as well as the abdomen to rule out visceral disease. In female athletes, a pelvic examination may be warranted, particularly if menstrual abnormalities are reported by the patient during the history. The neurologic examination should include assessment of motor strength, sensation, and deep tendon reflexes of the lower extremities.

Clearly, other components of a comprehensive physical examination need to be included as medically appropriate, as well. Consideration does need to be given to the potential for significant structural injury, including fracture, and the examination should always be modified appropriately for a given patient to elicit essential information and avoid further harm.

RADIOGRAPHIC EVALUATION OF THE ADOLESCENT SPINE

Spinal imaging should be considered as an additional diagnostic option to assist in establishing a specific diagnosis. There are a variety of different imaging modalities to assist in the diagnostic evaluation, and clinicians need to be familiar with the each of their strengths and limitations. In addition, the clinician should be comfortable with directly assessing the images. Given the relative sensitivities and specificities of the various diagnostic options, the clinician should develop a plan for which imaging modality would provide the most appropriate objective findings based on the formulated differential diagnosis. In addition, the clinician should also consider that the amount of exposure to radiation in the adolescent athlete is of particular concern. Therefore, specific radiographic options should include the risk assessment of radiation exposure versus the potential comparative benefit of the various diagnostic options. The imaging strategies vary based on clinical concerns of the presenting symptoms and findings during the history and physical examination and are discussed in greater detail with each specific spinal condition.[12]

SPECIAL CONSIDERATIONS IN THE ADOLESCENT ATHLETE

Treatment of adolescent athletes involves several specific considerations, as well. The state and demands of physiologic development of the athlete need to be taken into consideration when planning physical training. The psychosocial environment of an injured athlete may also pose challenges for treatment, and the psychological impact of injury can be difficult for athletes and their families. The use of medications may be problematic, as well. There are limited to no data on the effects on children and adolescents of several different medications commonly used to manage pain in adults. Care needs to be taken regarding weight and age in prescribing medications to young athletes, and clinicians need to be aware of any potential conflicts with substance use policies that may apply to an athlete's given sport or level of competition. There are also high rates of use of ergogenic aids and performance-enhancing supplements among adolescent athletes, which introduce the potential for medication interactions, among other problems.[55] The use of these supplements, legal or illegal, may not necessarily be reported to clinicians routinely, and the likelihood of this seems even lower if specific questions regarding their use are not asked.

SPECIFIC SPINAL CONDITIONS AND INJURIES

There are several specific clinical entities that are particularly important to understand in managing young athletes with low back pain. These entities include spondylolysis, spondylolisthesis, posterior element overuse syndrome, diskogenic injuries, vertebral body apophyseal avulsion fracture, Scheuermann kyphosis, SI pain, and other causes of low back pain. These individual conditions are discussed in greater detail in the following sections.[12]

Spondylolysis and Spondylolisthesis

Spondylolysis is a common cause of spinal disease in the adolescent spine and should be considered as a diagnostic possibility in almost every adolescent athlete with significant low back pain. However, it should be high on the differential diagnosis in all athletes who compete in sports involving repetitive extension and rotation, such as gymnastics, figure skating, and rowing.[12] Spondylolysis is definitively the most frequent diagnosis (47%) made in adolescent athletes presenting with low back pain.[9]

Spondylolysis refers to a defect in the pars interarticularis of the vertebral arch, a stress fracture caused by repetitive extension and torsion of the spine, and is most common at L5 and on the left side.[56] Bilateral spondylolysis at the same vertebral level can result in spondylolisthesis. Spondylolisthesis is a separate but related term referring to the anterior displacement of a vertebral body compared with its alignment with the adjacent vertebral body (**Fig. 1**).[12] Spondylolisthesis is graded using the Meyerding scale according to the percentage of slip: grade 1 is a slip of 0% to 25%, grade 2 is 25% to 50%, grade 3 is 50% to 75%, grade 4 is 75% to 100%, and grade 5 is more than 100%.[57]

Spondylolysis and spondylolisthesis are most frequently viewed under the categorization proposed by Wiltse and colleagues.[58] The term isthmic spondylolysis is used to identify those patients who have sustained a lesion in the pars. Isthmic

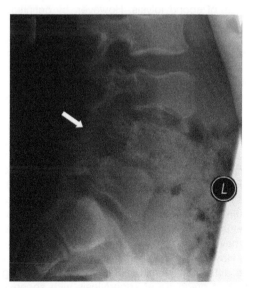

Fig. 1. Plain radiograph lateral view of lumbosacral spine of a young tennis player showing an isthmic spondylolisthesis with bilateral pars defects (*arrow*). (*From* Standaert CJ. Low back pain in the adolescent athlete. Phys Med Rehabil Clin N Am 2008;19(2):292; with permission.)

spondylolysis represents a pars lesion/defect that is believed to be a fatigue fracture of the bone. Most pars lesions identified in many studies occur at L5 (85%–95%).[39,40,42,58,59] In a study of 4243 young athletes with low back pain, Rossi and Dragoni[41] found that about one-half of those with spondylolysis also had concurrent spondylolisthesis. Significant progression of an associated spondylolisthesis is uncommon. There are data[60] to support that there is not any increased risk of progression of spondylolisthesis with sports participation. When there is an increase in the anterior translation of 1 vertebral body on the other, it is usually correlated with an adolescent growth spurt, and typically without any symptoms. Therefore, once spondylolisthesis is identified in the adolescent athlete, the affected individual needs to be monitored radiographically through adolescence to assess for any progression of the spinal disease.[12]

General population studies have shown pars lesions to be a common finding. In a prospective study of plain radiographs in 500 first-grade students, there was an overall prevalence of spondylolysis of 4.4% at age 6 years. All of these lesions identified in this study occurred without any symptoms. These diseases were then followed, and the number increased to 5.2% by age 12 years and 6% by adulthood.[39] Comparatively, another cadaveric study reviewed plain radiographs of 4200 cadaveric spines and found an overall prevalence of 4.2%.[40] However, the incidence of spondylolysis is different in adolescents who compete in athletics; large-scale studies[41,42] of adolescent athletes reported rates of 8% to 14%.

There is definitively a significant variance of the incidence of spondylolysis in athletes who participate in certain sports. Some of the sports with the highest reported frequencies of pars lesions include gymnastics, weight lifting, throwing track and field sports, diving, wrestling, cricket, and crew.[6,41,42,61,62] Sports that involve frequent flexion/extension motions of the lumbar spine, particularly when combined with rotation, may place athletes at more risk for pars fractures.

History and physical examination can be helpful in identifying a clinical pattern suggestive of the diagnosis of spondylolysis. However, by definition, additional spinal imaging is essential establish the diagnosis.

Athletes with spondylolysis typically present with insidious onset of extension-related low back pain.[8,11,12,63,64] The athlete frequently also has an associated reduction in hamstring flexibility. Symptomatic spondylolysis typically presents with axial low back pain without radiation into the legs; however, the athlete may occasionally have radiating pain, numbness, or weakness if the disease affects the nerve roots.[12] The pain typically occurs acutely after a specific traumatic event but may also occur after a relatively mundane event or may progress over time. The typical pain pattern associated with spondylolysis is usually worsened by activity and improved with rest.[12] The athlete may complain of pain with impact, such as running or jumping. It is common for the symptoms to begin to develop toward the end of 1 sports season, subside after the season while the athlete is no longer stressing the area of disease, and then return once the athlete starts training for the next season. The distribution of pain varies depending on whether the lesion is unilateral or bilateral but can lateralize to the side of the unilateral lesion or be more generalized in the low back.[12]

It is uncommon to have associated leg pain, paresthesias, or neurologic loss with isolated spondylosis. However, the presence of these symptoms does not eliminate spondylosis from the differential diagnosis. Rather, these findings should suggest the potential concomitant presence of spondylosis with spondylolisthesis or other diagnoses such as disk herniation in adolescent athletes.[11] There are no pathognomonic findings on physical examination for spondylolysis; however, pain with extension and rotation may suggest disease of the posterior elements such as a pars lesion or facets. A special test to assess for potential spondylolysis is the 1-legged hyperextension maneuver. This maneuver is performed by having the patient stand on 1 leg and leaning backward.[12] The maneuver has been proposed as a means of identifying the presence of a pars lesion, but a recent study of this test[65] concluded that it had low sensitivity and specificity.

Several diagnostic imaging modalities are available for evaluating the pars in an athlete with suspected spondylolysis.[12] However, there is significant controversy regarding the optimal imaging strategy, because of potential risks of radiation exposure in the growing adolescent spine. Given the relatively high prevalence of asymptomatic pars lesions in both the general population of adolescents and adolescent athletes, it is not enough just to visualize a pars lesion. Ideally, there is a clinical picture that is suggestive of disease of the pars, which is supported by the radiographic findings. Optimally, any radiographic pars defect needs to be identified as the source of pain and should be assessed for the potential of the lesion to heal. Therefore, in practical application, the clinician needs to assess the risks of radiation exposure from multiple imaging studies with the benefits of initial diagnosis and subsequent evaluation of pars defect healing.[12]

Historically, plain radiography has been the primary imaging modality used in the identification, diagnosis, and observation of healing of pars lesions based on results of many published studies. The anteroposterior (AP) view may identify anatomic variants or developmental defects such as transitional vertebrae or spina bifida occulta, which is seen frequently in patients with spondylolysis.[66] The lateral view may show spondylolisthesis or a lytic lesion. Typically, a spondylitic lesion seen in plain radiographs appears as a lucency in the area of the pars (see **Fig. 1**).[12] Oblique views may show a stress reaction of the pars interarticularis and is identified as the pathognomonic neck of the Scotty dog lesion.[12] However, the routine use of oblique views is discouraged in adolescent athletes, because of the increased dose of radiation and because only one-third of stress fractures can be identified on plain radiographs.[63,64] Bone scan, single-photon emission computed tomography (SPECT), computed tomography (CT), and MRI have all been shown to be more sensitive than plain radiography in the identification of pars lesions.[67]

Plain radiographs should be followed by nuclear imaging with bone scan or SPECT. Radionuclide imaging, particularly SPECT, can be helpful in the diagnostic evaluation of adolescent athletes with low back pain. Bony lesions in which active bony turnover is occurring are indicated by increased uptake on the bone scan.[8,11,12,63–65] Numerous studies have shown bone scan and SPECT to be more sensitive than plain radiography in the diagnosis of spondylolysis, and it seems to be superior to MRI and CT in this regard, as well.[12,68–75] Multiple studies have also shown that a positive bone scan or SPECT scan correlates with a symptomatic pars lesion.[12,69,76–80] This finding makes SPECT a particularly useful and sensitive screening tool in adolescent athletes with low back pain. However, significant limitation in the use of radionuclide imaging is low specificity, because there are several other abnormalities seen in the posterior elements of adolescents on SPECT or bone scan that do not represent pars lesions.[12,67,71,73,81] Additional imaging, particularly with CT, is generally required to clarify the bony abnormality in a patient with a positive SPECT study (**Figs. 2** and **3A**).[12]

CT can be used to confirm the presence of a pars interarticularis stress fracture and monitor the progress of healing.[8,63] Along with clarifying a bony process identified on nuclear imaging, CT can distinguish between well-corticated fracture margins, termed chronic lesions or nonunions by various investigators, and differing stages of more recent or incomplete fractures.[12,67,75,81–83] The stage of the pars lesion on CT has also been found to be associated with the potential for bony healing.[74,81] In addition,

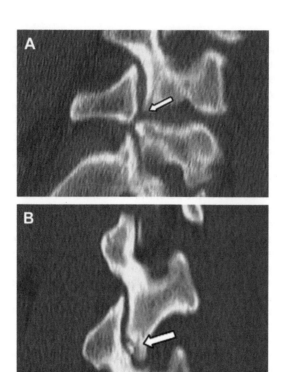

Fig. 2. CT oblique sagittal reformations. (*A*) A chronic pars lesion (*arrow*) with the classic appearance of the neck of the Scotty dog. (*B*) A spondylolytic lesion in the inferior articular process (*arrow*) in a young basketball player confirmed with SPECT. (*From* Standaert CJ. Low back pain in the adolescent athlete. Phys Med Rehabil Clin N Am 2008;19(2):295; with permission.)

in several studies,[12,61,73,75,81,83] several patients have been identified with increased activity in the area of the pars on SPECT but either an incomplete fracture or no fracture noted on CT. This finding seems most consistent with the presence of a stress reaction in the bone without overt fracture and shows the importance of correlating CT findings with nuclear imaging.[12,81] CT involves a higher level of radiation, and is of particular concern in the growing spine of the adolescent athlete. The risk for additional radiation must be weighed with the potential additional clinic benefit provided by CT. Therefore, many reserve CT scans for those not responding to treatment.[11]

Compared with the other imaging modalities, MRI has limitations that hamper its effectiveness as the primary imaging modality for adolescent athletes with low back pain. The main advantages of MRI include the lack of ionizing radiation and the ability to identify disk abnormalities and other types of disease. However, it can be difficult to appreciate cortical detail well at the pars on MRI compared with CT, and it is less sensitive for detecting spondylolysis compared with SPECT bone scan. The important diagnostic findings on MRI in patients with a potential pars lesion are those that are consistent with edema in the area of the pars or pedicle, suggestive of an acute

A **B**

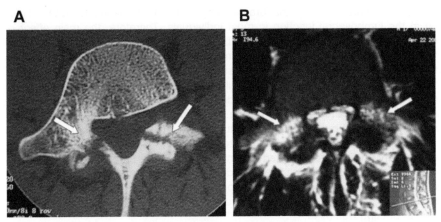

Fig. 3. (*A*) Axial view CT scan showing bilateral pars fractures (*arrows*). (*B*) Axial view CT scan shows unilateral pars fracture *(arrows)* with reactive sclerotic changes on the contralateral side. (*From* Standaert CJ. Low back pain in the adolescent athlete. Phys Med Rehabil Clin N Am 2008;19(2):296; with permission.)

fracture (see **Fig. 3**B).[12] There is a lack of evidence on the clinical implications of these MRI findings. In addition, studies have shown other significant limitations in the ability to identify and appropriately stratify pars lesions based on MRI.[12,65,74] A recent study comparing the relative usefulness of MRI compared with SPECT and CT found that MRI identified only 80% of the pars lesions seen on SPECT.[65] Therefore based on the lack of evidence, and comparative limitations to CT and SPECT, MRI does not seem to be an effective screening tool.[65,74]

Overall, the clinician should develop a definitive diagnostic approach to an adolescent athlete with low back pain who has signs or symptoms suggestive of a spondylolysis. Given the current review of literature, the adolescent athlete should initially be assessed with limited plain films, particularly isolated standing AP and lateral views to identify a spondylolisthesis or gross bony abnormalities, followed by a SPECT study. If the SPECT study is positive, a thin-cut CT (axial sequences 1 mm thick or less) should be obtained through the area of abnormality on SPECT to confirm the diagnosis and to stage the lesion for treatment. If the SPECT study is negative, it is highly unlikely that the athlete has a symptomatic pars defect, and other diagnoses should be considered.[8,11,12,63–75]

In an era of evidence-based medicine, it is interesting to know that there are no controlled trials on the treatment of spondylolysis in adolescent athletes.[12] However, there are several published case series that use a wide variety of treatment approaches. The essential element of care seems to be relative rest.[12] Activity modifications should occur to avoid any activities that cause pain, particularly extension activities. However, the ideal extent of activity restriction involved and the length of time out of sports is unclear.[12] An exercise program should include strengthening of the abdominal muscles, hip flexor and hamstring stretches, and antilordotic exercises.[3,11,49]

Bracing is a particularly controversial issue in the management of spondylolysis.[12] Several investigators[1,8,63,64,66,84,85] advocate the routine use of lumbosacral orthoses of a variety of types in the management of these patients in the early management to limit extension and rotation of the spine. Others[8,86] simply restrict activities without bracing, in conjunction with physical therapy. Biomechanical studies on the effects of lumbosacral bracing show that bracing results in an increase in intervertebral motion at the lumbosacral junction in most individuals. Therefore, the main effect of bracing seems to be a restriction in gross body motion rather than restricting interseg-mental mobility.[87,88] The results of outcome studies tend to be similar regarding rates of healing and return to play, regardless of the type or extent of bracing used. Studies[66,82,86,89,90] have shown bony healing with the use of a rigid brace, a soft brace, and no brace. The variance of these findings is what has made the use of specific bracing controversial. It is also surprising that in studies there is little correlation between the extent of bony healing and return to play. Most studies addressing these issues[12,66,83,90–92] show relatively high rates of return to play and lower rates of heal-ing. A recent study[89] that included patients treated with a brace as well as patients treated without a brace did not find any advantage for brace use in terms of achieving bony union. However, another study in young soccer players[93] showed that the best results were obtained with a period of rest from sport for 3 months, regardless of whether bracing was used.

Based on the current evidence, the best initial treatment of all athletes is rest. Ideally, rest should include avoidance of all physical activity and particularly sports beyond that needed for routine daily function.[12] Although there is no evidence showing any specific duration of activity restriction, the consensus is based on the individual clinical response and the appearance of their pars lesion on CT. If CT shows an early or progressive stage lesion, the athlete is advised to rest for 3 months, with subse-quent follow-up imaging.[12] However, if the pars lesion has chronic features on CT, the opportunity for bony union is diminished, and rest is advised until the low back pain has subsided.[12,82]

Although anecdotally advocated by some in clinical practice, the routine use of bracing is not uniformly supported by the literature. If bracing is used, bracing con-tinues until the athlete has resumed full activities without pain, and then the brace is gradually weaned until the athlete is participating fully without pain.[12,63,64] As a means of further restricting activity by providing a physical barrier to motion, a rigid brace may be used after 2 or 3 weeks of rest if symptoms are not resolving. After adequate rest for the stage of the lesion and restoration of pain-free range of motion, athletes can be placed in to a comprehensive rehabilitation program.[12]

Generally, rehabilitation for spondylolysis can be started early and progressed depending on symptoms, and generally return to play is about 6 to 8 weeks after the initial injury. The healing time for acute spondylolisthesis requires 2 to 4 months to complete followed by rehabilitation, resulting in return to sport approximately 4 to 6 months after diagnosis.[12] However, the return associated with minimally symptom-atic lesions may be sooner during the rehabilitation process.

A patient who has resumed full pain-free activities out of the brace is considered clinically healed. Patients with spondylolisthesis should be followed every 4 to 6 months with standing lateral films until skeletal maturity to assess for progression of slip.[12] Athletes are at low risk for worsening of spondylolisthesis. However, if the slip progresses beyond 50%, or if there are neurologic symptoms or persistent pain, surgical stabilization is indicated.[1,63]

Surgical intervention is rarely required to treat the pain associated with spondyloly-sis. However, there are potential indications for surgical intervention, including progressive slip, intractable pain, the development of neurologic deficits, and segmental instability associated with pain.[12] Surgical treatment is usually considered the best option for patients with a slip of 50% or greater, and these patients should all undergo surgical evaluation. There are several case series on athletes undergoing sur-gery with direct pars repair and returning to high-level sports, but considerations about return to play and long-term quality of life need to be factored into decisions on surgical intervention.[12]

As a routine issue, follow-up films are not necessary for patients with a unilateral pars lesion without a spondylolisthesis who do well with conservative treatment. Those with a spondylolisthesis need repeat plain films every 6 to 12 months during the adolescent growth spurts to monitor for possible slip progression. Similarly, this approach can be considered in those with bilateral pars defects, particularly if they are very young at the time of presentation.[12] Repeat imaging with CT can be helpful if it is necessary to determine the extent of healing or progression of the fracture; however, as noted earlier, the risk with additional radiation exposure needs to be assessed. Therefore, if the adolescent is no longer having any more clinical symptoms, the potential risk of increased radiation exposure exceeds the benefit of confirmed radiographic healing. Additional diagnostic evaluation should also be considered in patients who are not responding well to what seems to be appropriate treatment.

Posterior Element Overuse Syndrome

Posterior element overuse syndrome is a constellation of conditions involving muscle-tendon units, ligaments, facet joints, and joint capsules. It is a result from repeated extension and rotation of the spine. It is also called hyperlordotic low back pain, mechanical low back pain, or muscular low back pain.[1,8,9,49,85,94] Posterior element overuse syndrome is the most common cause after spondylolysis of low back pain in adolescents.[65]

Young athletes with posterior element overuse syndrome present with symptoms similar to those of spondylolysis. Pain is associated with extension of the spine and sometimes with rotation. There may be paraspinal muscle tenderness, as well as focal tenderness over the lower lumbar spine, adjacent to the midline. Imaging is typically negative, ruling out spondylolysis.

Management includes ice and nonsteroidal antiinflammatory drugs (NSAIDs) to relieve pain and inflammation. Pain-free activities are permitted, and extension of the spine is avoided. An exercise program emphasizing abdominal strengthening, antilordotic exercises, and hamstring and thoracolumbar stretches should be initiated at home or under the guidance of a physical therapist.[1,8,11,29,85] Although there is insufficient evidence of significant benefit, an antilordotic brace may be helpful in the short-term to provide support and protection.

Disk Disease

Low back pain secondary to disk disease is an uncommon problem in adolescent athletes; however, when it does occur, it can be a significant problem. Acute disk herniations of the nucleus pulposus are uncommon. Adolescents typically present with flexion-based back pain with associated paraspinal muscle spasms, hamstring tightness, and gluteal pain.[1,7,10,11] Compared with the adult population, traditional radicular symptoms are not often initially present.[6,49] In a study comparing adolescents with adults presenting to a sports medicine clinic, Micheli and Wood[9] attributed the low back pain secondary to disk abnormalities in about 50% of the adults compared with only about 10% of the adolescents. Kumar and colleagues[95] reviewed a series of 742 patients undergoing surgery for lumbar disk disease, and adolescents (age <20 years) accounted for only 3.5% of the cases.

Disk disease can result in isolated axial low back pain or radiating pain to the buttocks or lower extremities. The symptoms are generally considered to be worsened by activities involving flexion, rotation, or increases in intra-abdominal pressure.

However, there are no true pathognomonic aspects of the history for diskogenic pain. Similar symptoms can be seen with other types of spine disease, and disk problems can present with other patterns of symptoms. Disk protrusions associated with congenital canal stenosis may represent a distinct problem in athletes with back or leg pain, because there may be an increased risk of neurologic involvement and potentially a less favorable natural history.[7] These athletes may present with a history more consistent with spinal stenosis, including neurogenic claudication. As with all athletes with low back disorders, a comprehensive physical examination including a neurologic evaluation is essential in those with presumed diskogenic abnormalities, to appropriately treat these athletes.

Physical examination of low back pain associated with diskogenic disease shows a decrease in lumbar range of motion, particularly flexion, and positive neural tension signs such as straight leg raise, Lasègue sign, Lazarević sign, Bragard sign, and seated slump test.[54] It is possible to also see decreased reflexes and strength on the affected side of the correlating myotomes. However, the presentation can be variable, with the patient having only axial low back pain until undergoing the provocative examination.[29]

Disk abnormalities on imaging studies are less commonly identified in adolescents than in adults.[12] In a study of 439 13-year-old children from the general population, about one-third were noted to have diskogenic abnormalities on MRI, compared with more than 50% of 40-year-olds in a similar study.[96,97] Athletes who participate in specific sports have been found to have higher rates of degenerative disk changes than the general population.[31,37] Disk herniations in adolescent athletes may also be affected by genetic factors, and the rate of disk herniations occurring in individuals younger than 21 years is 5 times greater in those with a positive family history.[98]

Treatment options for disk injuries in adolescent athletes are similar to those in adults, although there are a few distinct considerations regarding sports participation and age that may be relevant.[12] Overall, almost 90% of patients improve with conservative management.[85,94] Conservative management and nonoperative care are clearly advised as the dominant form of treatment of most adolescent athletes with diskogenic pain.[7,12,47,51,99] Several nonoperative treatment modalities are available, although there is limited study of their effectiveness in the adolescent population. These modalities include physical therapy to address lumbar stability and neuromuscular control, therapeutic modalities, manipulative care, massage, bracing, medications, and interventional spine procedures (eg, epidural injections).[12] In general, it may be best to minimize the use of interventions, medications, and surgery in this population on reviewing the potentials risks versus benefits of some of these treatment options.

Surgical care is generally reserved for those with severe radicular pain who are not responding to optimal conservative management and nonoperative care, having saddle anesthesia or bowel/bladder incontinence as a result of cauda equina involvement, or progressive neurologic loss.[51] Before any consideration of surgical intervention, there should be definitive and clear imaging and other diagnostic findings such as electromyography and nerve conduction studies, which correlate disk and nerve root involvement in the same distribution as the athlete's symptoms. In the care of the adolescent athlete, the clinician and surgeon must take into consideration the balance between the long-term ramifications of surgical intervention on global and spinal health compared with the potential postoperative complications of surgery. Surgical intervention by itself does not guarantee clinical improvement or performance enhancement and should be reserved for clear definitive athletes who have failed conservative management, developed cauda equina symptoms, or have progressive neurologic deficits.[7] As with all other conditions, treatment of disk injuries needs to be directed toward the benefit of the whole individual.

A potential serious complication of disk herniation is cauda equina syndrome, which is caused by the compression of the nerve roots in the lower aspect of the spinal canal.[56] Symptoms of cauda equina syndrome include paralysis of the lower extremities and loss of bowel and bladder function. Cauda equina syndrome is a surgical emergency, and the deficits can remain permanent if not addressed promptly. For this reason, it is imperative to inquire about red flag symptoms in all patients.[11]

Athletes with disk herniation may return to activity once they have attained full pain-free range of motion and full strength and have progressed through sport-specific activities in a controlled setting.[1,49]

Vertebral Body Apophyseal Avulsion Fracture

Activities that involve repetitive flexion and extension of the spine can result in injury to the ring apophysis. Fractures of the cartilaginous ring apophysis may occur, with displacement posteriorly into the spinal canal, along with the intervertebral disk.[11,49] Avulsion fractures occur most often in sports such as gymnastics, wrestling, volleyball, and weight lifting.[11,49] Athletes present with lumbar pain on flexion of the spine. There are usually no associated neurologic symptoms. On examination, both spine flexion and extension are limited. There may be paraspinal muscle spasm. The neurologic examination is usually normal. Lateral radiographs of the lumbar spine may show an ossified fragment in the canal. CT can better identify the fractured apophysis and displaced piece of bone, which may be missed on MRI.[29] Management consists of rest, heat, NSAIDs, and possibly, massage for pain relief. If there are significant neurologic findings resulting from neural compression, the fragment may need to be surgically excised.[11,49,85]

Scheuermann Kyphosis

Another relatively frequent cause of low back pain in adolescents is Scheuermann kyphosis. Scheuermann kyphosis is a developmental condition of uncertain cause affecting the thoracic or thoracolumbar spine and was originally described by Scheuermann in 1921. It is defined by the presence of anterior wedging of at least 5° in 3 consecutive vertebrae, end-plate irregularities, disk space narrowing, and the presence of Schmorl nodes (**Fig. 4**).[12,100,101] The condition has an incidence reported to be 0.4% to 8.3% in the general population and may be more frequent in males than females.[100,101] The mean height in affected individuals tends to be greater than that in the overall population.[101] Although the cause is uncertain, several have been proposed, including mechanical injury, chronic anterior loading, osteoporosis, cartilage abnormalities, and a variety of genetic factors.[51,99,101]

The typical presentation of symptoms in patients with Scheuermann kyphosis is pain, fatigue, deformity, or poor posture. The location of the pain is usually in the area of the deformity and is worsened by activity. It is rare to have any neurologic symptoms or findings with Scheuermann kyphosis. Patients typically present during adolescence, and presentations before age 10 years are uncommon.[51,99–101] The natural history of the disorder is not well understood, but the symptoms often diminish as patients reach skeletal maturity. Adults with a deformity of less than 60° have little chance of having back pain beyond that noted in the general population.[99,101] Physical examination typically shows postural changes, such as lumbar hyperlordosis, and a forward head position caused by increased thoracic kyphosis. The kyphosis in Scheuermann kyphosis is rigid and does not typically correct with extension.[101]

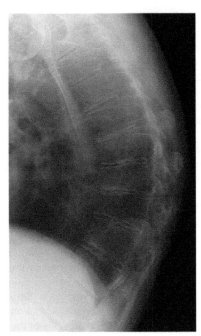

Fig. 4. Plain radiograph, lateral view of the thoracic spine showing the findings associated with Scheuermann kyphosis. Note the multilevel vertebral body wedging, end-plate irregularities, and disk height loss. (*From* Standaert CJ. Low back pain in the adolescent athlete. Phys Med Rehabil Clin N Am 2008;19(2):299; with permission.)

The treatment options for Scheuermann kyphosis depend on the extent of the symptoms and the degree of curvature. Patients with a curve of less than 50° to 60° typically respond well using flexibility and postural exercises in combination with relative rest, antiinflammatories, or bracing. For more substantial curves of 50° to 75° in a skeletally immature patient, bracing should be considered. For those with curves greater than 75°, bracing may no longer be effective and surgical treatment should be considered.[99–101]

Although the kyphosis generally occurs in the thoracic spine, a less common lumbar variant of Scheuermann kyphosis has been described, with end-plate changes, Schmorl nodes, and disk space narrowing as well as vertebral wedging, which occurs less frequently (**Fig. 5**).[12] The lumbar variant is presumed to have a more clearly defined mechanical basis than typical Scheuermann kyphosis and is seen more commonly in athletes participating in sports associated with rapid flexion/extension motions or with heavy lifting.[51,99–101] Although it is often thought of as simply a variant of thoracic Scheuermann kyphosis, some believe that this process may a be a different clinical entity.[101] Pain is typically located at the area of involvement in the thoracolumbar region and exacerbated by activity, particularly lumbar flexion. Examination of the thoracic and lumbar spine typically does not show any marked kyphotic deformity; however, there may be flattening of the lumbar lordosis. The natural history is typically nonprogressive, and treatment involves relative rest, antiinflammatory medication, lumbar stabilization, flexibility, postural training, time, and the use of an orthosis.[99–101]

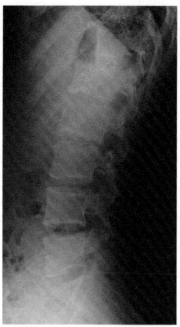

Fig. 5. Plain radiograph lateral view showing the findings associated with the lumbar variant of Scheuermann kyphosis. Again, note the end-plate irregularities, disk height loss, Schmorl nodes, and relative lack of vertebral body wedging. (*From* Standaert CJ. Low back pain in the adolescent athlete. Phys Med Rehabil Clin N Am 2008;19(2):300; with permission.)

SI Joint

The SI joint disperses the forces between the trunk and the lower extremities. This joint can be a source of pain in young athletes, as a result of excessive or reduced motion within the SI joint. Disease of the lumbar spine can alter the mechanics of the lumbar spine, resulting in stress to the SI joints.[11] Inflammation of the SI joint can also result in SI joint pain. SI joint inflammation can occur from infection, such as Reiter syndrome, as well as from seronegative spondyloarthropathies, such as Crohn disease, psoriatic arthritis, and juvenile ankylosing spondylitis. Another cause of SI joint pain is a stress fracture of the sacrum.[11] Athletes with SI joint pain present with extension pain, which is insidious in onset.[8,11]

On examination, pain is localized to the lumbar or buttock region with extension of the spine. They may have poor pelvic stability on Trendelenberg testing. There are several provocative tests that can elicit SI joint pain, including FABER test, Gaenslen, Gillet, and Fortin finger test.[52,53] Palpation elicits tenderness over the affected SI joint.[1,8,11]

Plain radiographs should be considered if symptoms have been present for more than 3 weeks; however, frequently, this imaging is normal. Bone scan may show a stress fracture of the sacrum. MRI can more precisely define the anatomic abnormality. However, the gold standard for diagnosis of SI joint pain is diagnostic intra-articular injection. If infection or a spondyloarthropathy is suspected, blood work, including erythrocyte sedimentation rate, C-reactive protein, rheumatoid factor, anti-nuclear antibody, and HLA-B27, should be obtained.[11]

Management of SI joint dysfunction includes ice, NSAIDs, activity modification, bracing, physical therapy, osteopathic manipulation, and injections. Ice and NSAIDs help alleviate pain and inflammation. Activities should be restricted to those that do not provoke pain. If a sacral stress fracture is present, protected weight bearing is necessary until pain resolves.[11] Bracing can help stabilize the joint. Physical therapy involves possible manipulation of the SI joint, pelvic stabilization exercises, and hip girdle and abdominal strengthening. SI joint injections, including corticosteroids, prolotherapy, and radiofrequency ablation, are effective in refractory cases.[1,3,8,11]

Other Causes of Low Back Pain

Injury is not the only cause of low back pain in young athletes.[1,11,84,94,102] Infection (diskitis or osteomyelitis), inflammation (seronegative spondyloarthropathies), and tumors (eg, osteoid osteoma, osteoblastoma, bone cysts, Ewing sarcoma, osteogenic sarcoma) can also cause back pain, as well as visceral disease, such as pyelonephritis. A high index of suspicion is necessary to avoid missing these potential reasons for low back pain. Systemic symptoms such as fever, night pain, weight loss, and malaise are red flags for more sinister causes of back pain and should prompt further investigation.[28]

REHABILITATION AND RETURN TO PLAY

Several investigators have described rehabilitation programs for adolescent athletes with low back pain caused by these various lumbar disorders. However, there is insufficient evidence advocating any specific rehabilitation protocols. Nonoperative rehabilitation programs tend to be empirically and anecdotally derived. However, more research into these various programs needs to be performed to determine the most effective means to facilitate recovery and improve function. One of the complexities of developing good evidence-based research on these rehabilitation programs is that both the disease process and the rehabilitation programs are multifactorial. Comprehensive rehabilitation generally addresses several factors affecting the injured athlete and may use additional therapeutic modalities to assist with the recovery and facilitate return to play. Therefore in the clinical setting, it is imperative to establish an early and accurate diagnosis, initiate appropriate acute treatment of injured structures, perform a full assessment of the kinetic chain and athletic technique, and identify environmental or psychosocial barriers to performance.[12] Rehabilitation should progress through a structured, sport-specific program with a focus on specific motions, postures, and activities required in the performance of the athlete's chosen sport. Specific activities, timing, and progression of training in a given athlete depend heavily on the nature of any acute injury and subsequent treatment as well as individual factors related to the athlete that affect performance.[7,12,47,103]

Return to play after injury is allowed when the athlete has been given sufficient time to recover from their acute injury and progressed through a sport-specific rehabilitation program, which also addresses spinal awareness and dynamic postural control. Return to play criteria include full, pain-free range of motion, appropriate aerobic conditioning, normal strength, and a proven ability to perform sports-related skills without pain.[12,104]

When an injured athlete is returning to sport, recommendations must take into account the diagnosis, the sport or activity, the age and skeletal maturity of the child, and the amount of cooperation of the athlete, parents, and coaches in allowing activity modifications during healing.[11,29,49] In general, relative rest is indicated to allow for healing. Activities that cause pain should be avoided until the patient is pain free.

Most athletes are able to continue in their sport with modifications of the activity. Once the athlete has attained pain-free range of motion with all activities and has obtained normal strength, they can return to full sport participation.[29]

SUMMARY

Low back pain is frequently encountered in adolescent athletes. The adolescent athlete is at risk for significant structural injuries as well as nonmechanical problems. Adolescent athletes who present with low back pain are more likely to have structural injuries and therefore should be investigated fully. Any athlete with severe, persisting, or activity-limiting symptoms needs to be evaluated thoroughly. It is imperative to complete a comprehensive evaluation of back pain, and a cause such as muscle strain should be a diagnosis of exclusion. Clinicians must have knowledge of the growth and development of the adolescent spine and the subsequent injury patterns and other spinal conditions common in the adolescent athlete. The management and treatment of spinal injuries in adolescent athletes require a coordinated effort between the clinician, patients, parents/guardians, coaches, therapists, and athletic trainers. Treatment should not only help alleviate the current symptoms but also address flexibility and muscle imbalances to prevent future injuries by recognizing and addressing risk factors. Return to sport should be a gradual process once the pain has resolved and the athlete has regained full strength.

REFERENCES

1. d'Hemecourt PA, Gerbino PG II, Micheli LJ. Back injuries in the young athlete. Clin Sports Med 2000;19:663–79.
2. Gerbino PG II, Micheli LJ. Back injuries in the young athlete. Clin Sports Med 1995;14(3):571–90.
3. George SZ, Delitto A. Management of the athlete with low back pain. Clin Sports Med 2002;21:105–20.
4. Hutchison MR. Low back pain in elite rhythmic gymnasts. Med Sci Sports Exerc 1999;31:1686–8.
5. Kolt GS, Kirkby RJ. Epidemiology of injury in elite and subelite female gymnasts: a comparison of retrospective and prospective findings. Br J Sports Med 1999; 33:312–8.
6. Semon RL, Spengler D. Significance of lumbar spondylolysis in college football players. Spine 1981;6:172–4.
7. Watkins RG. Lumbar disc injury in the athlete. Clin Sports Med 2002;21:147–65.
8. Kraft DE. Low back pain in the adolescent athlete. Pediatr Clin North Am 2002; 49:643–53.
9. Micheli LJ, Wood R. Back pain in young athletes. Arch Pediatr Adolesc Med 1995;149:15–8.
10. Trainor TJ, Trainor MA. Etiology of low back pain in athletes. Curr Sports Med Rep 2004;3:41–6.
11. Zetaruk M. Lumbar spine injuries. In: Micheli LJ, Purcell LK, editors. The adolescent athlete. New York: Springer; 2007. p. 109–40.
12. Standaert CJ. Low back pain in the adolescent athlete. Phys Med Rehabil Clin N Am 2008;19(2):287–304.
13. Ferguson RL. Thoracic and lumbar spinal trauma of the immature spine. In: Herkowitz HN, Garfin SR, Eismont FJ, et al, editors. Rothman-Simeone the spine. 5th edition. Philadelphia: Saunders; 2006. p. 603–12.

14. Clark P, Letts M. Trauma to the thoracic and lumbar spine in the adolescent. Can J Surg 2001;44(5):337–45.

15. Commandre FA, Gagnerie G, Zakarian M, et al. The child, the spine and sport. J Sports Med Phys Fitness 1988;28(1):11–9.

16. Cyron BM, Hutton WC. The fatigue strength of the lumbar neural arch in spondylolysis. J Bone Joint Surg Br 1978;60-B:234–8.

17. Malina R. Growth and maturation: applications to children and adolescents in sports. In: Birrer RB, Griesemer BA, Cataletto MB, editors. Pediatric sports medicine for primary care. Philadelphia: Lippincott Williams & Wilkins; 2002. p. 39–58.

18. Burton AK, Clarke RD, McClune TD, et al. The natural history of low back pain in adolescents. Spine 1996;21(20):2323–8.

19. Harreby M, Nygaard B, Jessen T, et al. Risk factors for low back pain in a cohort of 1389 Danish school children: an epidemiologic study. Eur Spine J 1999;8(6):444–50.

20. Kovacs FM, Gestoso M, Gil del Real MT, et al. Risk factors for non-specific low back pain in schoolchildren and their parents: a population based study. Pain 2003;103:239–68.

21. Salminen JJ, Erkintalo M, Laine M, et al. Low back pain in the young. A prospective three-year follow-up study of subjects with and without low back pain. Spine 1995;20(19):2101–7.

22. Taimela S, Kujala UM, Salminen JJ, et al. The prevalence of low back pain among children and adolescents: a nationwide, cohort-based questionnaire survey in Finland. Spine 1997;22(10):1132–6.

23. Troussier B, Davoine P, de Gaudemaris R, et al. Back pain in school children: a study among 1178 pupils. Scand J Rehabil Med 1994;26:143–6.

24. Auvinen J, Tammelin T, Taimela S, et al. Associations of physical activity and inactivity with low back pain in adolescents. Scand J Med Sci Sports 2008;18:188–94.

25. Mogensen AM, Gausel AM, Wedderkopp N, et al. Is active participation in specific sport activities linked with back pain? Scand J Med Sci Sports 2007;17(6):680–6.

26. Wedderkopp N, Leboeuf-Yde C, Andersen LB, et al. Back pain in children. No association with objectively measured level of physical activity. Spine 2003;28(17):2019–24.

27. McBeth J, Jones K. Epidemiology of chronic musculoskeletal pain. Best Pract Res Clin Rheumatol 2007;21(3):403–25.

28. Hestbaek L, Leboeuf-Yde C, Kyvik KO, et al. The course of low back pain from adolescence to adulthood: eight-year follow-up of 9600 twins. Spine 2006;31(4):468–72.

29. Purcell L, Micheli L. Low back pain in young athletes. Sports Health 2009;1(3):212–22.

30. Kujala UM, Taimela S, Erkintalo M, et al. Low back pain in adolescent athletes. Med Sci Sports Exerc 1996;28(2):165–70.

31. Hickey GJ, Fricker PA, McDonald WA. Injuries to elite rowers over a 10-yr period. Med Sci Sports Exerc 1997;29(12):1567–72.

32. Hosea TM, Gatt CJ. Back pain in golf. Clin Sports Med 1996;15(1):37–53.

33. Iwamoto J, Abe H, Tsukimura Y, et al. Relationship between radiographic abnormalities of lumbar spine and incidence of low back pain in high school rugby players: a prospective study. Scand J Med Sci Sports 2005;15:163–8.

34. Sward L, Hellstrom M, Jacobsson B, et al. Disc degeneration and associated abnormalities of the spine in elite gymnasts. A magnetic resonance imaging study. Spine 1991;16(4):437–43.

35. Sward L, Hellstrom M, Jacobsson B, et al. Back pain and radiologic changes in the thoraco-lumbar spine of athletes. Spine 1990;15(2):124–9.

36. Goldstein JD, Berger PE, Windler GE, et al. Spine injuries in gymnasts and swimmers: an epidemiologic investigation. Am J Sports Med 1991;19:463–8.

37. Bennett DL, Nassar L, DeLano MC. Lumbar spine MRI in the elite-level female gymnast with low back pain. Skeletal Radiol 2006;35:503–9.

38. Iwamoto J, Abe H, Tsukimura Y, et al. Relationship between radiographic abnormalities of lumbar spine and incidence of low back pain in high school and college football players. Am J Sports Med 2004;32(3):781–6.

39. Fredrickson BE, Baker D, McHolick WJ, et al. The natural history of spondylolysis and spondylolisthesis. J Bone Joint Surg Am 1984;66:699–707.

40. Roche MA, Rowe GG. The incidence of separate neural arch and coincident bone variations: a survey of 4,200 skeletons. Anat Rec 1951;109:233–52.

41. Rossi F, Dragoni S. The prevalence of spondylolysis and spondylolisthesis in symptomatic elite athletes: radiographic findings. Radiography 2001;7:37–42.

42. Soler T, Calderon C. The prevalence of spondylolysis in the Spanish elite athlete. Am J Sports Med 2000;28:57–62.

43. Lundin O, Hellstrom M, Nilsson I, et al. Back pain and radiologic changes in the thoraco-lumbar spine of athletes: a long-term follow-up. Scand J Med Sci Sports 2001;11:103–9.

44. Teitz CC, O'Kane JW, Lind BK. Back pain in former intercollegiate rowers; a long-term follow-up study. Am J Sports Med 2003;31(4):590–5.

45. Tsai L, Wredmark T. Spinal posture, sagittal mobility, and subjective rating of back problems in former female elite gymnasts. Spine 1993;18:872–5.

46. Anderson SJ. Assessment and management of the pediatric and adolescent patient with low back pain. Phys Med Rehabil Clin N Am 1991;2(1):157–85.

47. Bono CM. Low-back pain in athletes. J Bone Joint Surg Am 2004;86:382–96.

48. Hosalkar H, Dormans J. Back pain in children requires extensive workup. Biomechanics 2003;10(6):51–8.

49. Simon LM, Jih W, Buller JC. Back pain and injuries. In: Birrer RB, Griesemer BA, Cataletto MB, editors. Pediatric sports medicine for primary care. Philadelphia: Lippincott Williams & Wilkins; 2002. p. 306–25.

50. Standaert CJ, Herring SA, Cole AJ, et al. The lumbar spine and sports. In: Cole AJ, Herring SA, editors. The low back pain handbook. 2nd edition. Philadelphia: Hanley & Belfus; 2003. p. 385–404.

51. Mason DE. Back pain in children. Pediatr Ann 1999;28(12):727–38.

52. Hoppenfeld S. Physical examination of the lumbar spine. In: Hoppenfeld S, editor. Physical examination of the spine and extremities. Upper Saddle River (NJ): Prentice Hall; 1976. p. 237–63.

53. Fortin JD, Falco FJ. The Fortin finger test: an indicator of sacroiliac pain. Am J Orthop 1997;26(7):477–80.

54. De Luigi AJ, Fitzpatrick KF. Physical examination in radiculopathy. Phys Med Rehabil Clin N Am 2011;22(1):7–40.

55. Dodge TL, Jaccard JJ. The effect of high school sports participation on the use of performance-enhancing substances in young adulthood. J Adolesc Health 2006;39:367–73.

56. Gregory PL, Batt ME, Kerslake RW, et al. Single photon emission computerized tomography and reverse gantry computerized tomography findings in

patients with back pain investigated for spondylolysis. Clin J Sport Med 2005; 15:79–86.

57. Meyerding HW. Spondylolithesis. Surg Gynecol Obstet 1932;54:371–7.
58. Wiltse LL, Newman PH, Macnab I. Classification of spondylolysis and spondy-lolisthesis. Clin Orthop Relat Res 1976;117:23–9.
59. Wiltse LL, Widell EH, Jackson DW. Fatigue fracture: the basic lesion in isthmic spondylolisthesis. J Bone Joint Surg Am 1975;57:17–22.
60. Muschik M, Hahnel H, Robinson PN, et al. Competitive sports and the progres-sion of spondylolisthesis. J Pediatr Orthop 1996;16:364–9.
61. Gregory PL, Batt ME, Kerslake RW. Comparing spondylolysis in cricketers and soccer players. Br J Sports Med 2004;38:737–42.
62. McCarroll JR, Miller JM, Ritter MA. Lumbar spondylolysis and spondylolisthesis in college football players: a prospective study. Am J Sports Med 1986;14: 404–6.
63. d'Hemecourt P, Zurakowski D, Kriemler S, et al. Spondylolysis: returning the athlete to sports participation with brace treatment. Orthopedics 2002;25:653–7.
64. McTimoney CA, Micheli LJ. Current evaluation and management of spondyloly-sis and spondylolisthesis. Curr Sports Med Rep 2003;2:41–6.
65. Masci L, Pike J, Malara F, et al. Use of the one-legged hyperextension test and magnetic resonance imaging in the diagnosis of active spondylolysis. Br J Sports Med 2006;40:940–6.
66. Steiner ME, Micheli LJ. Treatment of symptomatic spondylolysis and spondylo-listhesis with the modified Boston brace. Spine 1985;10:937–43.
67. Harvey CJ, Richenberg JL, Saifuddin A, et al. Pictorial review: the radiological investigation of lumbar spondylolysis. Clin Radiol 1998;53:723–8.
68. Jackson DW, Wiltse LL, Dingeman RD, et al. Stress reactions involving the pars interarticularis in young athletes. Am J Sports Med 1981;9:304–12.
69. Elliott S, Hutson MA, Wastie ML. Bone scintigraphy in the assessment of spon-dylolysis in patients attending a sports injury clinic. Clin Radiol 1988;39: 269–72.
70. Anderson K, Sarwark JF, Conway JJ, et al. Quantitative assessment with SPECT imaging of stress injuries of the pars interarticularis and response to bracing. J Pediatr Orthop 2000;20:28–33.
71. Bellah RD, Summerville DA, Treves ST, et al. Low back pain in adolescent ath-letes: detection of stress injury to the pars interarticularis with SPECT. Radiology 1991;180:509–12.
72. Bodner RJ, Heyman S, Drummond DS, et al. The use of single photon emission computed tomography (SPECT) in the diagnosis of low back pain in young pa-tients. Spine 1988;3:1155–60.
73. Congeni J, McCulloch J, Swanson K. Lumbar spondylolysis: a study of natural progression in athletes. Am J Sports Med 1997;25:248–53.
74. Campbell RS, Grainger AJ, Hide IG, et al. Juvenile spondylolysis: a comparative analysis of CT, SPECT, and MRI. Skeletal Radiol 2005;34:63–73.
75. Stretch RA, Botha T, Chandler S, et al. Back injuries in young fast bowlers–a radiologic investigation of the healing of spondylolysis and pedicle sclerosis. S Afr Med J 2003;93:611–6.
76. Lowe J, Schachner E, Hirschberg E, et al. Significance of bone scintigraphy in symptomatic spondylolysis. Spine 1984;9:653–5.
77. Collier BD, Johnson RP, Carrera GF, et al. Painful spondylolysis or spondylolis-thesis studied by radiography and single photon emission computed tomogra-phy. Radiology 1985;154:207–11.

78. Itoh K, Hashimoto T, Shigenobu K, et al. Bone SPECT of symptomatic lumbar spondylolysis. Nucl Med Commun 1996;17:389–96.
79. Lusins JO, Elting JJ, Cicoria AD, et al. SPECT evaluation of lumbar spondylolysis and spondylolisthesis. Spine 1994;19:608–12.
80. Raby N, Mathews S. Symptomatic spondylolysis: correlation of CT and SPECT with clinical outcome. Clin Radiol 1993;48:97–9.
81. Gregory PL, Batt ME, Kerslake RW, et al. The value of combining single photon emission computerised tomography and computerised tomography in the investigation of spondylolysis. Eur Spine J 2004;13:503–9.
82. Fujii K, Katoh S, Sairyo K, et al. Union of defects in the pars interarticularis of the lumbar spine in children and adolescents: the radiologic outcome after conservative treatment. J Bone Joint Surg Br 2004;86:225–31.
83. Miller SF, Congeni J, Swanson K. Long-term functional and anatomical follow-up of early detected spondylolysis in young athletes. Am J Sports Med 2004;32:928–33.
84. King HA. Back pain in children. Orthop Clin North Am 1999;30:467–74.
85. Brown TD, Micheli LJ. Spinal injuries in children's sports. In: Maffuli N, Chan KM, Macdonald R, et al, editors. Sports medicine for specific ages and abilities. London: Churchill Livingstone; 2001. p. 31–44.
86. Standaert CJ, Herring SA. Spondylolysis: a critical review. Br J Sports Med 2000;34:415–22.
87. Axelsson P, Johnsson R, Stromqvist B. Effect of lumbar orthosis on intervertebral mobility. Spine 1992;17:678–81.
88. Calmels P, Fayolle-Minon I. An update on orthotic devices for the lumbar spine based on a review of the literature. Rev Rhum Engl Ed 1996;63:285–91.
89. Ruiz-Cotorro A, Balius-Matas R, Estruch-Massana AE, et al. Spondylolysis in young tennis players. Br J Sports Med 2006;40:441–6.
90. Blanda J, Bethem D, Moats W, et al. Defects of pars interarticularis in athletes: a protocol for nonoperative treatment. J Spinal Disord 1993;6:406–11.
91. Iwamoto J, Takeda T, Wakano K. Returning athletes with severe low back pain and spondylolysis to original sporting activities with conservative treatment. Scand J Med Sci Sports 2004;14:346–51.
92. Sys J, Michielsen J, Bracke P, et al. Nonoperative treatment of active spondylolysis in elite athletes with normal X-ray findings: literature review and results of conservative treatment. Eur Spine J 2001;10:498–504.
93. Rassi GE, Takemitsu M, Woratanarat P, et al. Lumbar spondylolysis in pediatric and adolescent soccer players. Am J Sports Med 2005;33:1688–93.
94. Sponseller PD. Evaluating the child with back pain. Am Fam Physician 1996;54:1933–41.
95. Kumar R, Kumar V, Das NK, et al. Adolescent lumbar disc disease: findings and outcome. Childs Nerv Syst 2007;23(11):1295–9.
96. Kjaer P, Leboeuf-Yde C, Sorensen JS, et al. An epidemiologic study of MRI and low back pain in 13-year-old children. Spine 2005;30(7):798–806.
97. Kjaer P, Leboeuf-Yde C, Korsholm L, et al. Magnetic resonance imaging and low back pain in adults: a diagnostic imaging study of 40-year-old men and women. Spine 2005;30(10):1173–80.
98. Ala-Kokko L. Genetic risk factors for lumbar disc disease. Ann Med 2002;34:42–7.
99. Waicus KM, Smith BW. Back injuries in the pediatric athlete. Curr Sports Med Rep 2002;1:52–8.

100. Karol LA. Back pain in children and adolescents. In: Herkowitz HN, Garfin SR, Eismont FJ, et al, editors. Rothman-Simeone the spine. 5th edition. Philadelphia: Saunders; 2006. p. 493–506.
101. Shah SW, Takemitsu M, Westerlund LE, et al. Pediatric kyphosis: Scheuermann's disease and congenital deformity. In: Herkowitz HN, Garfin SR, Eismont FJ, et al, editors. Rothman-Simeone the spine. 5th edition. Philadelphia: Saunders; 2006. p. 565–85.
102. Hollingworth P. Back pain in children. Br J Rheumatol 1996;35:1022–8.
103. Standaert CJ, Herring SA, Pratt TW. Rehabilitation of the athlete with low back pain. Curr Sports Med Rep 2004;3(1):35–40.
104. Herring SA, Kibler WB. A framework for rehabilitation. In: Kibler WB, Herring SA, Press JM, et al, editors. Functional rehabilitation of sports and musculoskeletal injuries. Gaithersburg (MD): Aspen; 1998. p. 1–8.

Managing Hip Pain in the Athlete

Heidi Prather, DO*, Berdale Colorado, DO, MPH, Devyani Hunt, MD

KEYWORDS

- Hip • Pain • Athlete • Groin

KEY POINTS

- Hip and groin pain is commonly experienced by athletes.
- The differential diagnosis is extensive and should include both intra-articular and extra-articular sources for pain and dysfunction.
- Evaluation for the underlying disorder can be complicated.
- A comprehensive history and physical examination can guide the evaluation of hip pain and the potential need for further diagnostics such as imaging or diagnostic hip injection.
- Treatment of athletes with hip disorders includes education, addressing activities of daily living, pain-modulating medications or modalities, exercise and sports modification, and therapeutic exercise.

INTRODUCTION

Hip and groin pain is commonly experienced by athletes of all ages and activity levels. Groin pain accounts for 10% of all visits to sports medicine centers and groin injuries account for up to 6% of all athletic injuries.[1,2] Hip and groin injuries occur in 5% to 9% of high school athletes.[3] Sports involving increased amounts of acceleration and deceleration, as well as cutting movements, seem to have increased incidences. A study of high school soccer injuries reported that 13.3% of all injuries sustained by girls involved the hip and thigh.[4] Causes of hip and groin pain can often be complicated by the overlapping signs and symptoms of other disorders, as well as the complex anatomy and biomechanics of the hip. Furthermore, many hip and groin injuries have multiple components or coexisting injuries.[5] This article reviews the causes of hip pain in athletes, provides a clinical approach for accurate diagnosis, and discusses treatment options for common hip disorders.

Disclosures: None declared.
Department of Orthopaedic Surgery, Washington University School of Medicine, 660 South Euclid Avenue, Campus Box 8233, St Louis, MO 63110, USA
* Corresponding author.
E-mail address: pratherh@wudosis.wustl.edu

Phys Med Rehabil Clin N Am 25 (2014) 789–812
http://dx.doi.org/10.1016/j.pmr.2014.06.012
1047-9651/14/$ – see front matter © 2014 Elsevier Inc. All rights reserved.

DIFFERENTIAL DIAGNOSIS

The differential diagnosis for athletes presenting with hip pain is extensive and can span multiple medical specialties and disciplines. For example, an athlete whose technique of running has altered because of a hip injury may begin to experience pain in other areas, including the pelvic girdle, lumbar spine, and knee. Both musculoskeletal and nonmusculoskeletal sources of hip pain must be considered (**Box 1**). These nonmusculoskeletal sources may include visceral structures of the abdomen and pelvis.

It is important for the sports medicine provider to distinguish between intra-articular versus extra-articular sources of hip pain (see **Box 1**), which is accomplished through a complete evaluation, including a thorough history and physical examination, along with appropriate diagnostic testing.

History

The medical history for a patient presenting with hip pain should include age, onset (and mechanism of injury, if applicable), distribution, quality, severity, progression, exacerbating factors, alleviating factors, and other associated signs/symptoms.

The differential diagnosis for hip pain can vary based on the age of the athlete. In the pediatric and adolescent athlete presenting with hip and groin pain, consideration should be given to apophyseal injuries, Legg-Calve-Perthes disease, and slipped capital femoral epiphysis. In contrast, older athletes are often affected by osteoarthritis (OA) of the hip.

Hip pain with acute onset has a distinct differential diagnosis from hip pain that is chronic or of insidious onset. A detailed mechanism of injury should be elicited with hip pain of acute onset. For example, sudden forceful muscle contractions (particularly eccentric) often result in muscle strains or tears in adults and apophyseal avulsions in adolescents. The adductor muscles are often involved, particularly in soccer, football, and hockey athletes. Adductor strain is the most common cause of groin pain in athletes.[6] Further, fracture should be considered in athletes with sudden onset of pain associated with a specific event. The event may not have seemed to be significant enough to cause a bony fracture, but athletes with an underlying bone mineralization deficit may become symptomatic with a seemingly benign event.

The distribution of hip pain is wide and variable but should be assessed by the health care provider to assist in making a diagnosis and to reassess following treatment. Anterior groin pain is often associated with intra-articular hip disorders. These disorders include femoral or acetabular fracture, avascular necrosis, OA, synovitis, ligamentum teres tear, and prearthritic hip disorders (isolated acetabular labral tears, developmental hip dysplasia [DDH], and femoroacetabular impingement [FAI] with and without acetabular labral tears). Extra-articular sources associated with anterior groin pain include the pubic rami, iliopsoas, adductor group, and abdominal muscles. Sports hernia typically involves injury to the abdominal muscles, particularly the external oblique muscle and aponeurosis, with possible injury to the adductors. In addition to the muscles and surrounding soft tissues, higher lumbar radiculopathy should also be considered as a source of an athlete's groin pain.

Lateral hip pain can be associated with intra-articular hip disorders, including all of those listed for anterior distribution of pain. In isolation, lateral hip pain is often associated with extra-articular disorders, including greater trochanteric bursitis or greater trochanteric pain syndrome, which may include gluteus medius or minimus tendinopathy, or pain related to tensor fascia lata/iliotibial band dysfunction. Lumbar spine disorders, particularly those involving the L4 to L5 distribution, can present with lateral hip pain.

Box 1
Differential diagnosis of hip pain

Musculoskeletal hip pain disorders:

  Intra-articular

    Ligamentum teres tear

    Hip dislocation/subluxation/capsular injury

    Fracture/stress fracture

    Synovitis

    Infection

    Osteonecrosis of femoral head

    Osteochondritis dissecans

    Legg-Calve-Perthes disease

    Slipped capital femoral epiphysis

    Femoroacetabular impingement

    Developmental hip dysplasia

    Acetabular labral tear

    Osteoarthritis

  Extra-articular

    Hip

    Bursitis

    Muscle strain/tendinopathy/tear: gluteus medius/minimus, piriformis, adductors, rectus femoris, iliopsoas, rectus abdominis, proximal hamstrings, tensor fascia lata

    Greater trochanteric pain syndrome

    Snapping hip syndrome

  Regional musculoskeletal

    Pubic ramus stress fracture/osteitis pubis

    Sports hernia/pubalgia

    Lumbar spine: facet joint pain, lumbosacral radiculopathy

    Sacroiliac joint dysfunction

    Peripheral nerve entrapment: genitofemoral, iliohypogastric, ilioinguinal, lateral femoral cutaneous, obturator, pudendal, superior and inferior gluteal

Nonmusculoskeletal hip pain disorders:

  Gastrointestinal: appendicitis, diverticulitis, lymphadenitis, inflammatory bowel disease, inguinal/femoral hernia

  Genitourinary: endometriosis, prostatitis, urinary tract infection, pelvic inflammatory disease, ovarian cysts, nephrolithiasis, ectopic pregnancy

  Pelvic tumor

Posterior pelvic pain is the area of great overlap between the hip, pelvic girdle, and lumbar spine and is not fully understood. Multiple structures contribute to posterior pelvic pain,[7] including the sacroiliac joints, ischial bursa, and the insertion of the proximal hamstring.[7] The European guidelines for evaluation and treatment of pelvic girdle pain continue to provide a comprehensive resource for understanding the relationships of the pelvic girdle and lumbar spine and include diagnostic and therapeutic evidence-based reviews.[8] Increased tone, fatigue, or dysfunction of the hip abductors, extensors, lateral rotators, and the lumbopelvic fascia are confounding factors. Lumbar spine disorders also commonly present with pain in the posterior pelvis and can range from structural and physiologic changes of the intervertebral disc, facet joint, and central or foraminal canal, ranging from L1 to S1 myotome and dermatome levels. Less understood is the role of the hip in posterior pelvic pain. In a previous descriptive study, 20% of patients successfully treated with hip arthroscopy for acetabular labral tears in isolation with pain unresponsive to conservative treatment reported posterior pelvic pain as part of the distribution of pain before surgery.[9] In a series of descriptive studies, posterior pelvic pain was reported by patients before surgery in 17.3% of patients with DDH, 29% of patients with FAI, and 38% of patients with isolated acetabular labral tears.[10–12] Patients with FAI also reported a 23% incidence of low back pain and 12% incidence of posterior thigh pain.[11] Lumbar spine, pelvic girdle, and hip disorders can present with a variety of distributions of pain that overlap across regions. Recognizing this overlap in the distribution of symptoms enables the sports medicine provider to consider an underlying hip disorder in athletes with isolated groin pain as well as in the lumbopelvic region.

Pain quality, severity, progression, exacerbating factors, and alleviating factors provide additional information to narrow the differential diagnosis. Burning pain is often associated with a neuropathic cause. Pain with active contraction or passive stretch of a particular muscle suggests a tendinopathy or muscle strain/tear. Symptoms that are worse with coughing or sneezing and causing an increase in intra-abdominal and intraspinal pain may suggest an intervertebral disc or abdominal or inguinal hernia as a source of pain.

Specific motions or weight bearing associated with snapping, catching, or locking can be associated with extra-articular and intra-articular hip disorders. Snapping hip is commonly associated with hip pain and has been estimated to occur in 5% to 10% of the general population, but is especially seen in athletes such as soccer players, runners, weight lifters, and dancers who perform significant hip flexion and extension movements.[13–15] It is most commonly associated with snapping of the iliotibial band or the gluteus maximus over the greater trochanter[16] that occurs during return to full extension of the hip. Another common cause of anterior snapping hip is aberrant movement of the iliopsoas tendon snapping over the iliopectineal eminence.[16] This snapping often occurs while climbing stairs, getting out of a car, or rising from a chair.[17] Catching or locking symptoms are also associated with hip pain and can suggest acetabular labral tear or loose body.[18] In patients undergoing surgical treatment of acetabular labral tears, 53% report mechanical symptoms of popping or snapping, whereas 41% report true locking or catching.[10]

Neurologic deficits in strength and sensation imply nerve root damage (radiculopathy) or peripheral nerve entrapment. Affected nerves can include the obturator, pudendal, superior gluteal, inferior gluteal, genitofemoral, iliohypogastric, ilioinguinal, and lateral femoral cutaneous nerves. Past surgical history may often be associated with peripheral nerve entrapments.

Providers should be aware of signs and symptoms that may indicate nonmusculoskeletal sources of hip pain, including various gastrointestinal and genitourinary disorders. Further questioning regarding bowel and bladder function, sexual activity, and menstrual history should be considered.

Physical Examination

The physical examination for hip pain should be guided by each athlete's history. In general, it should include inspection, range of motion, palpation, a neurologic examination, and provocative hip testing.

Inspection should assess seated and standing postures, transfers, ability to bear weight, and gait. Areas of asymmetry, including muscle atrophy or masses, should be noted. Antalgic and asymmetric movements with transfers and gait should also be noted to help further characterize the underlying disorder. Foot position preference in standing and with ambulation should be noted because it is an initial indicator of pain, bony abnormality, and/or soft tissue adaptation or restriction. Observing a Trendelenburg gait gives the sports medicine provider an initial impression of gluteal weakness that has implications for dysfunctions across regions including the lumbar spine, pelvic girdle, and hip.

Active and passive range of motion of the hip should be performed, assessing for asymmetries from side to side and available end range. Hip range-of-motion parameters are variable in the literature. Age, gender, bony deformity, and soft tissue laxity and restrictions can all influence hip range of motion but are not consistently controlled for in studies assessing active and passive hip range of motion, which likely contributes to the variability of reported normal.[19–26] Asymptomatic elite female soccer athletes showed variability in hip passive range of motion by age and experience.[27] Specific hip disorders have been found to be associated with patterns of reduced hip range of motion. Patients with FAI have reduced hip flexion and internal rotation,[11] whereas those with hip OA may first experience reduced hip internal rotation and progress to a loss of motion in all planes. Active range of motion of the lumbar spine should be performed to assess whether pain is provoked in a specific direction, which may help determine whether a spine disorder is contributing to the constellation of symptoms associated with a hip disorder.

Palpation of relevant anatomic structures (as described earlier) of the lumbar spine, posterior pelvis, lateral hip, and anterior groin can help identify underlying disorders when pain is provoked or asymmetries are palpated in the bony and soft tissue structures. Dynamic palpation tests can also be used, such as palpation of the inguinal canal during coughing in the setting of a possible inguinal hernia. Abdominal hernia can be assessed by palpation of the abdominal muscle insertion in the midline on the superior pubis insertion during lower abdominal contraction. If an asymmetrical fullness is noted with pain at the time of contraction versus at rest, abdominal hernia becomes a consideration. Palpation of the iliopsoas tendon with concentric and eccentric contraction may elicit the pain and the snap. Likewise, palpation of the iliotibial band during hip flexion and abduction may provoke a painful snap.

Evaluation of strength and length in the muscles about the hip can identify areas of movement system breakdown that may be contributing to the patient's hip pain. For example, extra-articular muscle imbalances between posterior hip abductors and external rotators in combination with shortened hip flexors and iliotibial band can lead to groin and lateral hip pain.[28]

A neurologic examination consisting of sensory, motor, reflex, and neural tension provocative tests can further assess neurologic involvement in the patient's hip pain. If any of the neurologic examination tests are positive, regional sources for pain in the pelvis and lumbar spine should be considered.

Several provocative hip tests can help assess intra-articular versus extra-articular hip disorders (**Table 1**). None are specific enough to be used in isolation but collective

Table 1
Provocative tests of the hip

Name of Test	Purpose	Sensitivity/Specificity	Description of Test
Anterior hip impingement test	To assess hip disorder, impingement, or anterior superior labral tear	0.59–1.00/0.05–0.75[29]	Patient lies supine. Examiner passively flexes hip and knee, internally rotates and adducts hip. A positive test reproduces anterior or lateral hip pain
Patrick test or FABER test	To discern between hip, sacroiliac joint, and low back disorders	0.42–0.81/0.18–0.75[29]	Patient lies supine. Examiner places the ankle of the test leg just above the opposite knee in the position shown in **Fig. 4.** The opposite ASIS is stabilized with one hand and the other hand applies pressure to the test leg's knee toward the table. A positive test for sacroiliac joint or low back disorder reproduces posterior pelvic pain
Resisted straight leg raise test or Stinchfield test	To assess hip disorder	0.59/0.32[29]	Patient lies supine and actively flexes hip with knee extended to 30° against resistance. A positive test reproduces anterior or lateral hip pain
Log roll test	To assess hip disorder	Unavailable	Patient lies supine with hips and knees extended. Examiner passively internally and externally rotates test leg while stabilizing knee and ankle so that motion occurs at the hip. A positive test reproduces anterior or lateral hip pain
Posterior hip impingement test	To assess hip disorder, posterior labral test	0.97/0.11[29]	Patient lies prone with hip and knee extended. Examiner passively extends, adducts, and externally rotates hip. A positive test reproduces anterior hip or posterior pelvic pain

Test	Purpose	Sensitivity/Specificity	Description
Ober test	To assess iliotibial band posterior fiber length	0.41/0.95[30]	Patient lies on side. Lower leg is flexed at the hip and knee. Examiner passively extends the patient's upper leg with the knee flexed at 90°. While supporting the knee, the examiner slowly lowers the leg. If the iliotibial band is shortened, the leg remains abducted and does not fall to the table
	To assess iliotibial band anterior fiber length	0.41/0.95[30]	Patient lies on side. Lower leg is flexed at the hip and knee. Examiner passively flexes the patient's upper limb hip with the knee flexed at 90°. While supporting the knee, the examiner slowly lowers the leg. If the iliotibial band is shortened, the leg remains abducted and does not fall to the table
Thomas test	To assess hip flexor contracture	0.89/0.92[29]	Patient sits at the edge of table. Patient flexes 1 knee to chest and rolls onto back while allowing test leg to remain extended at the hip off the edge of the table. If the hip does not fully extend, this indicates hip flexion contracture. If the leg abducts, this indicates iliotibial band tightness
Trendelenburg sign	To assess hip abductor strength	0.23–0.97/0.77–0.96[29]	Patient is standing. Examiner places hands on top of the iliac crests and monitors. Patient stands on the affected leg in a single-leg stance. Test/sign is positive if pelvis droops on the unaffected side, which indicates hip abductor weakness on the side of the stance leg

Abbreviation: FABER, flexion, abduction, external rotation.

assessment can help direct further diagnostic evaluation and treatment. The log roll test, anterior hip impingement, and flexion, abduction, external rotation (FABER)/Patrick test have been shown to have high inter-rater agreement in asymptomatic young adults (**Figs. 1** and **2**).[31]

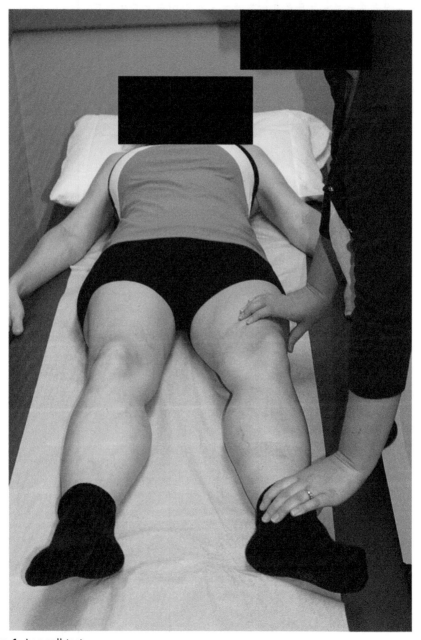

Fig. 1. Log roll test.

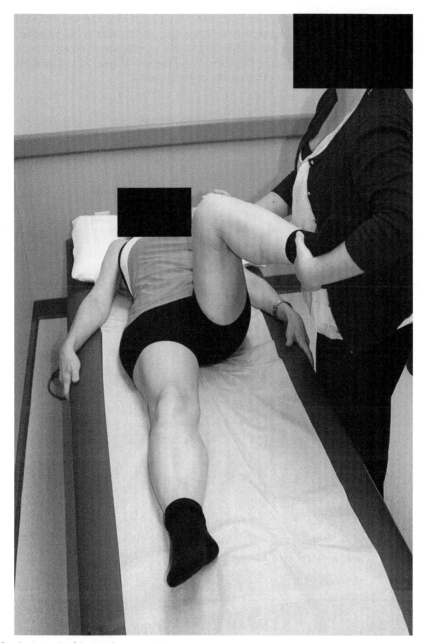

Fig. 2. Anterior hip impingement test.

DIAGNOSTIC IMAGING

Many hip disorders are diagnosed by history and physical examination. However, imaging can confirm a diagnosis and reveal or rule out other possible structural entities. Plain radiographs are typically the first-line imaging method to assess hip pain. They are useful for detecting osseous abnormalities, including fractures, OA, and intra-articular bodies. Radiographic views that best evaluate the hip include anteroposterior (AP) pelvis, false-profile, Dunn, frog-lateral, and cross-table lateral views.[32,33] In general, the AP pelvis (**Fig. 3**) and false-profile views provide the most information regarding acetabular morphology, and the lateral and Dunn (**Fig. 4**) views provide the most information regarding the proximal femur.[32]

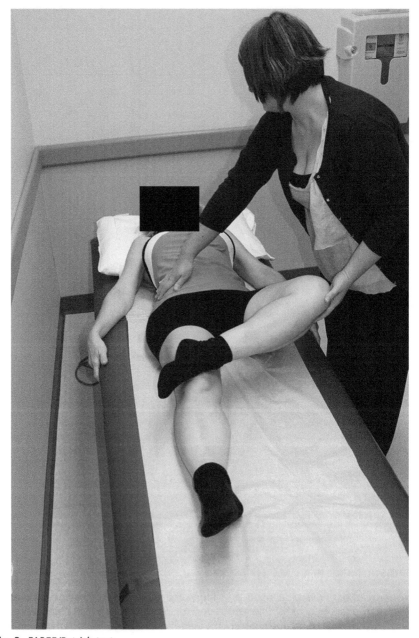

Fig. 3. FABER/Patrick test.

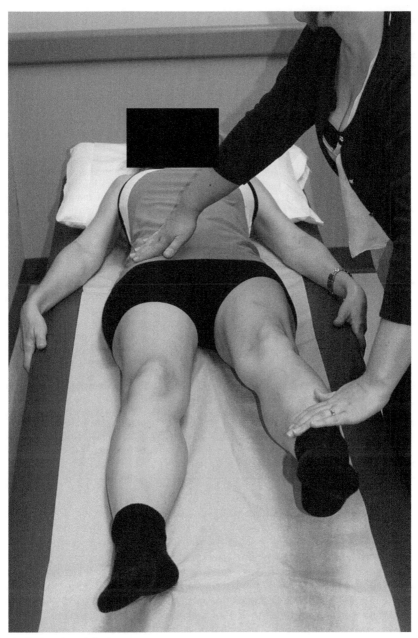

Fig. 4. Resisted straight leg test.

Radiographs remain the best way to assess bony hip structure. There are several measurements used to describe bony structure and hip deformity (**Box 2**). Examiners should be aware that these measurements can be adequately assessed only with standardized, high-quality radiographs with proper positioning of the patient.[32] Examples of measurements including the alpha angle, femoral head and neck offset

---

Box 2
Radiographic measurements in FAI

Name of Measurement or Sign	Purpose	Abnormal Values	Description of Measurement
Alpha angle	To detect cam-type deformity	$\geq63°$	First, determine best-fit circle to the femoral head. First arm of the angle is drawn from the center of the femoral neck to the center of the femoral head. Second arm is drawn from the center of the femoral head to the point where the femoral head-neck junction extends beyond the margin of the circle
HNO	To detect cam-type deformity	≤8 mm	First, determine axis of the femoral neck. Then, 2 parallel lines are drawn to the femoral neck axis at the anterolateral edge of the femoral head and at the anterolateral aspect of the femoral neck. The distance between these 2 lines define the femoral HNO
Crossover sign	To detect acetabular retroversion	Presence of sign	Sign is present when the anterior wall projects lateral to the posterior wall before converging at the lateral acetabular sourcil
Posterior wall sign	To detect acetabular retroversion	Presence of sign	Sign is present when the center of the femoral head is located lateral to the posterior wall
Ischial spine sign	To detect acetabular retroversion	Presence of sign	Sign is present when any portion of the ischial spine projects within the pelvic brim

Abbreviation: HNO, head-neck offset.

---

ratio, and cross-over sign are shown in **Figs. 5–8**. Hip expert examiners from different practices have not shown high inter-rater reliability for these common measurements, but inexperienced examiners trained by one expert showed good inter-rater reliability.[34] The cutoff points for normal range of measurements and deformity have varied in the past but a recent consensus review by an international group of hip experts[33] suggested the current range of cutoffs for FAI and hip OA (see **Box 2**). Using this range of cutoffs for specific measurements, an estimated 8% to 13% of asymptomatic male patients and 2% to 7% of asymptomatic female patients[33,35] have measurements on hip radiographs consistent with FAI. As a result, the determination of hip deformity does not uniformly determine the athlete's source of pain and dysfunction. OA found on plain radiographs of the hip has important implications on counseling and management of the athlete with intra-articular hip pain. The Tonnis grade or Kellgren-Lawrence scale are commonly used to describe the extent of OA based on the presence and degree of joint space narrowing, osteophytes, sclerosis, and subchondral cysts. It is important to delineate the extent of degenerative change in an athlete's hip. Athletes with a Tonnis grade 2 or higher are poor candidates for hip preservation surgery.[35,36]

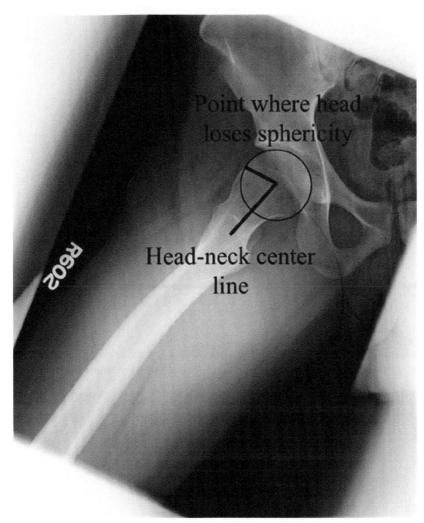

Fig. 5. Lateral frog leg of the hip.

For FAI, the maximal bony deformity is commonly located at the anterosuperior head-neck junction.[37,38] The 45° Dunn view best profiles this location.[39] The standing AP pelvis, false-profile, and Dunn views are the preferred series in the young athletic population. This combination allows the practitioner to make the appropriate measurements to assess for FAI and DDH with the least amount of radiation.[32,33] The quantitative radiographic measurements used most commonly for detecting a cam-type deformity in FAI are the alpha angle (see **Fig. 3**) and the head-neck offset ratio (see **Fig. 4**).[33] The radiographic evaluation of pincer-type deformity in FAI focuses on the detection of acetabular retroversion with the presence or absence of a cross-over sign (see **Fig. 5**), posterior wall sign, and prominent ischial spine sign.[32,33] Global acetabular coverage, a form of pincer-type FAI, is evaluated with measurement of the lateral center edge angle as well as the presence or absence of acetabular protrusion or coxa profunda.[33]

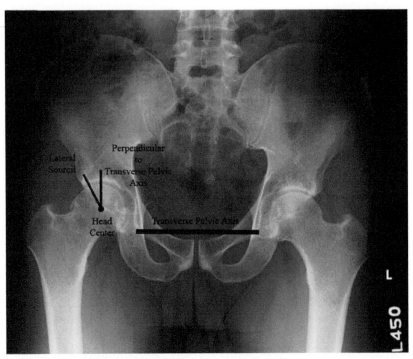

Fig. 6. AP view of the pelvis showing the center of edge angle of Wiberg.

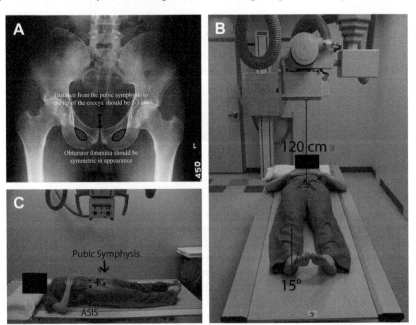

Fig. 7. (*A*) AP view of the pelvis, which allows appropriate hip measurements. (*B*) Appropriate positioning for AP view of the pelvis with attention to positioning of the lower extremities. (*C*) Appropriate positioning for anterior posterior view of the pelvis with attention to positioning of the anterior superior iliac spine (ASIS).

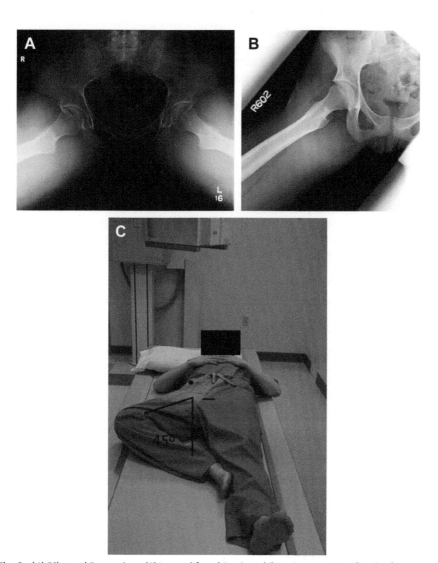

Fig. 8. (*A*) Bilateral Dunn view. (*B*) Lateral frog hip view. (*C*) Patient position for the frog view.

Magnetic resonance imaging (MRI) can detect abnormal soft tissue disorders of a tendon, muscle, or bursa and can assess the degree of degenerative changes or early avascular necrosis to a greater extent than radiographic imaging. It is also becoming the imaging study of choice for the evaluation of bony stress injuries.[40] With intra-articular contrast administration (magnetic resonance arthrography [MRA]), cartilage lesions and labral tears can adequately be assessed.[41] A meta-analysis comparing conventional MRI with MRA in the detection of acetabular labral tears found MRA superior to MRI, with a sensitivity of 87% and specificity of 64% for MRA compared with a sensitivity of 66% and specificity of 79% for MRI.[42] The health care provider must keep in mind that MRI is especially limited. One study showed 22% sensitivity[43] in its ability to detect acetabular cartilage flaps or delamination lesions, which often accompany labrochondral junction injuries. MRI provides a description of the anatomy of the acetabulum, including acetabular version, acetabular depth, labral size,[44] labral integrity, and labral ossification/acetabular rim bony apposition.[45] Biochemical MRI and delayed gadolinium-enhanced MRI of cartilage are being investigated to detect early changes in cartilage, and these are likely to lead to more detailed diagnostic information.[46,47]

Ultrasonography, or sonography, evaluates superficial tendons, muscles, and bursa about the hip.[48] The dynamic real-time potential of ultrasonography, including sonopalpation, is an advantage compared with static plain radiographs and MRI. This advantage may be particularly helpful in the case of a snapping hip. However, ultrasonography has difficulty with evaluating deep structures in which visibility can be reduced based on patient size. Ultrasonography has lesser diagnostic ability than MRA in the detection of anterosuperior acetabular labral tears. One study found the sensitivity and specificity of ultrasonography to be 82% and 60%, respectively, whereas the sensitivity and specificity of MRA were 91% and 80%, respectively.[49] Despite this reduced specificity and sensitivity, using ultrasonography in the athletic population can be useful in the acute setting of symptoms because of its low cost and potential ease of access. However, if symptoms persist and a cause remains undetermined or requires confirmation, more sensitive and specific imaging modalities should be used.

DIAGNOSTIC INTRA-ARTICULAR HIP INJECTION

A diagnostic hip injection should be considered to confirm an intra-articular process. A positive response to an intra-articular diagnostic injection is 90% predictive of intra-articular disorder found at arthroscopy.[41] A diagnostic (anesthetic only) injection that provides relief in symptoms and resolution of provocative hip tests paired with MRI/MRA that shows deformity with or without a labral tear can help confirm the intra-articular source of pain.

MANAGEMENT

Management of select hip disorders encountered in athletes (divided by intra-articular and extra-articular processes) is presented later. In general, the treatment of hip pain involves reduction of pain, activity modification, movement retraining, and progression to return to sport with implementation of a maintenance program.[28,50]

INTRA-ARTICULAR PROCESSES
Prearthritic Hip Disorders

There are limited data on the outcomes of comprehensive conservative care of athletes with prearthritic hip disorders that include symptomatic DDH and FAI with and without acetabular labral tears. A recent systematic review of nonoperative treatment of symptomatic FAI by Wall and colleagues[51] found only 5 studies that reviewed treatment, and 2 of the 5 specifically described treatment. The investigators concluded that, with limited experimental data, there is a suggestion that physical therapy and activity modification are of benefit to patients. One of the studies that specifically described treatment described patients with history, physical examination, and imaging findings consistent with intra-articular hip disorders with and without mild deformity.[52] The 52 patients in the study underwent comprehensive conservative treatment including patient education, activity modification, a standardized physical therapy protocol[53] that allowed for individualization, and intra-articular hip injection as indicated for pain control. Patients were followed for 1 year. Pain, function, and progression to surgery were measured. Patients treated with conservative treatment alone compared with those who chose to have surgical intervention following conservative treatment showed similar improvements in pain and function at 1 year. Baseline pain, function, and degree of deformity did not affect outcome at 1 year. The only statistically significant differences between the two groups were that the group of patients who chose surgery was more active at baseline.[52] Specific therapeutic exercises have not been determined or fully studied for these disorders. Some therapeutic approaches for treatment are designed to reduce anteriorly directed forces on the hip by addressing the patterns of recruitment of muscles that control hip motion, by correcting the movement patterns during exercises such as hip extension and gait, and by instruction in the avoidance of pivotingmotions in which the acetabulum rotates on the femur, particularly under load. In particular, the control of the hip abductor, deep lateral rotator, gluteus maximus, and iliopsoas muscles should be optimized and dominant involvement of the quadriceps femoris and hamstring muscles should be corrected.[53] The specifics of appropriate conservative treatment have not been definitively determined. However, athletes with prearthritic hip disorders need education regarding the mechanisms involved in the disorder. Activity modification plays a major role and includes activities other than exercise and sports. Evaluation of the athlete's technique is imperative in modifying symptoms during sports. Although image-guided intra-articular corticosteroid injections can help modify pain in athletes with early OA, steroid injections should be avoided in this prearthritic population to minimize potential damage to chondrocytes.[54]

When comprehensive conservative management of the athlete has been attempted without satisfactory improvement, surgical intervention should be considered. With recent advances in hip arthroscopy techniques, more is known about the surgical options for these patients.[33] When mixed deformity is present, arthroscopy may not be an option and more extensive hip preservation surgery such as surgical dislocation or periacetabular osteotomy may be indicated.[55,56] The inherent goals of these surgical procedures are to reduce pain, improve function, and correct bony deformity with the hope of reducing the progression of hip OA. However, as expected with new interventions, patient selection is imperative[33] and the inadequacies of surgical intervention will be realized with time and experience.[57]

OA

Research has shown a higher prevalence of hip arthritis in former track athletes compared with age matched control groups.[58] This association has also been found in former long distance runners.[59] The cause of this association remains to be determined, but theories include repetitive trauma and underlying hip deformity[60] contributing to the development of secondary hip OA. However, the literature remains inconclusive about a causal relationship between running and OA.[61] Athletes with intra-articular hip pain, hip deformity, and secondary arthritis of Tonnis grade 2 or more have poor outcomes with hip preservation surgery. Therefore optimizing conservative measures is the first choice of treatment. Activity modification to avoid painful range of motion during sport, activities of daily living, and therapeutic exercise is essential. These patients may also benefit from a trial of glucosamine and chondroitin, medication regimens for pain control including acetaminophen and nonsteroidal antiinflammatory drugs, and intra-articular image-guided corticosteroid injections to modify pain and therefore improve function. Surgical intervention with hip resurfacing or total hip arthroplasty is a viable option in athletes with end stage arthritis not controlled with conservative measures.

Femoral Neck Stress Fracture

The major focus of treatment of femoral stress fractures is to avoid preventable complications. In one report of a series of athletes treated for femoral stress fractures, 30% had a complication, including nonunion, malunion, osteonecrosis, and development of OA.[62] Treatment of the stress fracture is determined by the location. Stress fractures on the tension side of the femoral neck, involving the superior portion, often require internal fixation because of potential instability and high rate of complications.[63] Compression side stress fractures involving the inferomedial femoral neck are typically treated conservatively with reduction in weight bearing for 6 to 8 weeks and graded return to activity. Frequent radiographic monitoring is recommended for possible progression, given the high rate of complications, and to confirm healing.[63] Widening of cortical cracks, displacement of fractures, or fractures that do not respond to conservative treatment generally require surgical stabilization.[64,65]

During the period of rest following diagnosis of stress fracture, use of crutches may be indicated initially if ambulation is antalgic. Oral analgesics may be required. Once the patient has achieved pain-free activities of daily living, then a gradual return to sport may be initiated. Treatment of the stress fracture should also include addressing any predisposing or contributing factors, such as low bone mineral density, menstrual dysfunction, and low energy availability (including inadequate calcium and vitamin D intake), especially in the female athlete.[66] In addition, any related training errors and biomechanical factors should be addressed.

Hip Dislocation/Subluxation

Although rare, dislocation of the hip may be caused by a collision in contact sports or in snow skiing.[64] Most cases are posterior dislocations, accounting for 87% to 93% of all dislocations.[67] The dislocated hip requires emergent treatment in order to minimize the risk of complications. The most common complication is osteonecrosis, but nerve injury, acetabular labral tears, and chondral injuries may also occur.[64,68] The incidence of osteonecrosis increases by as much as 20-fold if the time from injury to reduction is more than 6 hours.[68] After neurovascular assessment, closed reduction under conscious sedation is the initial treatment. In some cases, general anesthesia may be required. Open reduction is indicated if closed reduction is unsuccessful after 2 or 3 attempts, or if loose intra-articular osteochondral fragments or interposed soft tissue are present.[64,68,69] Following reduction, treatment involves protected weight bearing with crutches, followed by gradual range of motion, strengthening, and return to activity for a total of 6 to 8 weeks.[64,68,69]

EXTRA-ARTICULAR HIP DISORDERS
Greater Trochanteric Pain Syndrome

Greater trochanteric pain typically responds to conservative measures, including activity modification, physical therapy, antiinflammatory medications, ice/heat, and corticosteroid injection. Success rates for these conservative measures, either alone or in combination, can exceed 90%.[70] However, recurrence is common. In these cases, further evaluation to investigate the mechanism of the breakdown in the musculoskeletal system is imperative to find a point of resolution or, at a minimum, a reliable maintenance program; this is especially the case for greater trochanteric pain, because it is commonly caused by more than an isolated trochanteric bursitis. Microtrauma leading to tears of the hip abductor tendons may be the leading cause of this syndrome.[71] Physical therapy should focus on addressing the altered lower extremity biomechanics that are associated with greater trochanteric pain as a result of tensor fascia lata/iliotibial band tightness or pain; hip external rotator strain; and OA of the spine, hip, or knee.[72] Corticosteroid injections at the greater trochanter and low-energy shock wave therapy have been found to be effective in multiple studies.[73,74] Tendon damage or rupture is a potential complication of corticosteroid injections, and possible short-term benefits from repeated injections should be weighed against potential long-term risks. Platelet-rich plasma (PRP) has gained attention in recent years for soft tissue injuries, especially in athletes. However, at this time there is no evidence to support their use for greater trochanteric pain.[75] Several surgical procedures are available for greater trochanteric pain that is unresponsive to conservative measures, such as iliotibial band release or lengthening, bursectomy, or trochanteric reduction osteotomy.[73,74]

Snapping Hip Syndrome

There is overlap between the treatment of greater trochanteric pain syndrome and extra-articular snapping hip syndrome. Most cases of extra-articular snapping hip can be treated conservatively with activity modification, physical therapy, and antiinflammatory medications. If conservative measures fail, corticosteroid injections targeting either the iliopsoas bursa or underneath the iliotibial band over the greater trochanter may be beneficial.[16] Ultrasonography guidance is often used with these injections because of ease of visualization of muscle tendon junctions and tendon insertion points. Surgical treatments are available for extra-articular snapping hip, if conservative measures and injections fail; however the surgical techniques described are limited because of the limited number of patients requiring surgery.[16]

Muscle Strain/Tear

Muscle strains or tears involving the hip and groin typically involve the hip adductor muscles, as well as the iliopsoas, quadriceps, and hamstring muscles. Initial treatment of muscle strains and partial tears includes rest, ice, compressive wrap, and antiinflammatory medications. Gentle range-of-motion exercises may begin after pain subsides, followed by strengthening exercises and gradual return to activity. Athletes with acute strains typically return to sport within 4 to 8 weeks, with recovery time as long as 6 months with chronic strains.[76] Progression of strains to partial tears, and partial tears to complete tears, may be a consequence of inadequate healing time. Surgical repair is typically indicated with complete tears.

Sports Hernia

Pain associated with posterior abdominal wall insufficiency and abnormalities is initially treated with conservative measures including rest from sport, followed by stretching and strengthening of the hip and lower abdomen.[64,69,76] Antiinflammatory medications are often used. Surgery may be considered after 6 to 8 weeks if these conservative measures fail.[69,76] Both laparoscopic and open surgical techniques have been described, with success in improving symptoms, primarily through reinforcement of the abdominal wall with mesh.[64] Treatment of the coexisting contracted or overdeveloped adductor longus muscle ipsilaterally may also be required via adductor muscle release, particularly if adductor muscle pain is noted.[64]

Osteitis Pubis

The initial treatment of this pubic bone stress injury includes conservative measures, including rest, stretching of the involved muscles/tendons, and antiinflammatory medications. A prolonged healing course of more than 3 months may be required, with occasional recurrence. Corticosteroid injection may be considered if conservative measures fail.[77,78] Surgical intervention, including curettage or wedge resection, may be of benefit if nonoperative measures fail.[76]

PRP

Musculoskeletal and sports medicine applications for the therapeutic use of PRP have received significant attention over the past decade. With regard to hip disorders, PRP has been proposed in the treatment of chronic ligamentous injury, chronic tendinopathy, and muscle tears, especially in the proximal hamstring, gluteal, and adductor muscles.[79] Although regenerative medicine is promising, the scientific literature on PRP remains in its infancy and the optimal injection technique and most efficacious injectate preparation remain uncertain. The role of PRP and other orthobiologics is discussed in further detail by Drs Mautner and Kneer elsewhere in this issue.

SUMMARY

Hip and groin pain is commonly experienced by athletes. The differential diagnosis is extensive and should include both intra-articular and extra-articular sources for pain and dysfunction. Further, evaluation for the underlying disorder can be complicated. A comprehensive history and physical examination can guide the evaluation of hip pain and the potential need for further diagnostics such as imaging or diagnostic hip injection. Treatment of athletes with hip disorders includes education, addressing activities of daily living, pain-modulating medications or modalities, exercise and sports modification, and therapeutic exercise. Advice on a graded return to exercise and sport is imperative for successful outcomes with athletes and reduction of recurrence of symptoms. Surgical techniques for prearthritic hip disorders are expanding and can offer appropriate patients a successful return to athletic endeavors when conservative measures are not effective. Further studies to determine appropriate conservative treatment are vital to improve patient outcomes, offer athletes more choices for treatment, and potentially improve overall surgical outcomes as patient selection becomes more focused.

REFERENCES

1. Minnich JM, Hanks JB, Muschaweck U, et al. Sports hernia: diagnosis and treatment highlighting a minimal repair surgical technique. Am J Sports Med 2011;39(6):1341–9.
2. Quinn A. Hip and groin pain: physiotherapy and rehabilitation issues. Open Sports Med J 2010;4:93–107.
3. DeLee JC, Farney WC. Incidence of injury in Texas high school football. Am J Sports Med 1992;20(5):575–80.
4. Yard EE, Schroeder MJ, Fields SK, et al. The epidemiology of United States high school soccer injuries, 2005-2007. Am J Sports Med 2008;36(10):1930–7.
5. Lovell G. The diagnosis of chronic groin pain in athletes: a review of 189 cases. Aust J Sci Med Sport 1995;27(3):76–9.
6. Morelli V, Smith V. Groin injuries in athletes. Am Fam Physician 2001;64(8):1405–14.
7. Stuge B, Garratt A, Krogstad Jenssen H, et al. The pelvic girdle questionnaire: a condition-specific instrument for assessing activity limitations and symptoms in people with pelvic girdle pain. Phys Ther 2011;91(7):1096–108.

8. Vleeming A, Albert HB, Ostgaard HC, et al. European guidelines for the diagnosis and treatment of pelvic girdle pain. Eur Spine J 2008;17(6):794–819. http://dx.doi.org/10.1007/s00586-008-0602-4.
9. Prather H, Hunt D, Fournie A, et al. Early intra-articular hip disease presenting with posterior pelvic and groin pain. PM R 2009;1(9):809–15.
10. Burnett RS, Della Rocca GJ, Prather H, et al. Clinical presentation of patients with tears of the acetabular labrum. J Bone Joint Surg Am 2006;88(7):1448–57.
11. Clohisy JC, Knaus ER, Hunt DM, et al. Clinical presentation of patients with symptomatic anterior hip impingement. Clin Orthop Relat Res 2009;467(3):638–44.
12. Nunley RM, Prather H, Hunt D, et al. Clinical presentation of symptomatic acetabular dysplasia in skeletally mature patients. J Bone Joint Surg Am 2011;93(Suppl 2):17–21.
13. Anderson SA, Keene JS. Results of arthroscopic iliopsoas tendon release in competitive and recreational athletes. Am J Sports Med 2008;36(12):2363–71.
14. Byrd JW. Evaluation and management of the snapping iliopsoas tendon. Instr Course Lect 2006;55:347–55.
15. Sammarco GJ. The dancer's hip. Clin Sports Med 1983;2(3):485–98.
16. Lee KS, Rosas HG, Phancao JP. Snapping hip: imaging and treatment. Semin Musculoskelet Radiol 2013;17(3):286–94.
17. Ilizaliturri VM Jr, Camacho-Galindo J. Endoscopic treatment of snapping hips, iliotibial band, and iliopsoas tendon. Sports Med Arthrosc 2010;18(2):120–7.
18. Plante M, Wallace R, Busconi BD. Clinical diagnosis of hip pain. Clin Sports Med 2011;30(2):225–38.
19. Aalto TJ, Airaksinen O, Harkonen TM, et al. Effect of passive stretch on reproducibility of hip range of motion measurements. Arch Phys Med Rehabil 2005;86(3):549–57.
20. Bierma-Zeinstra SM, Bohnen AM, Ramlal R, et al. Comparison between two devices for measuring hip joint motions. Clin Rehabil 1998;12(6):497–505.
21. Evan R. Illustrated orthopedic physical assessment. 2nd edition. St Louis, MO: Mosby; 2001.
22. Godges JJ, MacRae PG, Engelke KA. Effects of exercise on hip range of motion, trunk muscle performance, and gait economy. Phys Ther 1993;73(7):468–77.
23. Hoppenfeld S. Physical examination of the spine and extremities. Norwalk, CT: Prentice Hall; 1976.
24. Kendall F, McCreary K, Provance P, et al. Muscles: testing and function, with posture and pain. 5th edition. Baltimore, MD: Lippincott Williams & Wilkins; 2005.
25. Magee D. Orthopedic physical assessment. 4th edition. St Louis, MO: WB Saunders; 2002.
26. Simoneau GG, Hoenig KJ, Lepley JE, et al. Influence of hip position and gender on active hip internal and external rotation. J Orthop Sports Phys Ther 1998;28(3):158–64.
27. Prather H, Hunt D, Rho M, et al. Abnormal hip physical examination findings in asymptomatic female soccer athletes. Knee Surg Sports Traumatol Arthrosc 2013. [Epub ahead of print].
28. Hunt D, Clohisy J, Prather H. Acetabular labral tears of the hip in women. Phys Med Rehabil Clin N Am 2007;18(3):497–520, ix–x.
29. Reiman MP, Goode AP, Hegedus EJ, et al. Diagnostic accuracy of clinical tests of the hip: a systematic review with meta-analysis. Br J Sports Med 2013;47(14):893–902.

30. Fearon AM, Scarvell JM, Neeman T, et al. Greater trochanteric pain syndrome: defining the clinical syndrome. Br J Sports Med 2013;47(10):649–53.

31. Prather H, Harris-Hayes M, Hunt DM, et al. Reliability and agreement of hip range of motion and provocative physical examination tests in asymptomatic volunteers. PM R 2010;2(10):888–95. http://dx.doi.org/10.1016/j.pmrj.2010.05.005.

32. Clohisy JC, Carlisle JC, Beaule PE, et al. A systematic approach to the plain radiographic evaluation of the young adult hip. J Bone Joint Surg Am 2008; 90(Suppl 4):47–66.

33. Nepple JJ, Prather H, Trousdale RT, et al. Diagnostic imaging of femoroacetabular impingement. J Am Acad Orthop Surg 2013;21(Suppl 1):S20–6.

34. Carlisle JC, Zebala LP, Shia DS, et al. Reliability of various observers in determining common radiographic parameters of adult hip structural anatomy. Iowa Orthop J 2011;31:52–8.

35. Beck M, Leunig M, Parvizi J, et al. Anterior femoroacetabular impingement: part II. Midterm results of surgical treatment. Clin Orthop Relat Res 2004; 418:67–73.

36. Philippon MJ, Schroder ES, Briggs KK. Hip arthroscopy for femoroacetabular impingement in patients aged 50 years or older. Arthroscopy 2012;28(1):59–65.

37. Ito K, Minka MA 2nd, Leunig M, et al. Femoroacetabular impingement and the cam-effect. A MRI-based quantitative anatomical study of the femoral head-neck offset. J Bone Joint Surg Br 2001;83(2):171–6.

38. Rakhra KS, Sheikh AM, Allen D, et al. Comparison of MRI alpha angle measurement planes in femoroacetabular impingement. Clin Orthop Relat Res 2009;467(3):660–5.

39. Meyer DC, Beck M, Ellis T, et al. Comparison of six radiographic projections to assess femoral head/neck asphericity. Clin Orthop Relat Res 2006;445:181–5.

40. Kiuru M, Pihlajamaki HK, Hietanen H, et al. MR imaging, bone scintigraphy, and radiography in bone stress injuries of the pelvis and the lower extremity. Acta Radiol 2008;43(2):207–12.

41. Byrd JW, Jones KS. Diagnostic accuracy of clinical assessment, magnetic resonance imaging, magnetic resonance arthrography, and intra-articular injection in hip arthroscopy patients. Am J Sports Med 2004;32(7):1668–74.

42. Smith TO, Hilton G, Toms AP, et al. The diagnostic accuracy of acetabular labral tears using magnetic resonance imaging and magnetic resonance arthrography: a meta-analysis. Eur Radiol 2011;21(4):863–74.

43. Anderson LA, Peters CL, Park BB, et al. Acetabular cartilage delamination in femoroacetabular impingement. Risk factors and magnetic resonance imaging diagnosis. J Bone Joint Surg Am 2009;91(2):305–13.

44. Leunig M, Podeszwa D, Beck M, et al. Magnetic resonance arthrography of labral disorders in hips with dysplasia and impingement. Clin Orthop Relat Res 2004;418:74–80.

45. Corten K, Ganz R, Chosa E, et al. Bone apposition of the acetabular rim in deep hips: a distinct finding of global pincer impingement. J Bone Joint Surg Am 2011;93(Suppl 2):10–6.

46. Beaule PE, Kim YJ, Rakhra KS, et al. New frontiers in cartilage imaging of the hip. Instr Course Lect 2012;61:253–62.

47. Bittersohl B, Hosalkar HS, Kim YJ, et al. Delayed gadolinium-enhanced magnetic resonance imaging (dGEMRIC) of hip joint cartilage in femoroacetabular impingement (FAI): are pre- and postcontrast imaging both necessary? Magn Reson Med 2009;62(6):1362–7.

48. Blankenbaker DG, De Smet AA, Keene JS. Sonography of the iliopsoas tendon and injection of the iliopsoas bursa for diagnosis and management of the painful snapping hip. Skeletal Radiol 2006;35(8):565–71.
49. Jin W, Kim KI, Rhyu KH, et al. Sonographic evaluation of anterosuperior hip labral tears with magnetic resonance arthrographic and surgical correlation. J Ultrasound Med 2012;31(3):439–47.
50. Vasudevan JM, Smuck M, Fredericson M. Evaluation of the athlete with buttock pain. Curr Sports Med Rep 2012;11(1):35–42.
51. Wall PD, Fernandez M, Griffin DR, et al. Nonoperative treatment for femoroacetabular impingement: a systematic review of the literature. PM R 2013;5(5):418–26.
52. Hunt D, Prather H, Harris Hayes M, et al. Clinical outcomes analysis of conservative and surgical treatment of patients with clinical indications of prearthritic, intra-articular hip disorders. PM R 2012;4(7):479–87.
53. Lewis CL, Sahrmann SA. Acetabular labral tears. Phys Ther 2006;86:110–21.
54. Piper SL, Kramer JD, Kim HT, et al. Effects of local anesthetics on articular cartilage. Am J Sports Med 2011;39(10):2245–53.
55. Tippett SR. Returning to sports after periacetabular osteotomy for developmental dysplasia of the hip. N Am J Sports Phys Ther 2006;1(1):32–9.
56. van Bergayk AB, Garbuz DS. Quality of life and sports-specific outcomes after Bernese periacetabular osteotomy. J Bone Joint Surg Br 2002;84(3):339–43.
57. Jackson TJ, Watson J, Lareau JM, et al. Periacetabular osteotomy and arthroscopic labral repair after failed hip arthroscopy due to iatrogenic aggravation of hip dysplasia. Knee Surg Sports Traumatol Arthrosc 2014;22(4):911–4.
58. Vingard E, Sandmark H, Alfredsson L. Musculoskeletal disorders in former athletes. A cohort study in 114 track and field champions. Acta Orthop Scand 1995;66(3):289–91.
59. Marti B, Knobloch M, Tschopp A, et al. Is excessive running predictive of degenerative hip disease? Controlled study of former elite athletes. BMJ 1989;299(6691):91–3.
60. Nho S, Kymes S, Callaghan J, et al. The burden of hip osteoarthritis in the United States: epidemiologic and economic considerations. J Am Acad Orthop Surg 2013;21(suppl 1):S1–6.
61. Willick SE, Hansen PA. Running and osteoarthritis. Clin Sports Med 2010;29(3):417–28.
62. Johansson C, Ekenman I, Tornkvist H, et al. Stress fractures of the femoral neck in athletes. The consequence of a delay in diagnosis. Am J Sports Med 1990;18(5):524–8.
63. Harrast MA, Colonno D. Stress fractures in runners. Clin Sports Med 2010;29(3):399–416.
64. Anderson K, Strickland SM, Warren R. Hip and groin injuries in athletes. Am J Sports Med 2001;29(4):521–33.
65. Fullerton LR Jr. Femoral neck stress fractures. Sports Med 1990;9(3):192–7.
66. Nattiv A. Stress fractures and bone health in track and field athletes. J Sci Med Sport 2000;3(3):268–79.
67. Bastian JD, Turina M, Siebenrok KA, et al. Long-term outcome after traumatic anterior dislocation of the hip. Arch Orthop Trauma Surg 2011;131(9):1273–8.
68. Kovacevic D, Mariscalco M, Goodwin RC. Injuries about the hip in the adolescent athlete. Sports Med Arthrosc 2011;19(1):64–74.
69. Waite BL, Krabak BJ. Examination and treatment of pediatric injuries of the hip and pelvis. Phys Med Rehabil Clin N Am 2008;19(2):305–18, ix.

70. Brooker AF Jr. The surgical approach to refractory trochanteric bursitis. Johns Hopkins Med J 1979;145(3):98–100.

71. Klauser AS, Martinoli C, Tagliafico A, et al. Greater trochanteric pain syndrome. Semin Musculoskelet Radiol 2013;17(1):43–8.

72. Segal NA, Felson DT, Torner JC, et al. Greater trochanteric pain syndrome: epidemiology and associated factors. Arch Phys Med Rehabil 2007;88(8): 988–92.

73. Del Buono A, Papalia R, Khanduja V, et al. Management of the greater trochanteric pain syndrome: a systematic review. Br Med Bull 2012;102:115–31.

74. Lustenberger DP, Ng VY, Best TM, et al. Efficacy of treatment of trochanteric bursitis: a systematic review. Clin J Sport Med 2011;21(5):447–53.

75. Moraes VY, Lenza M, Tamaoki MJ, et al. Platelet-rich therapies for musculoskeletal soft tissue injuries. Cochrane Database Syst Rev 2013;(12):CD010071. http://dx.doi.org/10.1002/14651858.CD010071.pub2.

76. Tammareddi K, Morelli V, Reyes M Jr. The athlete's hip and groin. Prim Care 2013;40(2):313–33.

77. Holt MA, Keene JS, Graf BK, et al. Treatment of osteitis pubis in athletes. Results of corticosteroid injections. Am J Sports Med 1995;23(5):601–6.

78. O'Connell MJ, Powell T, McCaffrey NM, et al. Symphyseal cleft injection in the diagnosis and treatment of osteitis pubis in athletes. AJR Am J Roentgenol 2002;179(4):955–9.

79. Nguyen RT, Borg-Stein J, McInnis K. Applications of platelet-rich plasma in musculoskeletal and sports medicine: an evidence-based approach. PM R 2011;3(3):226–50.

Anterior Cruciate Ligament Injury

Mechanisms of Injury and Strategies for Injury Prevention

Judith R. Peterson, MD[a,b,*], Brian J. Krabak, MD, MBA[c,d]

KEYWORDS

- Knee • Anterior cruciate ligament • Sports injury • Injury prevention
- Lower extremity injury • Knee injury reduction

KEY POINTS

- Anterior cruciate ligament injuries are common in athletes.
- Anterior cruciate ligament injuries can have long-term consequences for the affected athlete.
- Widespread implementation of anterior cruciate ligament injury prevention programs has not occurred.
- This article reviews some strategies for prevention of anterior cruciate ligament injuries based on current research.

INTRODUCTION

Anterior cruciate ligament (ACL) injury is a common and severe sports injury. The female athlete is at particular risk for this type of injury. ACL injuries have immediate and long-term consequences for affected athletes.[1,2] Despite much medical literature concerning these injuries, widespread implementation of effective injury prevention programs has not occurred. The aim of this article is to review ACL injury epidemiology, including risk factors, mechanisms for injury, and strategies for ACL prevention based on current research.

[a] Department of Neurosciences, Sanford School of Medicine, University of South Dakota, 1400 West 22nd Street, Sioux Falls, SD 57105, USA; [b] Yankton Medical Clinic, 1104 West 8th Street, Yankton, SD 57078, USA; [c] Rehabilitation, Orthopedics, and Sports Medicine, University of Washington Sports Medicine, 3800 Montlake Boulevard Northeast, Box 354060, Seattle, WA 98195, USA; [d] Seattle Children's Sports Medicine, 4800 Sand Point Way Northeast, Seattle, WA 98145, USA
* Corresponding author. Yankton Medical Clinic, 1104 West 8th Street, Yankton, SD 57078.
E-mail address: judith.peterson@usd.edu

Phys Med Rehabil Clin N Am 25 (2014) 813–828
http://dx.doi.org/10.1016/j.pmr.2014.06.010
1047-9651/14/$ – see front matter © 2014 Elsevier Inc. All rights reserved.
pmr.theclinics.com

EPIDEMIOLOGY

ACL injury is a common sports injury that often occurs during adolescence and young adulthood. It often occurs from a noncontact knee injury, but can occur from direct trauma, such as a blow to the knee. It is estimated that year-round high-level female soccer and basketball participants have approximately a 5% risk of having an ACL tear.[3] Defining 1 athletic exposure (AE) as 1 athlete participating in 1 game or practice, studies at the high school level suggest football has the highest rate of knee injury at 6.29 per 10,000 AE. High school girls' soccer and girls' gymnastics are also huge contributors to knee injuries with 4.53 per 10,000 AE in girls' soccer and 4.23 per 10,000 AE in girls' gymnastics. When we examine the specific risk of ACL injury for girls compared with boys in sex-comparable sports at the high school level, we find that girls are generally at a profoundly higher risk of ACL injury with a relative risk (RR) of 2.38. This statement remains valid for softball versus baseball (RR, 4.99), basketball (RR, 4.54), and soccer (RR, 2.33)[4] Joseph and colleagues,[5] in a recent epidemiologic multisport comparison of high school athletics at 100 representative US high schools, found that 74.9% of ACL injuries occurred during competition versus practice. They found the highest injury rates per 100,000 AE in girl's soccer (12.2) followed by football (11.1) and girl's basketball. Interestingly, boy's basketball had a relatively low risk at 2.3.

Studies of collegiate athletes note that men's spring football and women's gymnastics have equal ACL injury rates per 1000 AE (0.33). The authors also note that 3 of the 4 collegiate sports with the highest ACL injury rate included women's gymnastics (0.33), women's soccer (0.28), and women's basketball (0.23).[6]

Given the above epidemiology and that ACL injuries frequently require surgery, the expense of these injuries becomes a significant public health concern.[4,7] A 2013 study of 2 prospective orthopedic cohorts estimated the costs for surgical repair and rehabilitative conservative care of ACL injuries. The Multicenter Orthopedics Outcomes Network cohort included 988 primary ACL tears followed up for a minimum of 6 years. The KANNON (knee anterior cruciate ligament, nonsurgical vs surgical treatment) cohort studied 121 patients for a minimum of 2 years. The societal costs of each type of treatment of this injury are significant. The lifetime cost estimate for ACL surgical repair was $38,121 compared with $88,538 for rehabilitative conservative care. The author's acknowledge that the long-term economic cost predictions were based on lower levels of evidence than level I. The authors additionally note that ACL tears may cause profound long-term issues for patients regardless of treatment approach, highlighting the importance of primary prevention.[7]

Although the above comments concern the long-term issues that arise after ACL injuries, there are immediate immense impacts of ACL injuries on health care expenditures. This serious injury necessitates physician evaluation, radiography, and rehabilitation in addition to potential surgical intervention and postoperative care; these represent a public health emergency. Given the huge health, economic, and societal tolls of ACL injury, it becomes imperative for physicians to better understand how to prevent this catastrophic injury. Third-party payer data on ACL injury costs are difficult to obtain. It is estimated, however, that up to 250,000 ACL injuries occur yearly in the United States, at a cost of more than $2 billion per year.[8] Given the above startling and troubling statistics, it is critical that physicians have a thorough understanding of the causes of ACL injuries and the ways in which ACL injuries can be prevented.

It is difficult to prevent acute knee injuries secondary to direct knee trauma because of the large contact forces on the joint encountered with direct knee impacts. In the United States, football participation is the leading cause of sports trauma overall and a common cause of injury to the ACL.[9] However, it is surprising that most sports-related ACL injuries are actually secondary to noncontact-related forces on the knee joint. Contact causes fewer ACL tears than cutting maneuvers or speed decelerations.[10]

Immediate morbidity and loss of function in the athlete are significant public health concerns. Larger public health concerns are the long-term sequelae of sports-related knee injuries. Of young adults with knee injuries, 13.9% will have knee osteoarthritis by age 65 compared with 6.0% in those without histories of knee injuries.[11,12] A study of female soccer players with a prior history of ACL injury found arthritic radiographic changes such as joint space narrowing or osteophytes in 82% of those examined radiographically 12 years after injury. Fifty-one percent of women fulfilled the radiographic requirements for radiographic knee osteoarthritis in the cohort with a median age of 31 years (range, 26 to 40 years old.) The cutoff for radiographic osteoarthritis in this study approximated grade 2 on the Kellgren/Lawrence scale. Seventy-five percent of respondents in this study noted symptoms affecting their knee-related quality of life. These symptoms resulted in lifestyle modifications in 50% of respondents.[13]

A study of male soccer players noted similar outcomes. Male soccer players with a history of ACL injuries were radiographically assessed 14 years after ACL injury. This radiographic examination documented abnormalities in 78% of evaluated knees with 41% of the injured knees showing findings of Kellgren/Lawrence grade 2 or higher. Surgical versus conservative treatment of these injured knees did not affect the radiographic outcome. Noninjured knees by contrast showed advanced changes in only 4% of knees. Study participants also responded to a questionnaire to further assess patient-relevant outcomes 14 years after ACL injury. Eighty percent of the study participants reported reduced activity level. Of these, 69% noted the knee injury as the cause of reduced activity. Thirty percent experienced severe changes in lifestyle.[14]

In addition to the physical toll of these injuries, the emotional functioning of otherwise healthy young people may be negatively affected. The long-term impact of the depression experienced by some of those who have an ACL injury remains to be determined.[15,16]

Anatomy

The cruciate ligaments are integral to knee joint stability (**Fig. 1**). The knee is described as having a screw-home mechanism where the tibia rotates as the knee flexes and extends through the tibiofemoral articulation. As the knee straightens, the tibia externally rotates. During this motion, contact points of the joint actually migrate anteriorly with knee extension. Knee ligaments become more taut with extension. The ACL is described as the primary structure preventing anterior tibial translation.[17] ACL strain injury occurs primarily through shear forces with additional contributions to injury from coronal and axial plane stress.[18,19] The ACL is actually 2 discrete anatomic bundles (**Fig. 2**). The anteromedial and posterolateral bundles begin from the posteromedial portion of the lateral femoral condyle and insert between and slightly anteriorly to the tibial intercondylar eminence. The bundles' names are descriptive of their relationship at this tibial insertion.[20] There are 2 bundles that comprise the ACL, which spiral and increase in tension with tibial internal rotation.[19] The bundles also have variable tension based on knee flexion angle and varus/valgus and rotational stress.[19,21,22] Because of this, the ACL is at particular risk with sidestepping or cutting maneuvers in knee flexion angles of 0° to 40°.[21,22]

The majority of the blood supply to the ACL is through the middle genicular artery, which derives from the popliteal artery. There are additional blood flow contributions

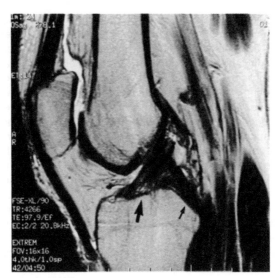

Fig. 1. Magnetic resonance imaging of normal knee with intact anterior cruciate ligament and posterior cruciate ligament. (*From* Snyder RR, Pacicca DM, Dewire P. Soft tissue injuries (Chapter 44). In: Becker JM, Stucchi AF, editors. Essentials of surgery. Philadelphia: Saunders Elsevier; 2006. p. 537; with permission. Copyright 2006, Elsevier Inc. All rights reserved.)

from the inferomedial and inferolateral genicular arteries, which traverse the anterior fat pad.[20] Tears of the ACL commonly result in permanent damage to the blood supply of the ligament, which impairs innate healing potential.[19]

Injury Risk Factors

Our knowledge of the various risk factors for a tear of the ACL and our ability to predict which athletes are at particularly high risk for this injury continue to evolve. Both

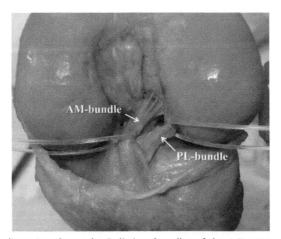

Fig. 2. Cadaveric dissection shows the 2 distinct bundles of the ACL. AM, anteromedial; PL, posterolateral. (*From* Hofbauer M, Muller B, Wolf M, et al. Contemporary ACL surgery anatomic double-bundle anterior cruciate ligament reconstruction. Oper Tech Sports Med 2013;21(1):47–54; with permission.)

extrinsic factors and intrinsic factors impact ACL injury risk. It remains unsettled, however, as to how all risk factors interplay and coalesce in each individual athlete to result in ACL injury.[1,3,10,23]

Several external and internal risk factors appear to predispose some athletes to ACL injury risk.[10,23] Playing American style football exposes the athlete's knee to large direct contact forces. Tackling or being tackled leads to most ACL injuries in football players. From 1987 to 2000, ACL reconstruction was the third most common orthopedic procedure incurred by National Football League prospects and the most common medical condition noted for players who received a medical fail with regard to their projected ability to play successfully in the National Football League.[24,25]

External ACL injury risk factors such as shoe type worn and type of playing surface have been evaluated. For example, football cleat design is found to have an impact on ACL injury risk.[26] A 3-year prospective study of high school football players found that wearing a shoe with an increased torsional resistance was associated with a significantly higher risk of ACL injury. In this study, the edge design of longer irregular cleats at the shoe sole periphery with smaller pointed cleats positioned interiorly was a higher-risk design than shoe designs with less torsional resistance.[26]

Playing surface coefficient of friction may also affect ACL injury risk. In a Norwegian handball study, the higher friction floor type increased the ACL injury risk for female handball players by a factor of 2.35. Their male counterparts did not accrue any statistically significant additional risk secondary to change in floor type.[27] A 3-year prospective study of game-related football injuries in college athletes evaluated the impact of FieldTurf, a polyethylene fiber blend with ground rubber infill versus natural grass turf. No significant difference in knee injuries was noted on FieldTurf versus natural grass.[28]

Intrinsic factors also play a role. There is a known familial predisposition to ACL tears. In a study by Flynn and colleagues,[29] 23.4% of individuals with an ACL tear were noted to have a first-degree relative with such an ACL injury compared with 11.7% of a control group of matched individuals without a history of an ACL tear. Posthumus and colleagues[30] noted that variants in matrix metalloproteinase genes on chromosome 11q22 were associated with increased risk of ACL tears.

Anatomic indices such as femoral intercondylar notch width, notch width index, (**Fig. 3**) and femoral intercondylar notch morphology are assessed as independent risk factors for ACL injury. Ireland and colleagues[31] evaluated the radiographs of 108 individuals (55 women, 53 men) with a history of ACL injury and compared the radiographic findings with those of 186 cases (94 women, 92 men) with an intact ACL. Small intercondylar notches were noted in those with ACL injury with a mean notch of 18.9±4.0 mm in those with ACL injury compared with 20.7±3.9 mm in those whose ACLs were intact. A smaller notch width index (ration of intercondylar notch width to width of distal femur) may also potentially increase ACL injury risk.[31]

The slope of the posterior tibia may also have an impact on ACL injury risk (**Fig. 4**).[10,32] The posterior tibial slope is the posterior inclination of the tibial plateau. The tibial slope is associated with an anterior position of the tibia.[33] In one study concerning those with chronic ACL rupture, each 10° increase in posterior tibial slope led to increased anterior laxity with a 6-mm increase in anterior tibial translation when the individual was in monopodal stance at 20° of flexion.[34]

The potential effect of hormones and oral contraceptives on ACL rupture risk also remains a matter for continued investigation. In a study by Bell and colleagues,[35] 30 women were studied to assess the effect of oral contraceptives on hamstring function in physically active female study participants. Oral contraceptive use did not alter muscle neuromechanics. Wild and colleagues[36] evaluated the role of the female

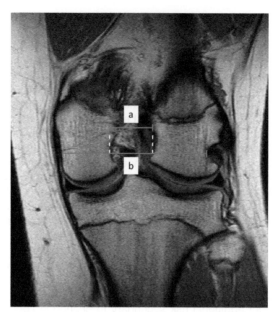

Fig. 3. Two-dimensional measurements of notch geometry. The NWI is the ratio of the inter-condylar notch width (a) to the bicondylar width of the distal femur (b) at the level of the popliteal groove. (*From* Swami VG, Mabee M, Hui C, et al. Three-dimensional intercondylar notch volumes in a skeletally immature pediatric population: a magnetic resonance imaging–based anatomic comparison of knees with torn and intact anterior cruciate ligaments. Arthroscopy 2013;29(12):1954–62; with permission. Copyright 2013 Arthroscopy Association of North America)

adolescent growth spurt with its large estrogen increases as a contributor to knee laxity and the risk of ACL injury. All participants were premenarchal 10- to 13-year-old girls to exclude cyclic hormone variation. Participants were biomechanically assessed up to 4 times during the 12-month period of the adolescent growth spurt. Interestingly, estradiol concentrations remained constant. Although quadriceps strength increased during the study, hamstring strength did not. The authors theorize that strength imbalance might place the ACL at injury risk. Passive knee joint laxity of study participants also increased during the testing period. It has also been observed that the peak velocity for lower limb growth precedes the peak height velocity. This growth rate discrepancy has an unclear biomechanical impact on lower extremity vulnerability.[37] Hormonal influences remain an area of intense interest. A recent symposium, ACL Research Retreat VI, highlighted the complexity of studying the effects of hormonal influences on mechanical properties of the ACL and ACL injury vulnerability.[38]

The injury predisposition in women may also be enhanced by properties of the ACL itself. The female ACL has an 8.3% lower tensile load to failure compared with the male ACL in one cadaveric study. The female ACL also had a 22.49% lower modulus of elasticity.[39] An additional cadaveric study found that the female ACL is shorter than the male ACL, with ACL mass correlating with height in women but not in men.[40] A retrospective cohort of subjects referred for knee magnetic resonance imaging noted that ACL volume correlated with height differences rather than gender.[41] The maximal ACL area is noted to be smaller in women than men when standardized for body weight.[42] A prospective study evaluating the effect of generalized joint laxity noted

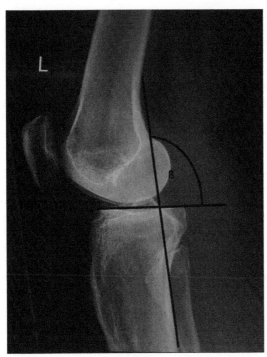

Fig. 4. Radiograph with 2 lines. (*From* Hohmann E, Bryant A, Reaburn P, et al. Does posterior tibial slope influence knee functionality in the anterior cruciate ligament–deficient and anterior cruciate ligament–reconstructed knee? Arthroscopy 2010;26(11):1496–502; with permission. Copyright 2010.)

that passive knee hyperextension and asymmetry of knee anterior-posterior laxity enhanced ACL injury risk.[43]

Research suggests that neuromuscular activation in a gender-specific pattern likely contributes to ACL injury risk. The proposed differences include female athletes landing differently from jumps than male athletes. Findings include landing from jumps with a relatively straight knees. A study of adolescent soccer players noted that female athletes exhibited decreased hip and knee flexion in jump tests.[44] Women have a greater vertical ground reaction force than is found in male athletes while performing jump tests. Knee valgus moments were significantly increased compared with those in male athletes for single and bilateral leg landings.[45] A retrospective analysis of 1718 athletes with ACL injury noted the dynamic alignment at time of injury in 1603 subjects (781 men, 822 women).The alignment of knee-in and toe-out was the most common, noted in 793 of 1603 with no significant difference in male and female subjects.[46]

The trunk also contributes to the ground reaction forces on the ACL. Relatively greater hip adduction, decreased hip abductor strength, and diminished trunk control can contribute to knee injury risk.[47] Proprioceptive deficiency has been correlated with knee injury in women but not in men. Impaired core proprioception in women was highly predictive of knee injury risk in this prospective study.[48] Another prospective study of 277 college athletes found that decreased trunk control was strongly predictive of knee injury in female athletes.[49]

The morphology of the knee joint articulation surface is also smaller in the female athlete.[11,50] magnetic resonance imaging of the joint surface of 18 healthy subjects found interesting differences in male and female joint anatomy. Compared with those in men, women's medial tibias had 32.9% less surface area and women's lateral tibias had 33.4% less lateral tibial surface area and 21% less femoral joint surface area.[50]

The quadriceps angle or Q angle is greater in women than in men (**Fig. 5**).[51] This measure of the femoral to tibial angle is an additional factor that may increase load on the ACL through increased lateral quadriceps pull.[17] Increased knee joint laxity has also been proposed to increase the risk of ACL injury in the athlete. As previously noted, the ACL is the principal restraint to anterior tibial translation. Anterior knee laxity in non–weight bearing is a test of ACL integrity. Shultz and colleagues[52] found that increased anterior knee laxity was in fact associated with increased anterior tibial translation, as the knee accepted weight.[52]

Athlete fatigue has been investigated as a potential risk factor for ACL injury. Fatigue may occur centrally, which causes reduction in muscle activity proximal to the neuromuscular junction, and peripherally, which adversely affects the muscle distal to the neuromuscular junction. In either case, fatigue may impair knee kinematics. In a study by McLean and Samorezov,[53] 20 female National Collegiate Athletic Association (NCAA) athletes had knee joint motion assessment during jump landings. A standardized fatigue protocol of 3 single-leg squats was followed by a landing trial, and the sequence was repeated until the athlete could not complete 3 sequential squats without assistance. Unilateral fatigue decreased initial contact knee flexion and

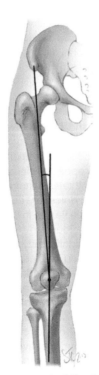

Fig. 5. Illustration depicting the measurement of the Q angle. The Q angle is measured by the intersection of a line drawn from the anterior superior iliac spine through the center of the patella and a line from the tibial tubercle through the center of the patella. (*From* Sherman SL, Plackis AC, Nuelle CW et al. Patellofemoral anatomy and biomechanics. Clin Sports Med 2014;33(3):397; with permission. Copyright 2014 Elsevier Inc.)

increased hip internal rotation. Unanticipated landings compared with anticipated landings in fatigued athletes provoked greater decreases in hip flexion and more hip internal rotation.[53]

Interestingly, fatigue also has a negative effect on knee laxity. Shultz and colleagues[54] examined the changes in knee joint laxity associated with strenuous exercise in the athlete. This study deliberately imitated the demands of a soccer match on athletes through a strenuous intermittent exercise protocol of 90 minutes' duration. Twenty-nine women and 30 males completed the study. Exercise-related increases in sagittal and frontal laxity were more pronounced in women than men. Compared with a control condition of no exercise, female athletes showed increased sagittal and frontal laxity with an intermittent exercise protocol, whereas male athletes did not show such increases ($P<.037$). Interestingly, male and female athletes showed increased transverse laxity with exercise ($P = .007$). However, 33% of women in this study and 10% of men showed increases in sagittal plane laxity $\geq$1.9 mm and frontal plane laxity $\geq$2.8 with exercise indicating that a small number of male athletes experience significant knee laxity changes with exercise.[54]

Prevention

Increasing awareness of the major public health implications and costs of ACL injuries has led researchers to devise programs that might help prevent these injuries. Effective ACL injury prevention seems even more critical when we reflect on the fact that once an athlete sustains an ACL injury and undergoes reconstructive surgery, that athlete's risk of additional knee injury remains elevated in both the affected extremity and the contralateral extremity.[55]

Mandelbaum and colleagues created the Prevent Injury Enhance Performance injury prevention program (PEP). The PEP program involves warm-up, stretching, strengthening, and plyometrics agility exercises and stretching.[56] Warm-up and cooling down are stressed. Warm-up includes exercises such as jogging forward and backward and shuttle runs. Strengthening includes walking lunges, Russian hamstring exercises, and repeated single-leg toe raises. Plyometric exercises emphasize landing technique and knee positioning. Plyometrics include forward, backward, and lateral hops over a 2-inch cone and single leg hops over a cone. Straight vertical jumps and scissors jumps are performed. Agility drills such as forward runs with decelerations, lateral diagonal runs, and bounding runs are completed. Finally, proper stretching technique is emphasized with a focus on calf muscles, quadriceps, hamstrings, inner thigh muscles, and hip flexors. The program in its entirety is designed to be completed in 15 to 20 minutes on the field without the use of specialized equipment or personnel. Year one of a study of PEP efficacy found 37,476 AEs for trained athletes and 68,580 AEs for the control athletes. Two ACL tears were noted in the protocol group, and 32 ACL tears were noted in control athletes. The authors note an 88% reduction in ACL tears for participants (1041 trained, 1905 controls). Year 2 of the study (844 trained, 1913 controls) again found striking decreases in ACL injury through training in the prevention program. A total of 30,384 AEs occurred in the trained group and 68,868 AEs occurred in the untrained group. Four ACL tears were noted in the treatment group, and 35 ACL tears were noted in the control group, representing a 74% ACL injury reduction in participants compared with controls.[56,57]

The Cincinnati SportsMedicine Research and Education Foundation program used preseason conditioning for 6 weeks to successfully reduce knee injury rates. The program involved training 3 days per week for 60 to 90 minutes per training session. An athletic trainer and physical therapist demonstrated proper stretching. Flexibility, plyometrics, and weight training were used to decrease the landing forces for athletes. A total of 1263 female athletes in soccer, volleyball, and basketball were studied. AEs were 23,138 in the untrained female group and 17,222 in the trained female group with 21,390 in the male control group. Knee injury incidence per 1000 athlete exposures was 0.12 in the trained group of female athletes and 0.43 in the untrained group of female athletes. The trained female group injury incidence of 0.12 was similar to that of the control males, with 0.09 the incidence of all knee injuries in the male controls. No trained female athlete suffered a noncontact ACL injury compared with 5 such injuries in untrained female athletes in this study.[58] Preseason and in-season neuromuscular training was found to decrease ACL injury risk factors in a follow-up study by Brent and colleagues.[59] The Cincinnati SportsMedicine Research and Education Foundation has developed a separate program of 20 exercises in 20 minutes called Warm-up for Injury Prevention and Performance (WIPP).[60] A study by Grandstrand and colleagues[61] evaluated the effects of this briefer program. WIPP was performed twice weekly for the 8-week duration of the soccer season by a girls youth soccer club (age 9–11 years). The WIPP program had to be modified to meet the athlete's abilities. The effect of this modified training was assessed using Sportsmetrics Software for the Analysis of Jumping Mechanics. Athletes failed to improve landing knee kinematics or maximum vertical jump height.[61]

A prospective study by Pfeiffer failed to show a reduction in ACL injuries in female athletes who participated in a twice-weekly program through the sports season.[62] The Knee Ligament Injury Prevention (KLIP) study compared 577 trained athletes with 862 controls. The PEP study involves athletes in training 3 times per week. This may explain the greater effect of the PEP program compared with the KLIP program. A new study by Waldén using a different protocol of 6 exercises performed twice weekly after a running warm-up did, however, show a positive impact on ACL injury reduction. This protocol, approximately 15 minutes in duration twice weekly, progressed through levels of difficulty and included single and 2-legged squats, pelvic lifts, the bench, and the lunge. Female soccer players age 12 to 17 experienced fewer injuries than the control group. A total of 2479 in the intervention group and 2085 in the control group fully participated in this study. Seven players in the group that did neuromuscular exercises experienced an ACL injury. Fourteen players in the control group experienced an ACL injury. AEs were not calculated in this study. Instead, this study calculated playing time through minutes of actual soccer sport participation including practices and matches.[63]

The effectiveness of these programs in ACL injury prevention is summarized in **Table 1**.

A meta-analysis by Sadoghi and colleagues[64] looked at the effectiveness of ACL prevention programs. These authors systematically reviewed the available literature and noted a pooled risk ratio of 0.38 (95% confidence interval, 0.20–0.72) representing a significant reduction in ACL injury secondary to prevention program adherence. The combined data from the studies in the meta-analysis show that athletes involved in prevention programs reduce ACL injuries by 62% compared with controls. The benefits of injury prevention programs apply to both male and female athletes. Risk reduction of an ACL injury through compliance with an ACL injury prevention program is 85% in male athletes and 52% in female athletes. An earlier meta-analysis of neuromuscular training by Hübscher and colleagues[65] noted that intervention, which could incorporate strengthening, stretching, and plyometrics, decreased risk of acute knee injuries by 54%. Compliance with the programs also affects outcomes. In one study, girls age 12 to 17 in football (soccer) with the highest compliance with a neuromuscular training program had an 88% decreased ACL injury rate compared with the players with lower compliance with the program.[66] It remains unclear which athlete groups will most benefit from an ACL injury prevention program.[3,67]

Table 1
ACL injury program effectiveness

Study	Description	No of Participants	Controls	ACL Injury in Treatment Group	ACL Injury in Control Group	Statistically Significant
Pfeiffer et al,[62] 2006	HS female athletes twice weekly for 20 min program	577	862	0.167 noncontact ACL injury per 1000 exposures. Player exposure defined as 1 player participating in 1 game or practice	0.078 noncontact ACL injury/athlete/1000 exposures	No
Mandelbaum et al,[57] 2005, year 1	Female soccer players age 14–18 Year 1 PEP program 3 times/wk	1041	1905	0.05 per 1000 exposures Exposure defined as participation in any practice or game in which athlete exposed to possibility of injury	0.47 injury/athlete/1000 exposures	Yes
Mandelbaum et al,[57] 2005, year 2	PEP program year 2	844	1913	0.13 injuries/athlete/1000 exposures	0.51 injuries/athlete/1000 exposures	Yes
Hewett et al,[58] 1999	High school soccer, volleyball, basketball, 6-wk preseason training	366 girls	463 girls 434 boys	0 noncontact ACL injuries in trained athlete/1000 exposures Exposure defined as 1 athlete participating in 1 practice or match	0.35 noncontact ACL injury in untrained girls; 0.05 noncontact ACL injuries in male controls	Yes
Waldén et al,[63] 2012	Exercises twice a week, progressive difficulty throughout season; female age 12–17; Swedish football	2479	2085	7 ACL injuries 149 214 h	14 ACL injuries 129 084 h	Primary outcome rate of ACL injury Yes

Given that youth athletic participation rates continue to increase in the United States, the optimal age at which to introduce neuromuscular training has been debated. Concerns regarding exposing athletes to the risk of overuse injuries are valid. Interestingly, poor physical conditioning is one of the principal risk factors for sports injury. Myer and coworkers[68] suggest that neuromuscular education be introduced before the growth spurt that occurs at age 12 in girls and at age 14 in boys. Quatman-Yates and colleagues[69] noted in a study the potentially adverse strength imbalances which emerge as girls mature from prepubertal status. Carter and Micheli[70] that training generally improves the overall health of the young athlete by increasing bone mass, improving cardiovascular fitness, assisting in injury prevention, and most likely enhancing self-esteem.[70]

Specific effects of neuromuscular training include positive effects on landing kinematics. Training improves the biomechanics of landing and may help reduce relative muscular strength imbalances that increase the ACL injury risk.[68,71] These benefits may accrue even to very young sports participants. Soccer players younger than 12 years (37 boys, 28 girls) were enrolled in a study that compared a conventional ACL prevention program (static flexibility with lower limb stretching, balance, strengthening, plyometrics, and speed drills) with a program designed specifically for a pediatric population. The pediatric ACL injury prevention program progressed through 3 phases over 9 weeks. One significant difference of the pediatric program was the inclusion of timing runs, which forced 2 participants to complete at the same time diagonal runs crossing another player. The goal of this exercise is to improve the processing of visual information on the playing field. Another difference in the pediatric program was an exercise that involved sustaining single-leg balance while a partner pushed the balancing athlete. The pediatric program also progressively increased the proportion of plyometric exercises completed as the training through the phases progressed. A total of 22 athletes (11 girls, 11 boys) completed the traditional program for 9 weeks. A total of 19 athletes (8 girls, 11 boys) completed the pediatric program of skills program. No injuries were reported in either group; the traditional ACL prevention program improved young athletes' vertical jump height and balance.[72] Despite the potential benefits of an ACL injury prevention program, integration of these programs in youth sports has not been universal. In a recent study of Utah girls soccer coaches, of athletes age 11 to collegiate, only 19.8% of survey respondents had adopted an ACL injury prevention program.[73]

SUMMARY

ACL injury is a common sports injury with severe negative consequences. Neuromuscular factors that increase risk, such as knee landing kinematics and fatigue-induced joint kinematic changes, may be ameliorated through training. Effective ACL injury prevention programs exist, although the ideal program is yet to be determined. It is imperative that athletes in high-risk sports participate in ACL injury prevention programs to reduce the risk of sustaining this injury. Effective ACL injury prevention programs would have positive effects on knee health and long-term knee quality of life for athletes.

REFERENCES

1. Quatman CE, Quatman CC, Hewett TE. Prediction and prevention of musculoskeletal injury: a paradigm shift in methodology. Br J Sports Med 2009;43:1100-7.
2. Sutton KM, Bullock JM. Anterior cruciate ligament rupture: differences between females and males. J Am Acad Orthop Surg 2013;21(1):41-50.

3. Prodromos CC, Han Y, Rogowski J, et al. A meta-analysis of the incidence of anterior cruciate ligament tears as a function of gender, sport, and a knee injury-reduction regimen. Arthroscopy 2007;23(12):1320–5.
4. Swenson DM, Collins CL, Best TM, et al. Epidemiology of knee injuries among U.S. High School Athletes, 2005/2006-2010/2011. Med Sci Sports Exerc 2013; 45(3):462–9.
5. Joseph AM, Collins CL, Henke NM, et al. A multisport epidemiologic comparison of anterior cruciate ligament injuries in high school athletics. J Athl Train 2013;48(6):810–7.
6. Hootman JM, Dick R, Agel J. Epidemiology of collegiate injuries for 15 sports: summary and recommendations for injury prevention initiatives. J Athl Train 2007;42(2):311–9.
7. Mather RC, Koenig L, Kocher MS, et al. Societal and economic impact of anterior cruciate ligament tears. J Bone Joint Surg Am 2013;95:1751–9.
8. Funded Injury Control Research Centers. Available at: http://www.cdc.gov/injury/erpo/icrc/2009/1-R49-CE001495-01.html. Accessed February 12, 2014.
9. Olson DE, Sikka RS, Hamilton A, et al. Football injuries: current concepts. Curr Sports Med Rep 2011;10(5):290–8.
10. Renstrom P, Ljungqvist A, Arendt E, et al. Non-contact ACL injuries in female athletes: an International Olympic Committee current concepts statement. Br J Sports Med 2008;42:394–412.
11. Bout-Tabaku S, Best TM. The adolescent knee and risk for osteoarthritis - an opportunity or responsibility for sports medicine physicians? Curr Sports Med Rep 2010;9(6):329–31.
12. Gelber AC, Hochberg MC, Mead LA, et al. Joint injury in young adults and risk for subsequent knee and hip osteoarthritis. Ann Intern Med 2000;133(5): 321–8.
13. Lohmander LS, Östenberg A, Englund M, et al. High prevalence of knee osteoarthritis, pain, and functional limitations in female soccer players twelve years after anterior cruciate ligament injury. Arthritis Rheum 2004;50(10):3145–52.
14. Von Porat A, Roos EM, Roos H. High prevalence of osteoarthritis 14 years after an anterior cruciate ligament tear in male soccer players: a study of radiographic and patient relevant outcomes. Ann Rheum Dis 2004;63:269–73.
15. Mainwaring LM, Hutchinson M, Bisschop SM, et al. Emotional response to sport concussion compared to ACL injury. Brain Inj 2010;24(4):589–97.
16. te Wierike SC, van der Sluis A, van den Akker-Scheek I, et al. Psychosocial factors influencing the recovery of athletes with anterior cruciate ligament injury: a systematic review. Scand J Med Sci Sports 2013;23:527–40.
17. Frankel VH, Nordin M, Walker PS. Biomechanics of the knee [Chapter 7]. In: Nordin M, Frankel VH, editors; Leger D, developmental editor. Basic biomechanics of the musculoskeletal system. 4th edition. Philadelphia: Wolters Kluwer/Lippincott Williams & Wilkins Health; 2012. p. 180–205.
18. Brophy RH, Silvers HJ, Mandelbaum BR. Anterior cruciate ligament injuries: etiology and prevention. Sports Med Arthrosc 2010;18(1):2–11.
19. Flandry F, Hommel G. Normal anatomy and biomechanics of the knee. Sports Med Arthrosc 2011;19(2):82–92.
20. Giuliani JR, Kilcoyne KG, Rue JH. Anterior cruciate ligament anatomy. A review of the anteriomedial and posterolateral bundles. J Knee Surg 2009;22:148–54.
21. Siegel L, Vandenakker-Albanese C, Siegel D. Anterior cruciate ligament injuries: anatomy, physiology, biomechanics, and management. Clin J Sport Med 2012; 22(4):349–55.

22. Besier TF, Lloyd DG, Cochrane JL, et al. External loading of the knee joint during running and cutting maneuvers. Med Sci Sports Exerc 2001;33:1168–75.

23. Griffin LY, Albohm MJ, Arendt EA, et al. Understanding and preventing noncontact anterior cruciate ligament injuries. A review of the Hunt Valley II meeting. Am J Sports Med 2006;34(9):1512–32.

24. Shah VM, Andrews JR, Fleisig GS, et al. Return to play after anterior cruciate ligament reconstruction in National Football League athletes. Am J Sports Med 2010;38(11):2233–9.

25. Brophy RH, Barnes R, Rodeo SA, et al. Prevalence of musculoskeletal disorders at the NFL combine-trends from 1987 to 2000. Med Sci Sports Exerc 2007;39(1): 22–7.

26. Lambson RB, Barnhill BS, Higgins RW. Football cleat design and its effect on anterior cruciate ligament injuries. A three-year prospective study. Am J Sports Med 1996;24(2):155–9.

27. Olsen OE, Myklebust G, Engebretsen L, et al. Relationship between floor type and risk of ACL injury in team handball. Scand J Med Sci Sports 2003;13(5): 299–304.

28. Myers MC. Incidence, mechanisms, and severity of game-related college football injuries on FieldTurf versus natural grass. A 3-year prospective study. Am J Sports Med 2010;38(4):687–97.

29. Flynn RK, Pedersen CL, Birmingham TB, et al. The familial predisposition toward tearing the anterior cruciate ligament. A case controlled study. Am J Sports Med 2005;33(1):23–8.

30. Posthumus M, Collins M, van der Merwe L, et al. Matrix metalloproteinase genes on chromosome 11q22 and the risk of anterior cruciate ligament (ACL) rupture. Scand J Med Sci Sports 2012;22:523–33.

31. Ireland ML, Ballantyne BT, Little K, et al. A radiographic analysis of the relationship between the size and shape of the intercondylar notch and anterior cruciate ligament injury. Knee Surg Sports Traumatol Arthrosc 2001;9:200–5.

32. Sonnery-Cottet B, Archbold P, Cucurulo T, et al. The influence of the tibial slope and the size of the intercondylar notch on rupture of the anterior cruciate ligament. J Bone Joint Surg Br 2011;93:1475–8.

33. Shelburne KB, Kim HJ, Sterett WI, et al. Effect of posterior tibial slope on knee biomechanics during functional activity. J Orthop Res 2011;29:223–31.

34. Dejour H, Bonnin M. Tibial translation after anterior cruciate ligament rupture. J Bone Joint Surg Br 1994;76:745–9.

35. Bell DR, Blackburn JT, Ondrak KS, et al. The effects of oral contraceptive use on muscle stiffness across the menstrual cycle. Clin J Sport Med 2011;21(6):467–73.

36. Wild CY, Steele JR, Munro BJ. Musculoskeletal and estrogen changes during the adolescent growth spurt in girls. Med Sci Sports Exerc 2013;45(1):138–45.

37. Tanner JM, Whitehouse RH, Marubini E, et al. The adolescent growth spurt of boys and girls of the Harpenden growth study. Ann Hum Biol 1976;3(2):109–26.

38. Shultz SJ, Schmitz RJ, Benjaminse A, et al. ACL research retreat VI: an update on ACL injury risk and prevention. J Athl Train 2012;47(5):591–603.

39. Chandrashekar N, Mansouri H, Slauterbeck J, et al. Sex-based differences in the tensile properties of the human anterior cruciate ligament. J Biomech 2006;39:2943–50.

40. Chandrashekar N, Slauterbeck J, Hashemi J. Sex-based differences in the anthropometric characteristics of the anterior cruciate ligament and its relation to intercondylar notch geometry: a cadaveric study. Am J Sports Med 2005; 33(10):1492–8.

41. Fayad LM, Rosenthal EH, Morrison MB, et al. Anterior cruciate ligament volume: analysis of gender differences. J Magn Reson Imaging 2008;27:218–23.
42. Anderson AF, Dome DC, Gautam S, et al. Correlation of anthropometric measurements, strength, anterior cruciate ligament size, and intercondylar notch characteristics to sex differences in anterior cruciate ligament tear rates. Am J Sports Med 2001;29(1):58–66.
43. Myer GD, Ford KR, Paterno MV, et al. The effects of generalized joint laxity on risk of anterior cruciate ligament injury in young female athletes. Am J Sports Med 2008;36(6):1073–80.
44. Yu B, McClure SB, Onate JA, et al. Age and gender effects on lower extremity kinematics of youth soccer players in a stop-jump task. Am J Sports Med 2005; 33(9):1356–64.
45. Pappas E, Hagins M, Sheikhzadeh A, et al. Biomechanical differences between unilateral and bilateral landings from a jump: Gender differences. Clin J Sport Med 2007;17(4):263–8.
46. Kobayashi H, Kanamura T, Koshida S, et al. Mechanisms of the anterior cruciate ligament injury in sports activitites: a twenty-year clinical researchof 1,700 athletes. J Sports Sci Med 2010;9(4):669–75.
47. Hewett TE, Myer GD. The mechanistic connection between the trunk, hip, knee, and anterior cruciate ligament injury. Exerc Sport Sci Rev 2011;39(4):161–6.
48. Zazulak BT, Hewett TE, Reeves NP, et al. The effects of core proprioception on knee injury: a prospective biomechanical-epidemiological study. Am J Sports Med 2007;35(3):368–73.
49. Zazulak BT, Hewett TE, Reeves NP, et al. Deficits in neuromuscular control of the trunk predict knee injury risk-A prospective biomechanical-epidemiologic study. Am J Sports Med 2007;35(7):1123–30.
50. Faber SC, Eckstein F, Lucasz S, et al. Gender differences in knee joint cartilage thickness, volume and articular surface areas: assessment with quantitative three-dimensional MR imaging. Skeletal Radiol 2001;30(3):144–50.
51. Tillman MD, Bauer JA, Cauraugh JH, et al. Difference in lower extremity alignment between male and females. Potential predisposing factors for knee injury. J Sports Med Phys Fitness 2005;45(3):355–9.
52. Shultz SJ, Schmitz RJ, Nguyen AD, et al. Knee joint laxity and its cyclic variation influence tibiofemoral motion during weight acceptance. Med Sci Sports Exerc 2011;43(2):287–95.
53. McLean SG, Samorezov JE. Fatigue-induced ACL injury risk stems from a degradation in central control. Med Sci Sports Exerc 2009;41(8):1661–72.
54. Shultz SJ, Schmitz RJ, Cone JR, et al. Multiplanar knee laxity increases during a 90-min intermittent exercise protocol. Med Sci Sports Exerc 2013;45(8):1553–61.
55. Wright RW, Dunn WR, Amendola A, et al. Risk of tearing the intact anterior cruciate ligament in the contralateral knee and rupturing the anterior cruciate ligament graft during the first 2 years after anterior cruciate ligament graft reconstruction. A prospective MOON cohort study. Am J Sports Med 2007; 35(7):1131–4.
56. The Santa Monica Sports Medicine Research Foundation. The PEP program: prevent injury and enhance performance. Available at: http://smsmf.org/files/PEP_Program_04122011.pdf. Accessed February 12, 2014.
57. Mandelbaum BR, Silvers HJ, Watanabe DS, et al. Effectiveness of a neuromuscular and proprioceptive training program in preventing anterior cruciate ligament injuries in female athletes: 2-year follow-up. Am J Sports Med 2005; 33(7):1003–10.

58. Hewett TE, Lindenfeld TN, Riccobene JV, et al. The effect of neuromuscular training on the incidence of injury in female athletes: a prospective study. Am J Sports Med 1999;27(6):699–706.

59. Brent JL, Klugman MF, Myer GD, et al. The effects of pre-season and in-season neuromuscular training on the tuck jump assessment: a test used to identify risk of ACL injury in female athletes. J Strength Cond Res 2011;25(Suppl 1):S120–1.

60. Warm-up for injury prevention and performance (WIPP). Available at: http://sportsmetrics.org/training-options/wipp/. Accessed February 12, 2014.

61. Grandstrand SL, Pfeiffer RP, Sabick MB, et al. The effects of a commercially available warm-up program on landing mechanics in female youth soccer players. J Strength Cond Res 2006;20(2):331–5.

62. Pfeiffer RP, Shea KG, Roberts D, et al. Lack of effect of a knee ligament injury prevention program on the incidence of noncontact anterior cruciate ligament injury. J Bone Joint Surg Am 2006;88(8):1769–74.

63. Waldén M, Atroshi I, Magnusson H, et al. Prevention of acute knee injuries in adolescent female soccer players: cluster randomized controlled trial. BMJ 2012;344:e3042.

64. Sadoghi P, von Keudell A, Vavken P. Effectiveness of anterior cruciate ligament injury prevention training programs. J Bone Joint Surg Am 2012;94:769–76.

65. Hübscher M, Zech A, Pfeifer K, et al. Neuromuscular training for sports injury prevention: a systematic review. Med Sci Sports Exerc 2010;42(3):413–21.

66. Hägglund M, Atroshi I, Wagner P, et al. Superior compliance with a neuromuscular training programme is associated with fewer ACL injuries and fewer acute knee injuries in female adolescent football players: secondary analysis of an RCT. Br J Sports Med 2013;47:974–9.

67. Alentorn-Geli E, Mendiguchía J, Samuelsson K, et al. Prevention of non-contact anterior cruciate ligament injuries in sports. Part II: systematic review of the effectiveness of prevention programmes in male athletes. Knee Surg Sports Traumatol Arthrosc 2014;22:16–25.

68. Myer GD, Faigenbaum AD, Ford KR, et al. When to initiate integrative neuromuscular training to reduce sports-related injuries and enhance health in youth? Curr Sports Med Rep 2011;10(3):157–66.

69. Quatman-Yates CC, Myer GD, Ford KR, et al. A longitudinal evaluation of maturational effects on lower extremity strength in female adolescent athletes. Pediatr Phys Ther 2013;25:271–6.

70. Carter CW, Micheli LJ. Training the child athlete for prevention, health promotion, and performance: how much is enough, how much is too much? Clin Sports Med 2011;30:679–90.

71. Beunen G, Malina RM. Growth and physical performance relative to the timing of the adolescent spurt. Exerc Sport Sci Rev 1988;16:503–40.

72. DiStefano LJ, Padua DA, Blackburn JT, et al. Integrated injury prevention program improves balance and vertical jump height in children. J Strength Cond Res 2010;24(2):332–42.

73. Joy EA, Taylor JR, Novak MA, et al. Factors influencing the implementation of anterior cruciate ligament injury prevention strategies by girls soccer coaches. J Strength Cond Res 2013;27(8):2263–9.

Foot and Ankle Problems in Dancers

Nancy Kadel, MD

KEYWORDS

- Dancer • Ankle sprains • Midfoot injuries • Heel pain • Hallux valgus
- Impingement syndromes

KEY POINTS

- The dancer's foot and ankle are subjected to high forces and unusual stresses in training and performance.
- To keep dancers healthy, the health care team and the dancer must work together.
- The physician must be an advocate for the dancer and work to provide an accurate diagnosis and an effective treatment strategy.
- Monitoring performance and rehearsal load, fitness, and general health of the dancer will help to maximize the dancer's healing potential.
- Creativity is needed to modify treatment plans to accommodate the dancer's need to maintain strength, flexibility, and fitness during recovery.

INTRODUCTION

Dance is a demanding art form requiring years of training, musicality, and motor control, often at the extremes of joint range of motion. Elite dancers are athletes whose rigorous training, rehearsal and performance schedules predispose them to injury. The stresses of dance can result in common overuse injuries as well as some injuries unique to dancers. Dance has many forms, including classical ballet, modern, contemporary, jazz, tap, break dance, hip-hop, musical theater, ballroom, Irish, African, Flamenco, folk, aerial and contact improvisation.

Reports on professional dancers show high rates of injury in ballet, modern, and Irish dancers.[1–7] In a Swedish study, 95% of the professional dancers sustained at least 1 injury during a 1-year study period.[8] The foot and ankle are the most frequently injured areas in dancers, with significantly higher rates reported in female ballet dancers.[5] The sur les pointes position requires maximal ankle, hindfoot, and midfoot plantar flexion, while placing high forces across those joints (**Fig. 1**). Dance injuries may be the result of acute trauma, such as landing from a leap or turn, or more commonly from repetitive microtrauma, usually after a rapid increase in training volume and intensity. Menstrual

Group Health Physicians, 125 16th Avenue East, Seattle, WA 98112, USA
E-mail address: nancykadelmd@gmail.com

Phys Med Rehabil Clin N Am 25 (2014) 829–844
http://dx.doi.org/10.1016/j.pmr.2014.06.003
1047-9651/14/$ – see front matter © 2014 Elsevier Inc. All rights reserved.

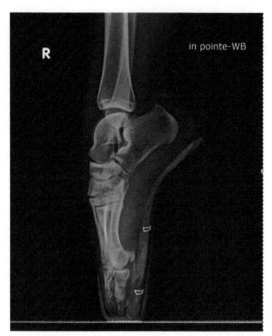

Fig. 1. Radiograph of a female ballet dancer's foot in the sur les pointes position.

irregularities, disordered eating, low energy availability, low vitamin D, and osteopenia may contribute to dancers' risk for injury or delayed healing.[9,10]

This article will review some common problems involving the foot and ankle in dancers, precipitating factors, clinical presentation, diagnostic tips, and treatment recommendations.

ANKLE SPRAINS

Ankle inversion injury is the most common traumatic injury in dance as it is in athletics.[1,3–5] Many authors report ankle sprains as the most frequent acute injury. The mechanism of injury is typically an inversion injury (rolling over the lateral border of the foot), often while en pointe or demi-pointe, or in a missed landing from a jump. The lateral ligaments are most frequently injured, with the anterior talofibular ligament (ATFL) the most commonly injured ligament. The ATFL is injured when the ankle is plantar flexed; the calcaneofibular ligament (CFL) is injured when the ankle (foot) is in dorsiflexion (neutral) and inverted.

A history of previous ankle sprain is the greatest risk factor for an ankle sprain injury.[11–13] Dancers and athletes who have had an ankle sprain have impaired dynamic postural control (more postural sway than controls or uninjured dancers). Even after return to full professional dance or sport participation, and without complaints of instability, measurable differences in postural sway can be demonstrated.[12–15]

Diagnosis includes physical examination revealing tenderness to palpation over the anterolateral ankle ligaments, swelling, and ecchymosis. Radiographs should be obtained if there is any bony tenderness over fibula, sinus tarsi, or fifth metatarsal. If symptoms do not improve in a week, a computed tomography (CT) scan or magnetic resonance imaging (MRI) scan should be obtained to identify possible osteochondral injury to the talus or occult fracture.

Most sprains resolve with conservative management. Early functional treatment of ankle sprains is recommended for dancers. Compression bandage, icing, ankle air-stirrup brace in athletic shoes outside of class, and limited class participation should be instituted as pain allows. Severe sprains may require use of a removable boot for 3 weeks. The boot should be worn for walking and sleeping, but removed for icing and range-of-motion exercises. Dancers with high-level sprains may need to do floor barre classes, Pilates or Gyrotonics before return to class and performance.

Note that dancers with generalized hypermobility may have a prolonged recovery compared with non-hypermobile dancers.[16]

Rehabilitation should include strengthening, edema control, and range of motion and proprioception exercises. Ballet dancers require full mobility of their hindfoot and midfoot joints to dance en pointe. An ankle sprain can lead to posterior ankle impingement if adequate care to achieve posterior talar glide and ankle dorsiflexion is not obtained, as the insufficient ATFL ligament allows the talus to move forward in the plantar flexed position, resulting in impingement of bone and/or soft tissues in the posterior ankle joint. It is important in dancers to encourage work on attaining full dorsiflexion at the tibiotalar joint following an ankle sprain; therapists should be encouraged to assist the dancer in posterior talar glide with manual therapy. Many dancers have a very flexible ankle with a moderately or highly arched (cavus) foot. They may have subtle hindfoot varus and are more prone to reinjury. One study found that fatigue-induced changes of dynamic postural control were more pronounced in those athletes with a history of ankle sprain, while changes in static sway velocity were similar for both groups.[13] Therefore, despite successful return to full dance after an ankle sprain, some sensorimotor control deficits remain, which can put the dancer at risk for reinjury of the ankle. Work on the entire kinetic chain is crucial for full recovery. Core strengthening, proprioception, and proximal hip strengthening exercises should be included in any dancer's rehabilitation from ankle sprain in addition to fibularis longus and brevis muscle strengthening. Work on unstable surfaces and balance tasks with eyes closed will help in assisting return of proprioception and full function. Practicing relevés in parallel position with a tennis ball held between the malleoli can help the injured dancer retrain ankle strength and motion in a neutral ankle position.

ACHILLES

Chronic Achilles tendinopathy, retrocalcaneal bursitis, and acute tendinitis may be seen in male and female dancers. Comin and colleagues[17] evaluated Achilles and patellar tendons in 79 professional ballet dancers and found a 12% prevalence of sonographic abnormalities in the Achilles and patellar tendons of asymptomatic dancers. Dancers who force their turnout, leading to increased pronation in the midfoot and hindfoot, are at risk for Achilles tendon problems. Failure of the dancer to land with his or her heels on the ground from jumps also can contribute to shortening of the Achilles tendon and risk for injury. In young dancers during periods of rapid growth, there is relative tightness and weakness of the gastrocnemius–soleus complex, placing them at risk for Achilles tendinitis. In a prospective study, Mahieu and colleagues[18] identified plantar flexion weakness and increased dorsiflexion excursion as significant predictors for Achilles tendon overuse injury. In the Comin study, only those dancers with hypoechoic changes seen on ultrasound later developed symptomatic Achilles tendinitis, suggesting that ultrasound in asymptomatic dancers may help identify those at risk.[17]

Tight ribbons around the ankle in ballet dancers may cause irritation. Ballet dancers may need adjustment of tight ribbons around the ankle, or the use of ribbons with elastic sewn in the area over the tendon to reduce pain.[19,20] Careful stretching and the use of a night splint while sleeping can alleviate most symptoms. Eccentric strengthening exercises, physical therapy with modalities such as Graston technique, or deep tissue massage may be beneficial. The use of a stretch box in the studio and back stage at the theater has been found to be a good preventative measure for some companies.

Achilles Tendon Rupture

Rupture of the Achilles tendon is unusual in female dancers, more commonly seen in male dancers over age 30. It typically presents as a sharp pain and inability to rise up on the toes to demi-pointe. Landing in hyperdorsiflexion or eccentric loading of the foot during push-off can result in an acute Achilles tendon rupture. Thompson test will be positive, and when examining the patient in the prone position with the knees flexed, the relaxed resting posture of the injured leg will demonstrate the foot in more dorsiflexion than the uninjured side. A palpable defect is usually present, but acute swelling may mask this finding.

Acute ruptures in dancers generally are treated with surgical repair, and any suspected rupture should be referred to an orthopedic surgeon.[19]

SEVER DISEASE

Sever disease (calcaneal apophysitis) is a common cause of posterior and or plantar heel pain in young dancers with open growth plates. There is a high incidence in Irish dancers, but it can also be seen in any child or adolescent dancer who complains of heel pain.[5] The dancer may complain of morning pain or pain with jumping, heel strike, and percussive movements. Radiographs usually are negative but may show relative widening of growth plate. On physical examination, the dancer will be tender over the apophyseal ossification center and calcaneal growth plate.

Treatment includes avoidance of painful activities, usually 3 weeks in removable boot cast, night splint for sleeping, and gentle Achilles stretches. The young dancer may need to continue the night splint for an additional month as symptoms subside. Return to dance includes relative rest such as avoidance of jumps and other painful activities until symptoms are resolved.

PLANTAR FASCIAL STRAIN

The plantar aponeurosis is a strong band of fascia extending from the base of the heel to the base of the toes. The plantar fascia may be strained, partially torn, or simply inflamed (plantar fasciitis). Occasionally there is an acute injury, most often insidious in onset after increased training intensity. Walls and colleagues[21] reported on MRI findings of the right ankles in 18 professional Irish dancers; insertional Achilles tendonopathy was observed in 14 dancers, and plantar fasciitis was seen in 7 dancers.

Dancers will usually have pain with their first few steps in the morning, may have tenderness over the plantar fascia, and rarely will have ecchymosis or swelling. Diagnosis is based on physical examination with tenderness over the palpation along the plantar fascia worse with dorsiflexion of the toes and decreased with plantar flexion of the toes. Calcaneal wall tenderness if present should alert the clinician to a possible calcaneal stress fracture (or Sever disease in a skeletally immature dancer) and need for further imaging.

Treatment should include relative rest, including avoiding painful activities, icing, calf stretches and plantar arch stretches, stiff soled shoes when not dancing (such as clogs or hiking boots), and use of a dorsiflexion night splint for sleeping.[22] In severe cases, a removable boot for walking for 3 to 6 weeks may be required. Many dancers get relief from taping the arch for dance until symptoms improve (**Fig. 2**).

ANKLE IMPINGEMENT SYNDROMES
Posterior Ankle Impingement

Posterior ankle impingement is a painful condition due to compression of the soft tissues between the posterior edge of the tibia and the calcaneus when the ankle is in plantar

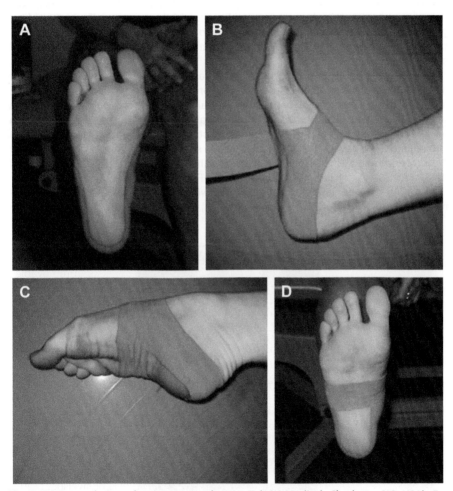

Fig. 2. Taping technique for dancers. Leukotape P (BSN Medical, Charlotte, NC, USA), Endura Sports tape (Patterson Medical, Warrenville, IL, USA), or similar nonflexible tape work best. Two pieces of tape are used. (*A*) The first is a u-shaped strap low on the foot from the base of fifth metatarsal to the base of the proximal 1st metatarsal. (*B*) The second longer piece starts in the middle of the plantar arch, then crosses over the dorsal midfoot angling toward and below the malleoli; this piece should touch the first strap on both sides. (*C*) This taping technique supports the arch and subtalar joint, while not limiting ankle motion. (*D*) Taping viewed from plantar surface of foot.

flexion. Bony impingement may be associated with an accessory bone of the ankle, called an os trigonum, or a prominent posterior lateral process of the talus called Steida process (**Fig. 3**).[23–34] Some authors have reported concurrent flexor hallucis longus (FHL) tenosynovitis secondary to an impinging os trigonum in dancers.[26] A fracture of the posterolateral process of the talus can also cause posterior ankle pain.

Dancers with posterior ankle impingement usually complain of recurrent pain posterior and lateral, behind the fibularis tendons and stiffness and limitation in plantar flexion. Pain is exacerbated by plantar flexing the foot and relevé. This condition may be mistaken for fibularis or Achilles tendonitis, and may follow an ankle sprain. Those with FHL tendonitis and os trigonum have posteromedial ankle tenderness and pain with flexion of the great toe against resistance. Crepitus may be palpated behind the medial malleolus with range of motion of the great toe. Triggering of the great toe may be present. Functional hallux rigidus may be present, as demonstrated by a limitation of great toe dorsiflexion with the knee fully extended and the ankle in full dorsiflexion.

The dancer complains of decreased active and passive plantar flexion, and may have difficulty achieving the full pointe position on the affected side. Swelling and tenderness may be present behind the lateral ankle joint anterior to the Achilles tendon. It is often exacerbated by forcing plantar flexion on the affected side to achieve as much range of motion as the unaffected side. Dancers with posterior ankle impingement will have a positive plantar flexion sign: pain with forced passive plantar flexion performed by the practitioner with the dancer's knee flexed at 90°. This test will not be positive in Achilles, fibularis, or isolated FHL tendinitis.[24,29,34]

Radiographs in maximal plantar flexion, or with the dancer en pointe, can demonstrate a bony block or os trigonum (**Fig. 4A**). MRI is helpful to identify posterior

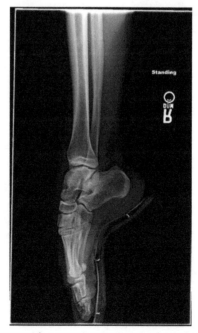

Fig. 3. Radiograph of dancer with a prominent posterior lateral process of the talus (Steida process).

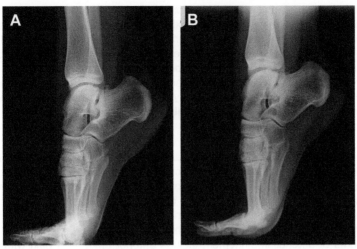

Fig. 4. (*A*) Radiograph of dancer with a symptomatic os trigonum on demi-pointe in maximal plantar flexion. Note this dancer has some limitation in plantar flexion. (*B*) Radiograph of same dancer after surgical excision of os trigonum. Note improved ankle plantar flexion on demi-pointe as demonstrated by better alignment of metatarsal and tibial shaft.

bone edema in the talus and calcaneus, and to identify fluid in the FHL tendon sheath.[31] An injection of lidocaine posterior to the fibularis tendons with pain relief can be diagnostic.[19,23,24]

Treatment consists initially of limitation of painful activities, including pointe work, and physical therapy to work on strengthening and mobilization of the ankle joint. The dancer should sleep with a night splint to help reduce stiffness and synovitis. Working on exercises to point the foot with a relaxed calf and intrinsic foot strength can reduce symptoms.[32] Surgery to remove the os trigonum and/or release of the FHL tendon sheath is reserved for those dancers who fail physical therapy and correction of technical errors (see **Fig. 4**B). Some dancers find benefit from changing their pointe shoe style and fit. A shoe with a half or three-quarter shank allows the dancer to achieve full pointe position with less compaction of the posterior structures.

FHL Tendinitis

Often called dancer's tendinitis, FHL tendinitis is common in dancers. It has been described in other athletes, but it is seen most frequently in the female ballet dancer.[19,23,24,26,35,36] A biomechanical study demonstrated that the muscles crossing the metatarsophalangeal joints work 2.5 to 3 times harder than those crossing just the ankle joint in dancers rising on to the full pointe position, placing these muscles and tendons (FHL, flexor digitorum longus [FDL]) at risk for overuse injuries.[37] The repetitive change in foot position from full plantar flexion of the en pointe position to plié with the ankle in dorsiflexion causes the FHL tendon to become inflamed, as it is compressed in its fibro-osseous tunnel along the posteromedial talus under the sustentaculum tali.

Dancers may complain of posteromedial ankle pain, swelling, or popping. Some dancers develop triggering or locking of the great toe; a nodule may form on the tendon. Crepitus can be palpated at the posteromedial ankle, and pain with resisted flexion of the hallux interphalangeal (IP) joint may be present. Functional hallux rigidus may be present, as demonstrated by a limitation of great toe dorsiflexion with the knee fully extended and the ankle in full dorsiflexion Thomasen test.[36]

Conservative treatment including temporary cessation of pointe work and jumps, physical therapy, and anti-inflammatory medication usually resolves the problem. In those dancers with triggering of the hallux or a nodule on the tendon, surgical release may be required. FHL tendinitis may be associated with posterior ankle impingement and an os trigonum, and the posterior bony block can be removed through a medial approach concurrent with release of the FHL sheath in those dancers who fail nonoperative treatment.

Anterior Ankle Impingement

Anterior impingement in dancers may be a consequence of hypertrophied soft tissues or osteophytes (talar neck and/or distal tibia) in the anterior ankle joint. The osteophytes are proposed to be a consequence of repeated ankle sprains or microtrauma from repetitive impact of loaded dorsiflexion.[38–40] Anterior impingement is more common in male dancers (more large jumps) and dancers with cavus feet.

Symptoms of anterior impingement include anterior ankle joint pain with landing jumps, plié, and limited ankle dorsiflexion. Some may have pain when descending stairs. Swelling may or may not be visible. Tenderness will be present to palpation of the anterior ankle joint. Pain with passive ankle dorsiflexion may be present, but this may be falsely negative in anterior impingement.[38,39]

Radiographs of the ankle and an oblique view of the foot will demonstrate osteophytes.

Treatment includes relative activity limitation, including avoiding jumps, avoiding forcing demi- plié, and use of a small felt heel pad to lift the heel in dance shoes and street shoes. Physical therapy to correct technical errors such as improper alignment in plié, pronation, or hindfoot supination, and taping the foot to support the subtalar joint and hindfoot may help to resolve symptoms (see **Fig. 2**; **Fig. 5**). A brief trial of a walking boot cast brace for 3 weeks and a night splint may help alleviate pain and inflammation. Judicious use of a single intra-articular corticosteroid injection may be used in select cases, followed by a walking cast brace for 3 weeks. If

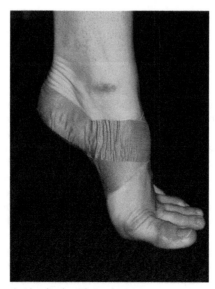

Fig. 5. Dancer in demi-pointe relevé with Leukotape.

pain persists, surgical treatment with arthroscopic or open debridement of osteo-phytes and soft tissue may be required.[41,42] Early postoperative care including Pilates and pool exercises (once incisions are healed) should be initiated early, with an increase of dance activity as pain allows. Full dance participation may take as long as 3 to 6 months.

Cuboid Subluxation

Acute cuboid subluxation may occur with ankle sprains or improper jump landings. The repetitive motions used rising up to and down from relevé position are associated with this injury when it is from overuse. The dancer will complain of lateral midfoot pain and an inability to roll through the foot correctly to achieve demi-pointe or the full pointe position. Some are unable to bear weight in acute injuries. Tenderness is usu-ally on the plantar surface of the cuboid. Mobility of the transverse tarsal joints may be diminished compared with the opposite foot. A step-off at the base of the fourth meta-tarsal may be palpable.

Diagnosis is largely clinical, as radiographs rarely identify this subtle injury. Treat-ment requires a manual reduction maneuver (cuboid whip) or passive mobilization of the rear and midfoot joints (cuboid squeeze); however, these maneuvers should not be performed repeatedly or with too much force. Taping is used to stabilize the midfoot, often with a small felt pad under the cuboid to help maintain the reduction initially. Fibularis longus tightness should be addressed, as this is associated with the condition.[43–47] Pointe work and jumps should be restricted for 1 to 2 weeks or until the dancer can comfortably roll through the foot. Dancers may require orthotics for their street shoes to control forefoot valgus if present.

METATARSAL
Fifth Metatarsal Fractures

Fractures of the fifth metatarsal can be seen in all forms of dance.

Missed landings from jumps and rolling over the outer border of the foot while on demi-pointe are 2 common mechanisms seen in dancers who sustain fifth meta-tarsal fractures. Lateral foot pain, tenderness, swelling, and ecchymosis are the usual presentation of dancers with these fractures. Physical examination will reveal tenderness over the metatarsal, but radiographs are needed for accurate diagnosis. Treatment for fracture of the fifth metatarsal is based on the location and type of fracture. Oblique spiral shaft fractures, known as a dancer's fracture, can be treated without surgery even when displaced.[48] A removable cast boot or similar immobilization is used until pain-free walking, usually 6 weeks. Pool exercises or gentle active range-of-motion exercises are begun out of the boot as soon as com-fort allows. Return to class and performance is done gradually along with a physical therapy program emphasizing proprioception and core and foot intrinsic strength training. The clinician should be careful to evaluate the ankle for instability or injury to the lateral ligaments, as both injuries may occur with this mechanism.

Avulsion fractures of the proximal fifth metatarsal are associated with an inversion injury and lateral ankle sprain. The fracture line is through the tuberosity and is usu-ally extra-articular. These fractures are treated symptomatically, with a stiff-soled shoe or removable cast boot. Surgical treatment is reserved for the unusual case of significant displacement or articular involvement. Jones fractures occur at the metaphyseal–diaphyseal junction of the fifth metatarsal. They are transverse, and because of poor blood supply in this area, they have a propensity for nonunion. These fractures are more common in modern dancers. Jones fractures can be treated in a short-leg cast for 6 to 8 weeks if the patient can avoid bearing weight, but in high-level dancers, surgical treatment and/or bone stimulator may be chosen to avoid prolonged immobilization.

Stress fractures of the proximal fifth metatarsal diaphysis are seen most commonly with repetitive adduction forces such as cutting or pivoting, again more common in modern dancers. The dancer may report a low level of chronic lateral foot pain followed by an acute event. Radiographs demonstrate cortical thickening, periosteal reaction, and a wider fracture line than the acute Jones fracture. These fractures require operative internal fixation, often with bone grafting and bone stimulator, as healing potential is poor just as in the acute Jones fracture.[19,48]

Stress Fracture

Bone remodeling is impaired when loading is increased too rapidly, weakening the bone and leaving it at risk for stress fracture. The cause of stress fractures is multifactorial; increased training intensity, hard floors, nutritional and hormonal factors, menstrual irregularities, and low energy availability have been implicated in stress fractures. Dancing more than 5 hours per day and amenorrhea greater than 90 days have been demonstrated as risk factors for stress fractures in female dancers.

Metatarsal stress fractures are the most common stress fracture reported in dancers.[49,50] Stress fractures in dancers have been reported in other bones, including the fibula, tibia, spine, and hip.

The dancer with a stress fracture often presents with a dull pain at the end of class or with specific activities such as jumps.

As symptoms progress, pain becomes more prevalent and may occur with walking and at night. Occasionally swelling is present, and at first pain is not well localized. Bony tenderness may be present. Initial radiographs may be unremarkable. Radionuclide bone scans are sensitive to stress fractures and can be positive only a few days after the injury, but MRI is recommended to make the diagnosis.

Dancers are at risk for an uncommon stress fracture at the base of the second metatarsal. Running athletes typically with have a stress fracture of the midshaft or more distal aspect of the metatarsal.[51] Due to the anatomy of the midfoot, the second metatarsal is recessed and locked in, and the second metatarsal–cuneiform joint is more proximal than the first or third metatarsal–cuneiform joints. The first and second metatarsals bear most of a dancers' weight, whether on demi-pointe, sur les pointes, or in landing from a jump, and those stresses are transmitted proximally to the midfoot.

A proximal second metatarsal stress fracture must be differentiated from synovitis of the second metatarsal–cuneiform joint. In the midfoot, synovitis of Lisfranc joints and a proximal second metatarsal stress fracture are difficult to distinguish with a bone scan.[50,52–54] Therefore, MRI has become the preferred test in a dancer with a suspected stress fracture and negative radiographs. Healing time is prolonged for the stress fracture (6–8 weeks) compared with synovitis (3 weeks); hence accurate diagnosis is important for managing these injuries.[55] Casting not usually required, but some dancers are more comfortable if a removable boot is worn for walking outside of class. Conditioning can be maintained with floor barre, Pilates, pool exercises, and exercise bicycle or elliptical trainer if there is no pain in the midfoot with those activities. Rehabilitation includes gradual return to class with avoidance of pointe work, jumps, turns, and demi-pointe until healing completed and tenderness resolved.

MIDFOOT INJURIES: LISFRANC SPRAIN/FRACTURE

Injuries to the midfoot in dancers are not common, but the physician treating dancers should have a high index of suspicion, because if this injury is not recognized or treated, it can be career ending. The ligaments of the tarso–metatarsal joints are required to support the medial and longitudinal arches of the foot. These injuries can be easily missed, as radiographic findings may be subtle, and the midfoot pain may be mistaken for possible stress fracture or synovitis. Usually these injuries have significant swelling when compared with a stress fracture or isolated synovitis. Plantar midfoot ecchymosis may be present, as is tenderness over the dorsal midfoot at the metatarsal–cuneiform joints (especially the base of first and second metatarsals).

Weight-bearing antero-posterior (AP) radiographs may show a diastasis between the first and second metatarsal bases. Lisfranc ligament is located between the medial cuneiform and the base of the second metatarsal. One may see an avulsed fragment of bone if the ligament is injured between the first and second metatarsal bases.

The mechanism of injury to Lisfranc joints in dancers has been described to include a fall off pointe position, missed jump landings, take-off for a jump when the foot sticks to the floor, and when a female dancer is pulled up onto full pointe by her partner and her foot catches a seam or irregularity in the floor.[56–58] These injuries occur in ankle plantar flexion, with or without rotation, often with the metatarsal–phalangeal joints in maximal dorsiflexion (demi-pointe).

Most Lisfranc injuries require surgical treatment, and only a simple sprain with no instability should be treated nonsurgically. Any suspected Lisfranc injury should be referred to an orthopedic surgeon for evaluation. Recovery is prolonged, and immobilization and avoidance of weight-bearing activities for 6 to 12 weeks are required, followed by a focused rehabilitation of the entire kinetic chain to return the dancer to full performance level.

HALLUX VALGUS

Although hallux valgus deformity is seen in dancers, conflicting data exist whether dancers have a higher incidence of bunions than the general population.[19,59–62] Dancers with flexible pes planus and those who force their turnout may exacerbate an existing bunion, but dancing en pointe alone does not cause bunion deformities. Young dancers who have hallux valgus often have congenital metatarsus primus varus.

Bunions in dancers should be managed conservatively. Surgery is reserved only for those dancers who have retired from performing, as any surgical correction may lead to loss of range of motion at the metatarsophalangeal (MTP) joint.[63] Use of horseshoe-type padding over the prominent medial MTP joint, toe spacers between the hallux and second toe, and intrinsic muscle strengthening exercises can help to make dancing en pointe more comfortable for those dancers with bunions. Careful fitting of the pointe shoe, with a higher vamp or wings to extend over the MTP joint to better support the hallux may reduce symptoms. Emphasis on proper alignment during training of young dancers can help to avoid exacerbation of bunion-prone feet.

HALLUX RIGIDUS

Hallux rigidus is an arthritic condition of the MTP joint. Dancers require 80° to 100° of dorsiflexion when performing relevé onto demi-pointe; therefore, loss of motion in this joint can be disabling. The stiffness in the joint causes the dancer to roll onto the lateral metatarsals in improper alignment (sickling) when rising to demi-pointe.

Dancers with this condition report stiffness and pain of the first MTP joint, and an inability to achieve full demi-pointe position. Dorsal fullness and a palpable osteophyte may be present, and limited dorsiflexion of the hallux. Radiographs reveal joint space narrowing or subchondral sclerosis, and dorsal osteophytes depending on the stage of the condition.

Early cases with stiffness, but few radiographic changes, should be treated with gentle traction and passive and active exercises that strengthen the intrinsic muscles of the foot. The dancer should avoid forcing the three-quarter pointe position, as this can exacerbate symptoms.

Surgical cheilectomy with resection of the dorsal one-third of the joint, including the osteophytes, can improve symptoms, but as this is a degenerative condition of the joint, the dancer must be warned that surgery will not restore normal function. Recovery time may be as long as 3 to 6 months, and despite a technically successful surgery, some dancers will not achieve the required range of motion of the great toe.[19,61]

Sesamoid Injuries

Sesamoid injuries are difficult problems seen in the dancer. Sesamoiditis, bursitis, osteonecrosis, osteoarthritis, and stress fractures are included in the differential diagnosis of plantar MTP joint pain.[19] Prolonged disability can result from these injuries. The sesamoids are small bones imbedded in the flexor hallucis brevis (FHB) tendons, and they articulate with the plantar aspect of the first metatarsal head. They are exposed to significant force when rolling through the foot onto demi-pointe or full pointe and in landing from a jump. Technical errors such as rolling in, pronation, or forcing turnout can cause excessive loading of the sesamoids, and these should be addressed primarily. Improper jump landings and walking with an out-toeing gait also can contribute to sesamoid disorders, as can hip and sacro–iliac joint dysfunction.[20]

The presenting symptoms are pain in the plantar forefoot under the first metatarsal head. Tenderness is present with palpation of the sesamoid; the tibial sesamoid is most involved commonly. On dorsiflexion of the hallux, the sesamoids move distally, as should the tenderness.

The bursa under the sesamoids can become swollen and inflamed, resulting in bursitis, usually palpable on physical examination. An injection of a small amount of local anesthetic will confirm the diagnosis. Bone scan and MRI may be needed to identify stress fractures or osteonecrosis. Plain radiographs or CT scans can identity osteoarthritis. Bipartite sesamoids are common, but rounded edges seen on a radiograph help to distinguish this from the sharply defined edges of an acute sesamoid fracture.

Treatment includes assessing and correcting alignment and technical problems. Sesamoid (dancer) pads can be used to off-load the area, and use of a stiff-soled shoe such as a clog or hiking boot outside of class to limit MTP joint motion may be helpful. A removable cast boot may be used if symptoms are severe. Corticosteroid injections in this area should be used only after technical errors are addressed. Sesamoid problems may take months to fully resolve, and need for surgical excision is rare.

SUMMARY

The dancer's foot and ankle is subjected to high forces and unusual stresses in training and performance. Most professional dancers employed for more than 1 year will have an injury, and the likelihood of that injury being in the foot or ankle is high.[5,8] To keep dancers healthy, the health care team and the dancer must work together. The physician must be an advocate for the dancer and work to provide an accurate diagnosis and an effective treatment strategy.

Monitoring performance and rehearsal load, fitness, and the general health of the dancer will help to maximize the dancer's healing potential. Adequate rest, fitness, recovery time, and nutrition are critical. Correction of muscle imbalances, attention to proper technique, sequential skill progression, and proper shoe fit may help limit acute injuries to the dancer.

The physician must not limit his or her examination to the foot and ankle, but the entire kinetic chain of the dancer must be assessed. Injury or pain in the foot may predispose the dancer to problems further up the kinetic chain, and these must be addressed for successful return to performance. The physician treating dancers must be sensitive to the fact that the dancer considers pain and injury a normal part of daily life. In their competitive world, dancers may fear treatments that could result in loss of rehearsal or performance time and possibly dance roles or position in the company. Creativity is needed to modify treatment plans to accommodate the dancer's need to maintain strength, flexibility, and fitness during recovery.

REFERENCES

1. Bronner S, Ojofeitimi S, Rose D. Injuries in a modern dance company: effect of comprehensive management on injury incidence and time loss. Am J Sports Med 2003;31(3):365–73.
2. Bowling A. Injuries to dancers: prevalence, treatment, and perceptions of causes. BMJ 1989;298:731–4.
3. Shah S, Weiss D, Burchette R. Injuries in professional modern dancers; incidence, risk factors, management. J Dance Med Sci 2012;16(1):17–25.
4. Noon M, Hoch A, McNamara L, et al. Injury patterns in female Irish dancers. PM R 2010;2(11):1030–4.
5. Wanke E, Arendt M, Mill H, et al. Occupational accidents in professional dance with focus on gender differences. J Occup Med Toxicol 2013;8:35.
6. Dobson R. Eight in ten dancers have an injury each year, survey shows. BMJ 2005;331(7517):594.
7. Byhring S, Bø K. Musculoskeletal injuries in the Norwegian National Ballet: a prospective cohort study. Scand J Med Sci Sports 2002;12:365–70.
8. Nilsson C, Leanderson J, Wykman J, et al. The injury panorama in a Swedish professional ballet company. Knee Surg Sports Traumatol Arthrosc 2001;9(4):242–6.
9. Lloyd T, Triantafyllou SJ, Baker ER, et al. Women athletes with menstrual irregularity have increased musculoskeletal injuries. Med Sci Sports Exerc 1986;18(4):374–9.
10. Warren MP, Brooks-Gunn J, Fox RP, et al. Persistent osteopenia in ballet dancers with amenorrhea and delayed menarche despite hormone therapy: a longitudinal study. Fertil Steril 2003;80(2):398–404.
11. Leanderson J, Eriksson E, Nilsson C, et al. Proprioception in classical ballet dancers. A study of the influence of an ankle sprain on proprioception in the ankle joint. Am J Sports Med 1996;24(3):370–4.
12. Lin C, Lee I, Liao J, et al. Comparison of postural stability between injured and uninjured ballet dancers. Am J Sports Med 2011;39(6):1324–31.
13. Steib S, Zech A, Hentschke C, et al. Fatigue-induced alterations of static and dynamic postural control in athletes with a history of ankle sprain. J Athl Train 2013;48(2):203–8.

14. Hiller CE, Refshauge KM, Beard DJ. Sensorimotor control is impaired in dancers with functional ankle instability. Am J Sports Med 2004;32(1):216–23.
15. Schmitt H, Kuni B, Sabo D. Influence of professional dance training on peak torque and proprioception at the ankle. Clin J Sport Med 2005;15(5):331–9.
16. Briggs J, McCormack M, Hakim AJ, et al. Injury and joint hypermobility syndrome in ballet dancers—a 5 year follow-up. Rheumatology (Oxford) 2009;48(12): 1613–4.
17. Comin J, Cook J, Malliaras P, et al. The prevalence and clinical significance of sonographic tendon abnormalities in asymptomatic ballet dancers: a 24 month longitudinal study. Br J Sports Med 2013;47:89–92.
18. Mahieu N, Witvrouw E, Stevens V, et al. Intrinsic risk factors for the development of Achilles tendon overuse injury: a prospective study. Am J Sports Med 2006; 34(2):226–35.
19. Hamilton WG, Hamilton LH. Foot and ankle injuries in dancers. In: Mann R, Coughlin M, editors. Surgery of the foot and ankle. 7th edition. St. Louis (MO): Mosby Incorporated; 1999. p. 1225–56.
20. Macintyre J, Joy E. Foot and ankle injuries in dance. Clin Sports Med 2000; 19(2):351–68.
21. Walls R, Brennan S, Hodnett P, et al. Overuse ankle injuries in professional Irish dancers. Foot Ankle Surg 2010;16(1):45–9.
22. Schwartz E, Su J. Plantar fasciitis: a concise review. Perm J 2014;18(1):e105–7.
23. Hamilton W. Posterior ankle pain in dancers. Clin Sports Med 2008;27:263–77.
24. Hamilton WG, Geppert MJ, Thompson FM. Pain in the posterior aspect of the ankle in dancers: differential diagnosis and operative treatment. J Bone Joint Surg Am 1996;78:1491–500.
25. Marotta J, Micheli LJ. Os trigonum impingement in dancers. Am J Sports Med 1992;20:533–6.
26. Kolettis GJ, Micheli LJ, Klein JD. Release of the flexor hallucis longus tendon in ballet dancers. J Bone Joint Surg Am 1996;78(9):1386–90.
27. Robinson P, White LM. Soft tissue and osseous impingement syndromes of the ankle: role of imaging in diagnosis and management. Radiographics 2002;22: 1457–71.
28. Kadel N. Excision of os trigonum. Oper Tech Orthop 2004;14:1–5.
29. Kadel N, Micheli L, Solomon R. Os trigonum impingement syndrome in dancers. J Dance Med Sci 2000;4:99–102.
30. Russell J, Kruse D, Koutedakis Y, et al. Pathoanatomy of posterior ankle impingement in ballet dancers. Clin Anat 2010;23:613–21.
31. Peace K, Hillier JC, Hulme A, et al. MRI features of posterior ankle impingement syndrome in ballet dancers: a review of 25 cases. Clin Radiol 2004;59(11): 1025–33.
32. Albisetti W, Ometti M, Pascale V, et al. Clinical evaluation and treatment of posterior impingement in dancers. Am J Phys Med Rehabil 2009;88(5):349–54.
33. Mouhsine E, Crevoisier X, Leyvraz PF, et al. Post-traumatic overload or acute syndrome of the os trigonum: a possible cause of posterior ankle impingement. Knee Surg Sports Traumatol Arthrosc 2004;12(3):250–3.
34. van Dijk C, Bergen C. Advancements in ankle arthroscopy. J Am Acad Orthop Surg 2008;16(11):635–46.
35. Sammarco GJ, Cooper PS. Flexor hallucis longus tendon injury in dancers and nondancers. Foot Ankle Int 1998;19:356–62.
36. Michelson J, Dunn L. Tenosynovitis of the flexor hallucis longus: a clinical study of the spectrum of presentation and treatment. Foot Ankle Int 2005;26(4):291–303.

37. Dozzi PA, Winter DA. Biomechanical analysis of the foot during rises to full pointe: implications for injuries to the metatarsal–phalangeal joints and shoe redesign. Kinesiology and Med for Dance 1993–1994;16(1):1–11. Available at: http://www.worldcat.org/title/biomechanical-analysis-of-the-foot-during-rises-to-full-pointe-implications-for-injuries-to-the-metatarsal-phalangeal-joints-and-shoe-redesign/oclc/36937111.
38. O'Kane J, Kadel N. Anterior impingement syndrome in dancers. Curr Rev Musculoskelet Med 2008;1:12–6.
39. van Dijk CN. Anterior and posterior ankle impingement. Foot Ankle Clin 2006; 11(3):663–83.
40. Kleiger B. Anterior tibiotalar impingement syndromes in dancers. Foot Ankle 1982;3(2):69–73.
41. Stretanski MF, Weber GJ. Medical and rehabilitation issues in classical ballet: literature review. Am J Phys Med Rehabil 2002;81:383–91.
42. Nihal A, Rose DJ, Trepman E. Arthroscopic treatment of anterior ankle impingement syndrome in dancers. Foot Ankle Int 2005;26(11):908–12.
43. Adams E, Madden C. Cuboid subluxation: a case study and review. Curr Sports Med Rep 2009;8(6):300–7.
44. Newell SG, Woodle A. Cuboid syndrome. Phys Sportsmed 1981;9(4):71–6.
45. Marshall P. The rehabilitation o overuse foot injuries in athletes and dancers. Clin Sports Med 1988;7(1):175–91.
46. Marshall P, Hamilton WG. Cuboid subluxation in ballet dancers. Am J Sports Med 1982;20(2):169–75.
47. Patterson SM. Cuboid syndrome: a review of the literature. J Sports Sci Med 2006;5:597–606.
48. O'Malley M, Hamilton W, Munyak J. Fractures of the distal shaft of the fifth metatarsal "dancer's fracture". Am J Sports Med 1996;24(2):240–3.
49. Kadel N, Teitz C, Kronmal R. Stress fractures in ballet dancers. Am J Sports Med 1992;20(4):445–9.
50. O'Malley MJ, Hamilton WG, Munyak J. Stress fractures at the base of the second metatarsal in ballet dancers. Foot Ankle Int 1996;17:89–94.
51. Micheli L, Sohn R, Solomon J. Stress fractures of the second metatarsal involving Lisfranc's joint in ballet dancers. J Bone Joint Surg Am 1985;67:1372–5.
52. Harrington T, Crichton K, Anderson I. Overuse ballet injury to the base of the second metatarsal a diagnostic problem. Am J Sports Med 1993;21:591–8.
53. Kadel N, Boenisch M, Teitz C, et al. Stability of Lisfranc joints in ballet pointe position. Foot Ankle Int 2005;26:394–400.
54. Nussbaum AR, Treves ST, Micheli L. Bone stress lesions in ballet dancers: scintigraphic assessment. AJR Am J Roentgenol 1988;150(4):851–5.
55. Albisetti W, Perugia D, De Bartolomeo O, et al. Stress fracture of the base of the metatarsal bones in young trainee ballet dancers. Int Orthop 2010;34:51–5.
56. DellaValle C, Su E, Nihal A, et al. Acute disruption of the tarsometatarsal (Lisfranc's) joints in a ballet dancer. J Dance Med Sci 2000;4(4):128–31.
57. Kadel N, Donaldson-Fletcher E. Lisfranc's fracture–dislocation in a male ballet dancer during take-off of a jump: a case report. J Dance Med Sci 2004;8(2):56–8.
58. Gillespie P, Robertson A, George B, et al. Acute Lisfranc joint disruption in a ballet dancer. Foot Ankle Surg 2005;11:105–8.
59. Einarsdottir H, Troell S, Wykman A. Hallux valgus in ballet dancers: a myth? Foot Ankle Int 1995;16(2):92–4.
60. van Dijk C, Lim L, Poortman A, et al. Degenerative joint disease in female ballet dancers. Am J Sports Med 1995;23(3):295–300.

61. Prisk V, O'Loughlin P, Kennedy J. Forefoot injuries in dancers. Clin Sports Med 2008;27:305–20.
62. Pique-Vidal C, Sole M, Antich J. Hallux valgus inheritance: pedigree research in 350 patients with bunion deformity. J Foot Ankle Surg 2007;46(3):149–54.
63. Jones C, Coughlin M, Grebing B, et al. First metatarsophalangeal joint motion after hallux valgus correction: a cadaver study. Foot Ankle Int 2005;26(8): 614–9.

Evaluation and Treatment of Injury and Illness in the Ultramarathon Athlete

Brian J. Krabak, MD, MBA[a,b,*], Brandee Waite, MD[c],
Grant Lipman, MD[d]

KEYWORDS

- Ultramarathon • Injury • Illness • Medical • Musculoskeletal • Hyponatremia

KEY POINTS

- In ultramarathoners, most musculoskeletal and skin-related issues are minor and can be treated successfully during the course of a race.
- Common medical illnesses, including hyperthermia and exercise-associated hyponatremia, require prompt assessment.
- Multistage ultramarathoners are more likely to experience hypernatremia than hyponatremia.
- Continued research should focus on preventative and optimal treatment strategies in hopes of preventing long-term complications in this unique athletic population.

INTRODUCTION

Ultramarathon races represent any foot race longer than 42 km; an estimated 70,000 runners participate yearly in running races throughout the world.[1,2] Most races are single-stage point-to-point continuous races occurring over a specific period (ie, 1 to 2 days). Multistaged races are point-to-point races that occur over 3 to 7 days. Ultramarathons typically occur in more extreme environments with variations in terrain

Conflicts of interest and source of funding: none.
[a] Rehabilitation, Orthopedics, and Sports Medicine, University of Washington Sports Medicine, 3800 Montlake Boulevard Northeast, Box 354060, Seattle, WA 98195, USA; [b] Seattle Children's Sports Medicine, 4800 Sand Point Way Northeast, Seattle, WA 98145, USA; [c] Physical Medicine and Rehabilitation, Sports Medicine, University of California Davis, 4860 Y Street, Suite 3850, Sacramento, CA 95817, USA; [d] Division of Emergency Medicine, Department of Surgery, Stanford University School of Medicine, 300 Pasteur Dr Alway Bldg M121 MC 5119, Stanford, CA 94305, USA
* Corresponding author. University of Washington Sports Medicine, 3800 Montlake Boulevard Northeast, Box 354060, Seattle, WA 98195.
E-mail address: bkrabak@uw.edu

Phys Med Rehabil Clin N Am 25 (2014) 845–863
http://dx.doi.org/10.1016/j.pmr.2014.06.006
1047-9651/14/$ – see front matter © 2014 Elsevier Inc. All rights reserved.

(mountains, snow, sand dunes, river crossings, slot canyons), temperature, and humidity. Ultramarathon runners require different equipment depending on the length and environment of the race. In multistage races, runners must be prepared to carry all their gear (eg, food, water, protective clothing) throughout the race.

Our knowledge of common injuries and illnesses in ultramarathon runners continues to increase. In the 1990s, studies focused on musculoskeletal injuries, noting that most running-related injuries were caused by Achilles tendinopathy (2%–18%) and patellofemoral pain (7%–15%).[2–4] In 2011, Krabak and colleagues'[5] prospective study of multistage ultramarathon runners suggested that 95% of injuries are minor and are caused by skin-related disorders (74.3%), musculoskeletal injuries (18.2%), and medical illnesses (7.5%) (**Table 1**). Other studies have focused on often asymptomatic but potentially injurious diseases, like exercise-associated hyponatremia (EAH) and acute kidney injury (AKI), reporting an EAH incidence of 8% to 50%[6,7] and AKI in more than 50% of the studied athletes.[8,9] Little is known about cardiovascular events during ultramarathon races.[10]

With the increase in ultramarathons come inherent challenges relating to the unique environments, training demands, nutritional preparation, and equipment. These challenges provide education and research opportunities for both physicians and athletes.

Table 1
Marathon and ultramarathon runners: medical encounters by diagnosis

Diagnosis	Marathon, n (%)	Multistage Ultramarathon Major, n (%)[a]	Minor, n (%)[a]
Medical illnesses			
Exercise-associated collapse[b]	863 (59.4)	35 (56.5)	43 (3.9)
Altitude sickness	—	0	11 (1.0)
Serious medical diagnosis[c]	2 (0.14)	1 (1.6)	1 (0.1)
Other medical diagnosis[d]	7 (0.48)	0	27 (2.4)
Musculoskeletal injuries			
Bursitis	—	1 (1.6)	11 (1.0)
Sprain	19 (1.3)	2 (3.2)	25 (2.3)
Strain	207 (14.3)	1 (1.6)	27 (2.4)
Tendonitis	—	7 (11.3)	115 (10.3)
Other[e]	4 (0.28)	3 (4.8)	29 (2.6)
Skin disorders			
Abrasion	27 (1.9)	0	43 (3.9)
Blister	289 (19.9)	10 (16.2)	642 (57.8)
Cellulitis	—	1 (1.6)	8 (0.7)
Hematoma (subungual)	—	1 (1.6)	106 (9.5)
Other[f]	—	00	23 (2.1)

[a] Major, unable to continue in race; minor, able to continue in race.
[b] Hyperthermia, normothermia, hypothermia.
[c] Hyponatremia, hematuria, renal stone.
[d] Blurry vision, conjunctivitis, diarrhea, dyspepsia, epistaxis, hematochezia, insect bite, neuropathy, pharyngitis, upper respiratory infections.
[e] Fracture, metatarsalgia, contusion, costochondritis, laceration, splinter.
[f] Callus, nail avulsion, rash, paronchyia, wart.
Adapted from Krabak BJ, Waite B, Schiff MA. Study of injury and illness rates in multiday ultramarathon runners. Med Sci Sports Exerc 2011;43(12):2315.

Ill-prepared athletes and physicians place the athlete at risk for injury and illness. By better understanding the ultramarathon athlete, the sports medicine physician can provide optimal care and it is hoped limit morbidity and mortality. In this article, the understanding of strategies for managing commonly encountered musculoskeletal injuries and medical illnesses in ultramarathon runners is reviewed.

MUSCULOSKELETAL INJURY

Injuries to the musculoskeletal system are common in running sports.[3,11–13] Reported musculoskeletal injury incidence varies depending on the methodology of the study. Musculoskeletal injury rates range from 2% to 18% in continuous single-stage ultramarathons[14] and 19% to 22% in multistage, multiday ultramarathons.[4,15] In multistage, multiday ultramarathons, musculoskeletal injuries accounted for 18% of the minor encounters (able to continue racing) and 22% of the major injury encounters (unable to continue racing) and are most likely to occur during stages 3 or 4 of a 7-stage race, highlighting the potential cumulative effect on the musculoskeletal system of running long distances. Although general muscle soreness affects most ultramarathoners, true musculoskeletal injuries, whether minor or major, may decrease performance and result in decreased training or medical withdrawal from a race.

Lower extremity injuries predominate, with the knee and ankle being most affected.[4,5,14,16] Evaluation and treatment of these injuries may differ in an acute setting during or immediately after a race compared with the subacute or chronic setting in a standard medical clinic setting. For the purposes of this article, the focus is the acute race or outpatient setting:

Achilles Tendinopathy/Tendonitis

Studies suggest a prevalence of 2.0% to 18.5%[2,14] and incidence of 10.8%.[17] The mechanism of injury is usually repeated or strained plantar flexion. Runners present for evaluation complaining of posterior heel or ankle pain. On physical examination, swelling or fullness may be visible in the affected Achilles region, although this is not always present. There is tenderness to palpation or squeezing of the tendon, most commonly at the midportion of the tendon, where there is a watershed vascular region of relatively low blood supply. Alternatively, the focus of tenderness may be at the insertion of the tendon at the posterior calcaneous, indicating that an enthesopathy or bursitis may be contributing to the pain. The runners may have pain with passive, manual stretch of the Achilles tendon. They usually have pain and possibly weakness with repeated single-leg toe raises and may be unable to perform full excursion for 5 to 10 repetitions. This method of testing strength is preferable to having them plantarflex against manual resistance, because their Achilles strength is greater than any examiner's upper extremity–provided resistance, meaning a manual test would miss all but the most severe cases. A Thompson test (passive manual calf squeeze showing plantar flexion if Achilles is intact) should be performed to rule out a significant tendon tear. Treatments in the acute setting include icing or cold compress for 15 to 20 minutes (repeated several times during the evening while not running), gentle stretching of the tendon, and providing an overnight dorsiflexion splint or bandage wrap. If elastic, stretchy tape is available, application of plantarflexion assist elastic tape can help during ambulation or continued running but should be removed at night in favor of dorsiflexion splinting. Topical antiinflammatory creams can be used at any time if the overlying skin is intact. Oral analgesics like acetaminophen can be used to help decrease pain. Current guidelines recommend that oral nonsteroidal antiinflammatory (NSAID) medications should be used only at the end of the day/race section when the runner can be adequately hydrated to prevent AKI associated with NSAID use. In the subacute setting, sports medicine clinical treatment strategies may include rest, physical therapy with a focus on eccentric exercises, peritendon steroid injections, intratendon autologous blood product injections, or referral to surgery for recalcitrant cases.

Anterior Tibialis Tendinopathy/Tendonitis

The mechanism of injury is usually repeated or strained dorsiflexion (particularly on a course that has prolonged, steep hills/inclines). Runners present for evaluation complaining of anterior ankle pain. On physical examination, swelling or fullness may be visible in the affected anterior tibialis tendon (**Fig. 1**A), although this is not always present. Occasionally, there is associated erythema in the anterior ankle as well (see **Fig. 1**B), and this must be closely followed to rule out a concurrent infection/cellulitis. They are tender to palpation of the tendon. They may have pain with passive, manual stretch of the anterior tibialis tendon, which is best elicited with combined passive ankle plantar flexion and passive great toe plantarflexion. The runners usually have pain and possibly weakness with repeated resisted ankle dorsiflexion, because they should be able to support the examiner's application of upper body weight (not simply the examiner's arm/hand strength) against dorsiflexed ankles. Treatments in the acute setting include icing or cold compress for 15 to 20 minutes (repeated several times during the evening while not running), and gentle stretching of the tendon. Topical anti-inflammatory creams can be used at any time if the overlying skin is intact. In multistage races, anecdotal cases of using an abundance of topical cream over the tendon with a bandage or occlusive dressing overnight has worked well, but it should be used with care and attention to possible skin reaction/allergy. Oral medications (analgesics and NSAIDs) follow the same guidelines as in the section on Achilles tendonitis. In the subacute setting, sports medicine clinical treatment strategies may include rest, physical therapy, peritendon steroid injections, intratendon autologous blood product injections, or referral to surgery for recalcitrant cases.

Plantar Fasciitis

Studies have suggested an incidence of 10.6%.[17] The mechanism of injury is repeated impact/shock absorption without proper arch support (either lack of support or too much support/pressure) or with higher-impact activities, even if arch support is correct for the corresponding anatomy and running style. Runners present for evaluation complaining of pain in the sole of the foot, frequently midarch, but it can be just proximal or distal to that. On physical examination, they are usually tender to palpation at the midarch or proximally along the plantar fascia toward the origin at the calcaneous. Pain may be reproduced with passive manual dorsiflexion, particularly if combined with toe extension. The runners may also have pain with resisted toe flexion in combination with ankle plantarflexed positioning. Treatment includes ice to the area, particularly ice massage by rolling a frozen or very cold water bottle underneath the arch after the day's running is complete. Passive manual stretch of the plantar fascia and dorsiflexion splinting at night can also help improve symptoms. The same medication guidelines given earlier for Achilles tendonitis hold true. In the subacute setting, strengthening intrinsic muscle of the foot, running gait evaluation/recommendations, and trials of varying levels of arch support/shoe style can help treat symptoms and prevent recurrence. Rest, physical therapy, corticosteroid injections, autologous blood product injections, and referral to surgery may also be used in an outpatient treatment setting.

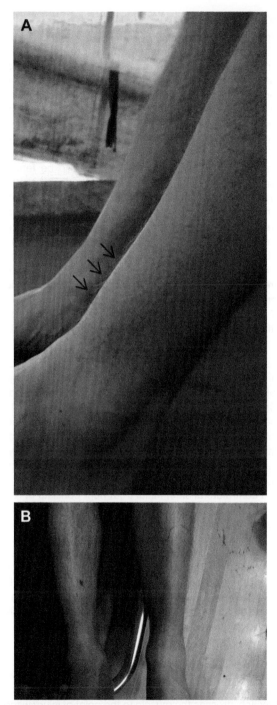

Fig. 1. (A) Acute anterior tibialis tendonitis (*arrows*) in the left distal tibia in an ultramarathon runner. (B) Acute anterior tibialis tendonitis presenting similar to a cellulitis.

Patellofemoral Syndrome

The prevalence in ultramarathon is 7.4% to 15.6%.[2,14] Incidence of knee issues is 24%,[17] although it is not clear how many of these are patellofemoral versus other knee issues (eg, meniscus tear, osteoarthritis). This injury tends to occur more often in the chronic setting but can occur as acute pain in ultradistance races. Mechanism of injury can be underlying structural anomaly of shallow femoral groove or lateralization of the patella versus inadequate quadriceps and core muscle strength for the demand distance running. Runners present with anterior knee pain. There are usually no symptoms of frank buckling or locking, but the injury can be associated with grinding sensation or crepitus. On physical examination, there is tenderness on the patellar facets, usually more on the medial aspect. There may also be tenderness along the patellar tendon, indicating a component of patellar tendonitis/tendinopathy as well. Pain may be reproduced with single-leg or double-leg squat or resisted knee extension. Acute treatment includes ice to the area and oral medications, as described earlier, taking care not to ice if the runner plans to continue running that day. A patellar tracking knee brace or band strap may help decrease pain with ambulation and running. Athletic tape can be used to fabricate a patellar band strap if none is readily available. If practitioners are trained in using kinesio tape for patellar tracking, that may also be helpful. In the subacute setting, physical therapy with attention to quadriceps and core strengthening can be used. Rest, steroid injections to the knee, viscosupplement injections if arthritis is associated, or referral to surgery for release of the lateral retinaculum or other interventions may also be used as treatment strategies.

Ankle Sprain

The incidence in ultramarathons is 10.8%.[17] The mechanism of injury is usually an inversion rolling of the ankle on uneven terrain, causing strain or tear of any of the anterolateral ligaments of the ankle. The runner presents with anterior or lateral ankle pain. There may be swelling or ecchymosis, and the athlete may or may not be able to fully bear weight. On physical examination, the athlete has tenderness to palpation over the affected ligaments. Tenderness over the bone/lateral maleolus may indicate a fracture. If able to bear weight, they may have increased pain or instability when standing on the toes with the ankles plantarflexed. An anterior drawer test may show laxity compared with the contralateral side. Initial treatment consists of rest, ice, compression, and elevation. If any instability or ecchymosis is noted, or if there is a high suspicion of fracture (based on Ottawa ankle rules), they should be removed from competition. Oral medications can be used as described in the section on Achilles tendonitis. If fracture is suspected, the patient must remain non–weight bearing until transported to a facility with radiograph services for further diagnostic evaluation. Medial-lateral ankle brace support or a rocker bottom boot should be used in cases of instability in which fracture is not suspected. A lace-up ankle brace or athletic taping of the ankle can be used for those who have no instability and are able to walk without a limp to allow them to continue if competition if desired.

Muscle Strain

The most common muscle strains involve the calf (incidence 13.1%) and hamstring (incidence 11.8%).[17] Mechanism of injury is usually an eccentric contraction or quick burst movement, which stresses the muscle to the point of injury without tearing a significant number of muscle fibers (although a small tear is difficult to differentiate from a strain). Most frequently involved muscles are those that cross 2 joints, like the hamstrings (crossing both hip and knee joints) and the gastrocnemius (crossing both knee and ankle joints)[18] Runners present with acute pain in the affected muscle. On physical examination, they may have pain with passive stretch or active contraction of the muscle. Initial treatment consists of rest, ice (after the day's competition is finished), compression, and elevation, as noted earlier. Oral medications can be used as described in the section on Achilles tendonitis. A runner may be able to continue in competition with a mild strain, but anything that causes limping or altered gait should be cause to consider removing the athlete from competition for risk of further injury. If a full tear of a muscle is suspected, then they should be removed from competition immediately and referred for further evaluation at a hospital or sports medicine clinic. In the subacute setting, if relative rest for 1 to 2 weeks along with oral antiinflammatory medication and the other treatments noted earlier do not resolve the issue, then, physical therapy or advanced imaging studies may be warranted.

Iliotibial Band Problem

The incidence is 15.8%.[17] Mechanism of injury is usually an overuse, more chronic presentation in runners but can be acute overuse in ultradistance running. The prevailing theory links this entity to impingement of the distal iliotibial band (ITB) at the lateral femoral condyle during the eccentric contraction just after heel strike.[19] Runners present with lateral knee pain at the lateral femoral condyle or just proximally or distally. They may have exacerbation of pain with compression of the band/tendon over the femoral condyle (Noble compression test) or with stretch of the ITB (Ober test). Treatment during competition consists of stretching the ITB and using topical antiinflammatory cream locally (if overlying skin is intact). Oral medications can be used, as described earlier. Icing should be used at the end of the day's competition, as described earlier. Cross-fiber friction massage can be used in the acute setting. In the subacute setting, rest, physical therapy, deep massage with foam roller, gait analysis, flexibility training, and core strengthening can be used for treatment. Other injections (eg, steroid, autologous blood products) may be considered if conservative treatment options fail.

Back Injuries

The incidence is 12.4%.[17] Mechanism of injury can be varied, from acute muscle strain, spasm or disk injury to chronic degenerative change in the lumbar spine. Runners presenting with acute axial back pain without trauma may be treated as a strain (rest, ice oral medications) or if believed to have palpable spasm, then application of heat and gentle stretching are appropriate treatments. If the presentation includes pain radiating into the thigh or lower leg, or if lower extremity numbness/tingling is associated, then, they may have an acute lumbar radiculopathy and should be removed from competition, given oral antiinflammatory medication, and referred for nonemergent evaluation at a hospital or clinic. Any presentation of back pain with notable lower extremity weakness, numbness/tingling in the groin/genitals/rectal area, or loss of control of bladder or bowel function should be treated as a spinal emergency and the patient should be transported to a hospital for immediate evaluation and treatment.

MEDICAL

Exercise-associated collapse (EAC) is the collapse of the conscious athlete after an exertional event who is unable to stand or walk unaided because of lightheadedness, faintness, or dizziness.[20–22] It is common in marathons, (59%–69% of all medical encounters at the finish line), resulting in 10.1 to 13.7 medical illnesses per 1000 runners.[23] EAC is less common during ultramarathons, representing 6.6% of all medical encounters during a multistage ultramarathon.[5] However, EAC accounted for 65% of medical illnesses for nonfinishers, resulting in 118 medical illnesses per 1000 runners.[5] Although EAC may have a variety of causes, including heat-related illness, electrolyte abnormalities, cardiovascular compromise, respiratory compromise, and seizures, it is primarily the result of transient postural hypotension caused by lower extremity blood pooling.[20] Once critical causes are ruled out, treatment is primarily symptomatic with rest in the Trendelenburg position, total body cooling, and if dehydrated, oral hydration (intravenous fluids are generally not needed).[20] This section focuses on common medical issues, heat-related illness, and EAH. The unique environment of the ultramarathon dictates the likelihood of other medical illnesses encountered.

HEAT-RELATED ILLNESS

Most heat-related illness is mild and responds to minimal interventions. However, more severe heat-related illness such as heat stroke can lead to significant morbidity and mortality. Identification of potential risk factors and environmental conditions are early interventions that are important to managing heat-related illnesses.[24,25]

Pathophysiology

Body temperature regulation occurs through the hypothalamus, which balances heat generation verses heat loss. Significant heat generation occurs with exercise, when skeletal muscles can increase their metabolic consumption by up to 20 times, with approximately 75% to 80% of that energy converted in to heat.[26] Heat lost to the environment occurs by 4 major methods: conduction, convection, radiation, and evaporation. Evaporation is the most important method of heat loss during exercise, and significant exercise can produce 1 to 2 L per hour of sweat loss,[27] with the evaporation of 1.7 mL of sweat consuming 1 kcal of heat.[28] High environmental humidity lowers the water vapor pressure difference between the skin and surrounding air, which hampers the ability of sweat to evaporate and subsequent heat loss. When the body senses an increase in core temperature, the thermal center of the hypothalamus increases cardiac output, triggers dilation of surface vessels, and increases sweating. Hyperthermia occurs when the natural ability of the body to maintain its core temperature is compromised, leading to an increase in body temperature.

Evaluation

Evaluation of an athlete suspected of heat-related illness lies in early recognition of presenting symptoms and signs. Symptom recognition is most important, because many hyperthermic endurance athletes remain asymptomatic despite increased core temperatures.[29] Mild forms of illness include heat rash (miliaria rubra), heat cramps, heat edema (painless swelling of limbs), or heat syncope, which is uncomfortable, but usually self-liming. Heat exhaustion, or exhaustion in the heat, is associated with temperatures that may normal or slightly increased (37°C –40°C), thirst, malaise, nausea, vomiting, headache, weakness, anxiety, dizziness, and an increased heart rate.[30] Sweating may be present or absent, and skin may or may not feel warm to touch. Mental status is preserved. Heat stroke is the third leading cause of death in athletes.[31] It is defined as a core temperature of at least 40°C, with central nervous system abnormalities, such as altered mental status, seizure, or unconsciousness. Vomiting, diarrhea, shortness of breath, increased heart rate, and multiorgan failure may occur, with mortality approaching 10%, when present with hypotension increasing to 33%.[31,32] In the hyperthermic individual with an altered sensorium, concern of heat stroke should not be dissuaded by a measurement value that may be lower than the diagnostic threshold of 40C.[25]

Treatment

Although there is scant evidence supporting treatments of mild to moderate heat-related illnesses, more treatments are anecdotal or extrapolated from more severe illnesses and confer minimal risk. Heat cramps, or exercise-associated muscle cramps, which are theorized to be caused by neuromuscular fatigue and altered control, are usually self-limited and rarely require hypertonic oral electrolyte solutions.[33] Heat edema is reversed by the Trendelenburg position or compression stockings. Heat syncope by definition is self-limiting. Heat exhaustion in mild forms usually resolves with removal of the athlete to a cool environment when possible, ceasing physical activity, and oral rehydration with isotonic fluids if hyperthermic, to optimize sweating and subsequent heat dispersion.[34] More severe heat exhaustion may require more aggressive cooling by evaporative and convective cooling: loosen clothing, spray or douse the patient with cold water to optimize the water vapor–skin interface, and maximize convection with fanning. Each athlete should be carefully assessed and fully recovered before returning to running.

The method and aggressiveness of cooling treatment depend on the type of heat-related illness. Regardless of the underlying cause, rapid reversal of the hyperthermia is critical, because the resulting morbidity is directly related to both the degree and duration of hyperthermia in heat stroke.[33–39] All treatment is first directed to stabilization of the patient's airway, breathing, and circulation before proceeding to more specific cooling therapy. Cold-water immersion therapy is the optimal and most rapid treatment for cooling heat stroke. It has been shown to provide twice the cooling rate of evaporative cooling,[37] with faster cooling by colder water.[40] Immersion takes advantage of the high thermal conductivity of water and resulting high thermal gradient between cold water and skin, with a resulting greater capacity for heat transfer. Cold-water immersion may be limited to a naturally occurring body of water (eg, lake, pond, or river). The person with heat stroke should have clothes and equipment removed, and their trunk and extremities should be submerged, ensuring protection against currents, aspiration, or drowning. If no cold water source is available, dousing with cold water is an acceptable alternative conductive cooling method. If immersion is unavailable, combined treatments of evaporative and convective cooling should be initiated, and the patient with heat stroke should be rapidly transported to a medical facility. In transferring care to emergency medical services, it is important to continue cooling the patient by the best available means en route to the receiving hospital.

HYDRATION AND EAH

Proper hydration management plays a crucial role in successfully completing an ultramarathon race. Studies suggest that athletes can lose up to 2 L per hour in sweat loss and body weight loss of 8% or greater without significant symptoms or consequences.[27,34,41,42] Some athletes experience a variety of symptoms relating to dehydration, including fatigue, nausea, vomiting, confusion, and weakness. The clinical diagnosis of dehydration is problematic, because these symptoms can occur with other medical illnesses.[43] Most cases respond to oral rehydration. Intravenous hydration should be considered in athletes who are not able to tolerate oral fluid intake and have evidence of significant hypovolemia (eg, orthostatis or resting tachycardia). If available, on-site point-of-care testing, (ie, iStat, Abbott Lab, IL, USA) should be used to confirm no evidence of hyponatremia. If point-of-care testing is not available or unfeasible (ie, remote locations with extreme temperatures outside the capabilities of the point-of-care equipment), the physician should proceed cautiously with rehydration, considering their clinical assessment of the cardiovascular/emergent needs of the athlete, and potential risk of exacerbating EAH.[43–47]

Epidemiology

EAH is defined as a serum sodium concentration of less than 135 mmol/L that occurs during or up to 24 hours after prolonged exercise.[6] Most runners who experience EAH are asymptomatic, although a smaller subset experience symptoms potentially leading to significant morbidity or even death. The incidence and prevalence of EAH vary, depending on the length of the running race. Studies of marathon runners have noted that 3% to 28% of runners experience some form of hyponatremia.[43–45] Studies of ultramarathon runners vary from an incidence of 5% to 50% for continuous single-stage[7,46] events to 1% to 12% for multistage events.[47] Although most EAH is often an asymptomatic biochemical diagnosis, there have been 12 documented fatalities.[45] Therefore, awareness in prevention and treatment of EAH is an important part of care for the ultramarathon athlete.

Pathophysiology

The pathologic mechanism of hyponatremia is mostly a result of fluid overload or impaired urinary water excretion resulting from inappropriate secretion of arginine vasopressin (AVP).[6,45,48] The primary cause of hyponatremia in the marathon runner is overhydration from excessive hydration.[42,45] Increased consumption of hypotonic solutions along the course of the race because of ease of access can lead to intravascular overload, resulting in lower sodium levels. Several studies of marathon runners have found a strong association between higher incidences of EAH and drinking volumes greater than 3 to 3.5 L during a marathon.[41,42,45] Other risk factors for marathon runners include slower race pace (>4 hours), female sex, and low body weight.[6,41]

The other major cause of EAH is inappropriate AVP secretion. In these cases, there is a failure to suppress AVP, which results in an inability of the kidneys to excrete the water load. This situation leads to an inability to produce diluted urine and resulting serum hyponatremia. Factors contributing to inappropriate AVP secretion include the response of the body to nonosmotic stimuli (prolonged exercise, stress, hypovolemia, fatigue, pain, and sleep deprivation), excessive sweating, or inadequate sodium supplementation.[6,7,41,42,49] A recent study of continuous single-stage ultramarathoners with EAH[7] noted that only 23.8% were classified as overhydrated, whereas 35.6% were dehydrated (weight change <−3%). The study noted a weak association between postrace sodium levels and change in body weight, with hyponatremia more common in runners with increased weight loss. In contrast, a recent study of dysnatremia in multistage ultramarathon runners[47] noted that hypernatremia (52.3%, rate of 0.15 per person-stage) was more common than hyponatremia (14.8%, rate of 0.03 per person-stage). In this study, runners became more dehydrated over the course of the race (22.5%–53.5%) and less overhydrated (44.9%–17.2%). The findings highlight the difference in dysnatremia and hydration status in marathon runners, continuous single-stage ultramarathon runners, and multistage ultramarathon runners. Each population needs to be treated in an appropriate manner, taking into account the differences noted earlier.

Evaluation

Recognizing the most common clinical symptoms of EAH is essential in avoiding more significant illness. Initial symptoms may include nausea, vomiting, sensation of bloating, puffiness, and headaches. All event support staff should be educated on EAH and instructed regarding appropriate treatment.[50] The symptoms should not be attributed to athlete fatigue and should prompt a thorough medical evaluation. As symptoms progress, athletes experience altered mental status, including confusion, disorientation, agitation, and delirium. Severe symptoms can lead to respiratory compromise, seizure, and death. Cases of suspected EAH or athletes undergoing intravenous rehydration should ideally have serum sodium levels measured by on-site point-of-care testing (ie, iStat) if available. As noted earlier, if point-of-care testing is not available or unfeasible (ie, remote locations with extreme temperatures outside the capabilities of the point-of-care equipment), the physicians should proceed cautiously with rehydration, considering their clinical assessment of the cardiovascular/emergent needs of the athlete and potential risk of exacerbating EAH.[44]

Treatment

Treatment of EAH depends on the clinical symptoms, as well as confirmation of serum sodium levels. In cases of EAH confirmed by blood analysis with absence of altered mental status, initial treatment should include an avoidance of hypotonic fluids.[6,42,45] Milder forms of EAH can be treated successfully with fluid restriction, close observation, and natural diuresis. If possible, small amounts of salty food or oral hypertonic solutions (concentrated broth) are appropriate.[51] For patients who cannot tolerate oral intake and present with neurologic compromise, isotonic fluids should be avoided, and athletes can be given 100 mL of 3% NaCl over 10 minutes × 2, with expedited transfer to a medical facility. In cases in which blood analysis confirmation is not available, caution should be exercised, because the symptoms and signs may represent dehydration and hypovolemia, as opposed to hyponatremia.[50] As noted earlier, the incidence of hyponatremia in continuous single-stage ultramarathon races is 31% to 50%, so treatment with fluid restriction or hypertonic saline solution is more likely to help.[6,50] However, in multistage ultramarathons, greater caution is warranted, because athletes are more likely to be hypernatremic and dehydrated over the course of the race. In these races, cavalier use of fluid restriction or hypertonic saline solution may be more harmful than helpful.[44,47]

Prevention strategies for hyponatremia focus on education of the ultramarathon runner. The primary strategy should be an avoidance of overhydration by adequate fluid consumption. Fluid ingestion based on the sensation of thirst during a race seems to be a safe relatively effective method for avoiding the extremes of overhydration and dehydration.[6,24,45,50] The American College of Sports Medicine position statement on fluid replacement recommends adequate fluid intake to prevent greater than 2% of body weight loss from dehydration and excessive changes in electrolyte balance based on an individualized program.[52] Studies[7,45] have suggested that most ultramarathon athletes should avoid weight gain and can afford a loss of 2% to 3% of their body weight without significantly affecting running performance. Athletes may consider measuring their hourly sweat rate and fluid consumption during training (ideally, similar to race environment) in preparation for a race. However, weight loss is not a reliable measure for excluding the diagnosis of EAH.[6,50,53] Food and hydration should be planned properly during the training schedule and should not significantly change during the course of the race. In multistage ultramarathon races, runners should be alerted that medical illnesses tend to occur during the first stage of the race, so fluid management should be minimally adjusted on the first day. Although many athletes use sodium supplementation, the exact role and impact of supplementation in preventing hyponatremia are not clear. All athletes should be educated regarding the typical symptoms of hyponatremia and need to seek medical evaluation, as appropriate.

FOOT CARE

Friction blisters are arguably the most common medical problem encountered in any endurance race. Blister rates vary by distance, ranging from 0.2% to 39% for marathons,[54] 32% to 45% for multistage adventure events,[31,55] and up to 70% of all medical visits in multiday ultramarathons.[5] For some, a foot blister may be considered merely a training nuisance; for others, it may an unavoidable injury that can ruin a run (**Fig. 2**), necessitate dropping out of an event, or even progress to cellulitis or sepsis, highlighting the importance of a thorough evaluation and optimal treatment. Blisters and foot issues remain the most often encountered injury in the endurance athlete.

Evaluation

Understanding the mechanism of a friction blister injury can assist in a thorough evaluation. The main cause is the repeated action of skin rubbing against another surface. As the external contact of either sock or footwear moves across the skin, the frictional force (F_f) opposes this movement. When horizontal shear forces overcome this resistance, repeated sliding at a friction point causes exfoliation of the stratum corneum and erythema in and around this zone.[56] This injury is experienced initially as a sensation of heat: the hot spot. Continued friction on a hot spot causes epidermal cells in the stratum spinosum to delaminate and split, leading to fluid accumulation and blister formation.[57] The intact superficial cells of the stratum corneum and stratum granulosum form the roof of the blister. A deeper injury involving the dermal plexus presents as a blood-filled blister, and an infected blister may contain cloudy fluid or surrounding erythema. Subungual hematomas present as a collection of blood underneath the nail bed or blister underneath the cuticle. The cuticle may be fluctuant with a large swollen vesicle, and the nail is often elevated, with dark blood underneath it. Blister evaluation is centered on appreciating the stage of the friction injury, which ranges from a hot spot to a torn-open or unroofed blister, and then, customizing the treatment to minimize friction to prevent reoccurrence or progression of injury.

Hot Spot Treatment

When treating a hot spot, the key to prevent blister formation involves decreasing shear forces on the skin. There are a few studies examining efficacy of various

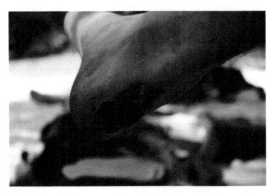

Fig. 2. Posterior heel blister during a multistage 250-km ultramarathon race.

products such as powders, antiperspirants, lubricants, or tapes. The concept of a friction prevention layer at a high friction spot is to have a layer over the skin such that the resulting shear occurs between the barrier and the footwear, not the footwear and the skin. The shelves of drugstores and running stores are stocked with products. Ideally, taping products should be thin, easy to apply, adhere well, and provide limited seams, which may themselves be friction points. Paper tape is anecdotally useful, and although not ideal in overly wet conditions, because of its low cost, ease of use, and silky feel, it is our first-line product to treat a hot spot to prevent blister formation.

Antiperspirants and powders have been proposed as other measures to decrease the amount of moisture at the foot-sock interface. The largest antiperspirant trial[58] found antiperspirant to be effective in prevention of blisters, but its high incidence in skin irritation (57% vs 6% of controls) likely limits its usefulness to those suffering from hyperhydrosis. Despite widespread marketing of powder compounds, there is no published scientific evidence to suggest that these products prevent foot blisters. Lubricants ostensibly prevent blister formation by decreasing friction at the foot–contact material interface. Several studies have shown that after applying lubricating substances to skin, there is an initial decrease of the coefficient of friction, but that within an hour, it returns to baseline with a subsequent increase in friction 35% higher than baseline over the next 4 to 6 hours.[59,60] The studies suggest that with prolonged exercise, the use of lubricants might contribute to blister formation, so if used, they need to be reapplied frequently.

Treating a blister as soon as possible improves outcome, reduces pain, and minimizes complications from either subsequent tissue damage or infection. In the early stages of blister formation, the presence of a sensation of warmth from the hot spot is a warning sign. Prompt attention and rapid treatment can stop the abrasive process to prevent progressive blister formation.[61,62] Proper blister care is not complicated, yet, it may be time intensive, depending on the extent of damage to the feet. Individuals should become familiar with techniques before heading outside and facing a blister predicament. Our medical experiences with ultraendurance races have shown that implementation of mandatory personal foot care kits for competitors and the expectation of self-care take a huge burden off the medical team.

Blister Treatment

Any tape used for blister treatment should be applied as smoothly as possible. The tape ideally acts as a second layer of skin, so rubbing acts on the tape, not on the underlying skin. Any folds or wrinkles in the tape should be avoided, because they may lead to high pressure and friction areas. Cutting the tape corners to round them and avoiding dog-ears helps in avoiding further blisters. All tape should be cut long enough to extend well beyond the border of the blister and any blister pads underneath the tape. Constriction through overlapping of tape and circumferential wrapping of the feet should be avoided, because it may lead to venous congestion and subsequent swelling.

Before taping, the skin should be clean of dirt and grit and as dry as possible, which enhances natural adhesion of tape. Using an adhesive substance, such as benzoin (liquid, squares, or spray), should be considered, to ensure security of the applied dressing. As a rule, blister tape should not be removed unless it is peeling off or there is increasing discomfort at the tape site. Ideally, soaking the bandages before removal loosens adhesion and minimize chances of ripping the roof off of intact blisters.

The pain from a blister is caused by pressure on an incompressible fluid between skin layers. As abrasion and pressure build, there is further pain and separation of skin layers and increasing potential for rupturing the blister, which leaves exposed raw and sensitive skin. The best protection for a blister is its own roof, so efforts should be taken to maintain this natural skin protection. If the skin is not intact, it should be removed before dressing (**Fig. 3**A). Small friction blisters that are not causing significant discomfort can be left intact. If the blister is punctured with a needle and drained, it often refills within a few hours. If a large hole is made that allows continuous fluid drainage, there is the risk of losing integrity of the blister, and having the blister's roof tear off, leaving a large damaged area. Our recommendation is to use a safety pin or similar-sized needle to create an optimum-sized hole.

Prepare the blister skin and safety pin with an alcohol pad. Puncture the blister with the prepared pin at a distal point, allowing natural foot pressure to continually squeeze out fluid. If more drainage is required, use several small holes rather than 1 large hole, limiting risk of deroofing the blister. Gently blot out the expressed fluid, cover the flattened blister with paper tape, which is cut to overlap the edge of the blister. This important step protects the roof of the blister when the overlying tape is removed. If the roof of the blister is ripped open, trim off the devitalized skin, apply a hydrocolloid layer of a Spenco 2nd Skin pad over the exposed base, and finish as described earlier (see **Fig. 3**B). Cover paper tape with a benzoin-type adhesive and allow it to become tacky (see **Fig. 3**C). As a final layer, apply shaped adhesive tape (ie, Elastikon) over the paper-taped blister (see **Fig. 3**D). Blisters that recur under intact tape can be drained with a prepared safety pin through the tape.

Subungual hematomas are relieved by trephination of the nail bed, a necessary step, because the collection of fluid leads to pressure, which makes this condition painful. It is common to acquire a subungual hematoma on downhill hikes or runs

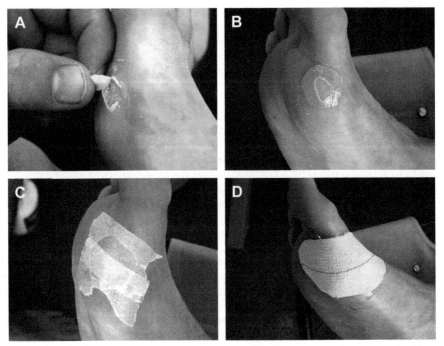

Fig. 3. (*A*) Open blister at the metatarsal region. (*B*) Placement of 2nd Skin over the blister after removal of the open cover. (*C*) Placement of paper tape over the blister. (*D*) Placement of external bandage.

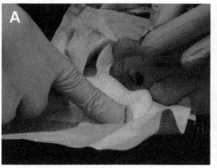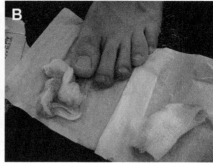

Fig. 4. (A) Subungual hematoma drainage. (B) Subungual hematoma, resolved.

when the toes are repetitively jammed into the toe box. Subungual hematomas are easily treated. An 18-gauge hypodermic needle is held perpendicular to the proximal nail bed over the area of greatest fullness (**Fig. 4**A). With gentle downward pressure, rotate the needle between the thumb and first finger; as it is twirled back and forth, it easily drills into and through the nail, releasing the hematoma. The release of blood under pressure through the 18-gauge hole may be dramatic, causing it to squirt, so appropriate universal precautions should be used. The 18-gauge needle should be re-capped and may need to be reused for the same patient, because these blisters have a tendency to recur. Treating a cuticle blister is a simple treatment, as described earlier (see **Fig. 4**B). As with all toe blisters, only paper tape should be used to wrap the injured digit, because any other tape with texture has the potential to rub on neigh-boring toes and cause adjacent intertriginous blisters.

There is no one correct way to care for feet. For every technique and product mentioned, there are several different options. We recommend avoiding draining of blood-filled blisters, because these are a potential route for bacteria to enter the wound and bloodstream, which can lead to cellulitis or sepsis. Blood blisters should be left intact, unless they are large, fluctuant, extremely painful, or at risk for sponta-neous rupture. To drain, use a providone-iodine preparation, clean gloves, and instru-ments with the techniques described earlier. Likewise, blisters deep to a callus should not be drained. These blisters are painful to access, yield little blister fluid, and quickly refill after drainage. A blister with murky hazy fluid or pus may be infected. The blister should be opened (deroofed), irrigated with providone-iodine, and then, antiseptic or antibiotic ointment should be applied to the cavity before being covered with the open blister technique. If the individual begins to show signs of worsening surrounding er-ythema, streaking, or systemic symptoms (eg, chills, fevers, nausea, or generalized weakness), definitive care, including oral or intravenous antibiotics, should be used to avoid sepsis. The goals of blister treatment are to optimize comfort for continued activity, minimize progression of disease, assist with epidermal recovery, and prevent further blister enlargement when resting and staying off the feet is not an option.

SUMMARY

Physicians and athletes participating in ultramarathons need to be prepared for a va-riety of injuries and illnesses that may occur during a race. Most musculoskeletal and skin-related issues are minor and can be treated successfully during the course of a race. Common medical illnesses, including environmental illnesses and EAH, require prompt assessment and appropriate treatment in hopes of avoiding significant morbidity and mortality. Continued research should focus on preventative and optimal treatment strategies in hopes of preventing long-term complications in this unique athletic population.

REFERENCES

1. Krabak BJ, Waite BW, Lipman G. Injury and illnesses prevention for ultra-marathoners. Curr Sports Med Rep 2013;12(3):183–9.
2. Khodaee M, Ansari M. Common ultramarathon injuries and illnesses: race day management. Curr Sports Med Rep 2012;11(6):290–7.
3. Van Gent RN, Siem D, van Middelkoop M, et al. Incidence and determinants of lower extremity running injuries in long distance runners: a systematic review. Br J Sports Med 2007;41(8):469–80 [discussion: 480].
4. Fallon KE. Musculoskeletal injuries in the ultramarathon: the 1990 Westfield Sydney to Melbourne run. Br J Sports Med 1996;30(4):319–23.
5. Krabak BJ, Waite B, Schiff MA. Study of injury and illness rates in multiday ultramarathon runners. Med Sci Sports Exerc 2011;43(12):2314–20.
6. Hew-Butler T, Ayus JC, Kipps C, et al. Statement of the Second International Exercise-Associated Hyponatremia Consensus Development Conference, New Zealand, 2007. Clin J Sport Med 2008;18(2):111–21.
7. Hoffman MD, Hew-Butler T, Stuempfle KJ. Exercise-associated hyponatremia and hydration status in 161-km ultramarathoners. Med Sci Sports Exerc 2013; 45:784–91.
8. Lipman GS, Krabak BJ, Waite BL, et al. A prospective cohort study of acute kidney injury in multi-stage ultramarathon runners: the Biochemistry in Endurance Runner Study (BIERS). Res Sports Med 2014;22(2):185–92.
9. Hoffman MD, Stuempfle KJ, Fogard K, et al. Urine dipstick analysis for identification of runners susceptible to acute kidney injury following an ultramarathon. J Sports Sci 2013;31(1):20–31.
10. Kim JH, Malhotra R, Chiampas G, et al. Cardiac arrest during long-distance running races. N Engl J Med 2012;366(2):130–40.
11. Satterthwaite P, Norton R, Larmer P, et al. Risk factors for injuries and other health problems sustained in a marathon. Br J Sports Med 1999;33(1):22–6.
12. Yeung EW, Yeung SS. Interventions for preventing lower limb soft-tissue injuries in runners [review]. Cochrane Database Syst Rev 2001;(3):CD001256.
13. Van Middelkoop M, Kolkman J, Van Ochten J, et al. Prevalence and incidence of lower extremity injuries in male marathon runners. Scand J Med Sci Sports 2008; 18(2):140–4.
14. Lopes AD, Hespanhol Júnior LC, Yeung SS, et al. What are the main running-related musculoskeletal injuries? A systematic review. Sports Med 2012; 42(10):891–905.
15. Scheer BV, Murray A. Al Andalus ultra trail: an observation of medical interventions during a 219-km, 5-day ultramarathon stage race. Clin J Sport Med 2011; 21(5):444–6.
16. Fields KB, Sykes JC, Walker KM, et al. Prevention of running injuries [review]. Curr Sports Med Rep 2010;9(3):176–82.
17. Hoffman MD, Krishnan E. Health and exercise-related medical issues among 1,212 ultramarathon runners: baseline findings from the ultrarunners longitudinal tracking (ULTRA) Study. PLoS One 2014;9(1):e83867.
18. Noonan TJ, Garrett WE Jr. Muscle strain injury: diagnosis and treatment. J Am Acad Orthop Surg 1999;7(4):262–9.

19. Baker RL, Souza RB, Fredericson M. Iliotibial band syndrome: soft tissue and biomechanical factors in evaluation and treatment. PM R 2011;3(6):550–61.

20. Asplund CA, O'Connor FG, Noakes TD. Exercise-associated collapse: an evidence-based review and primer for clinicians [review]. Br J Sports Med 2011;45(14):1157–62.

21. Childress MA, O'Connor FG, Levine BD. Exertional collapse in the runner: evaluation and management in fieldside and office-based settings. Clin Sports Med 2010;29:459–76.

22. Roberts WO. Exercise-associated collapse care matrix in the marathon. Sports Med 2007;37:431–3.

23. Roberts WO. A 12-yr profile of medical injury and illness for the Twin Cities Marathon. Med Sci Sports Exerc 2000;32(9):1549–55.

24. Armstrong LE, Casa DJ, Millard-Stafford M, et al. American College of Sports Medicine position stand. Exertional heat illness during training and competition. Med Sci Sports Exerc 2007;39(3):556–72.

25. Lipman GS, Eifling KP, Ellis MA, et al. Wilderness Medical Society practice guidelines for the prevention and treatment of heat-related illness. Wilderness Environ Med 2013;24(4):351–61.

26. Maugham RJ, Watson P, Shirreffs S. Heat and cold. What does the environment do to the marathon runner? Sports Med 2007;37:396–9.

27. Kenefick RW, Cheuvront SN, Sawka MN. Thermoregulatory function during the marathon. Sports Med 2007;37:312–5.

28. Nelson NA, Eichna LW, Horvath SM, et al. Thermal exchanges of man at high temperatures. Am J Physiol 1947;151:626–52.

29. Byrne C, Lee JK, Chew SA, et al. Continuous thermoregulatory responses to mass-participation distance running. Med Sci Sports Exerc 2006;38(5):803–12.

30. Noakes TD. A modern classification of the exercise-related heat illnesses. J Sci Med Sport 2008;11(1):33–9.

31. McLaughlin KA, Townes DA, Wedmore IS, et al. Pattern of injury and illness during expedition-length adventure races. Wilderness Environ Med 2006;17:158–61.

32. Centers for Disease Control and Prevention (CDC). Heat-related deaths–United States, 1999-2003. MMWR Morb Mortal Wkly Rep 2006;55(29):796–8.

33. Schwellnus MP. Cause of exercise associated muscle cramps (EAMC)–altered neuromuscular control, dehydration or electrolyte depletion? Br J Sports Med 2009;43(6):401–8.

34. Sawka MN, Latzka WA, Matott RP, et al. Hydration effects on temperature regulation. Int J Sports Med 1998;19(Suppl 2):S108–10.

35. Bedno SA, Li Y, Han W, et al. Exertional heat illness among overweight US Army recruits in basic training. Aviat Space Environ Med 2010;81:107–11, 40.

36. Biery JC Jr, Blivin SJ, Pyne SW. Training in ACSM black flag heat stress conditions: how US Marines do it. Curr Sports Med Rep 2010;9:148–54, 41.

37. Armstrong LE, Crago AE, Adams R, et al. Whole-body cooling of hyperthermic runners: comparison of two field therapies. Am J Emerg Med 1996;14:355–8, 42.

38. Hadad E, Rav-Acha M, Heled Y, et al. Heat stroke: a review of cooling methods. Sports Med 2004;34:501–11, 44.

39. Shapiro Y, Seidman DS. Field and clinical observations of exertional heatstroke patients. Med Sci Sports Exerc 1990;22:6–14.

40. Proulx CI, Ducharme MB, Kenny GP. Effect of water temperature on cooling efficiency during hyperthermia in humans. J Appl Physiol (1985) 2003;94:1317–23.

41. Almond CS, Shin AY, Fortescue EB, et al. Hyponatremia among runners in the Boston Marathon. N Engl J Med 2005;352(15):1550–6.
42. Noakes TD, Sharwood K, Speedy D, et al. Three independent biological mechanisms cause exercise-associated hyponatremia: evidence from 2,135 weighed competitive athletic performances. Proc Natl Acad Sci U S A 2005;102:18550–5.
43. McGarvey J, Thompson J, Hanna C, et al. Sensitivity and specificity of clinical signs for assessment of dehydration in endurance athletes. Br J Sports Med 2010;44(10):716–9.
44. Lipman GS. Clinical practice guidelines for treatment of exercise-associated hyponatremia. Wilderness Environ Med 2013;24(4):466–8.
45. Noakes T. The biology of EAH in waterlogged: the serious problem of overhydration in endurance sports. Champaign (IL): Human Kinetics; 2012. Acad Sci U S A 2005;102(51):241–92.
46. Knechtle B, Gnädinger M, Knechtle P, et al. Prevalence of exercise-associated hyponatremia in male ultraendurance athletes. Clin J Sport Med 2011;21(3): 226–32.
47. Krabak BJ, Lipman G, Rundell SD, et al. Exercise associated hyponatremia and body weight changes among runners in a 250 km multi-stage multi-stage ultramarathon. Presented at 2014 American Society for Sports Medicine Annual Conference, New Orleans, LA. April 7, 2014.
48. Siegel AJ, Verbalis JG, Clement S, et al. Hyponatremia in marathon runners due to inappropriate arginine vasopressin secretion. Am J Med 2007;120:461.e11–7.
49. Hew-Butler T, Jordaan E, Stuempfle KJ, et al. Osmotic and nonosmotic regulation of arginine vasopressin during prolonged endurance exercise. J Clin Endocrinol Metab 2008;93:2072–8.
50. Bennett BL, Hew-Butler T, Hoffman MD, et al. Wilderness Medical Society practice guidelines for treatment of exercise-associated hyponatremia. Wilderness Environ Med 2013;24(3):228–40.
51. Speedy DB, Thompson JM, Rodgers I, et al. Oral salt supplementation during ultradistance exercise. Clin J Sport Med 2002;12:279–84.
52. Sawka MN, Burke M, Eichner ER, et al. Exercise and fluid replacement: the American College of Sports Medicine Position Stand. Med Sci Sports Exerc 2007;39:377–90.
53. Lebus DK, Casazza GA, Hoffman MD, et al. Can changes in body mass and total body water accurately predict hyponatremia after a 161-km running race? Clin J Sport Med 2010;20:193–9.
54. Mailler EA, Adams BB. The wear and tear of 26.2: dermatological injuries reported on marathon day. Br J Sports Med 2004;38:498–501.
55. Townes DA, Talbot TS, Wedmore IS, et al. Event medicine: injury and illness during an expedition-length adventure race. J Emerg Med 2004;27:161–5.
56. Naylor P. The skin surface and friction. Br J Dermatol 1955;67:239–48.
57. Sulzberger MB, Cortese TA, Fishman L, et al. Studies on blisters produced by friction. I. Results of linear rubbing and twisting technics. J Invest Dermatol 1966;47:456–65.
58. Knapik JJ, Reynolds K, Barson J. Influence of an antiperspirant on foot blister incidence during cross-country hiking. J Am Acad Dermatol 1998;39:202–6.
59. Nacht S, Close J, Yeung D, et al. Skin friction coefficient: changes induced by skin hydration and emollient application and correlation with perceived skin feel. J Soc Cosmet Chem 1981;32:55–65.
60. Comaish S, Bottoms E. The skin and friction: deviations from Amonton's laws and the effect of hydration and lubrication. Br J Dermatol 1971;84:37–43.

61. Herring KM, Richie DH Jr. Friction blisters and sock fiber composition. A double-blind study. J Am Podiatr Med Assoc 1990;80:63–71.
62. Dai XQ, Li Y, Zhang M, et al. Effect of sock on biomechanical responses of foot during walking. Clin Biomech (Bristol, Avon) 2006;21:314–21.

Treatment of Tendinopathies with Platelet-rich Plasma

Ken Mautner, MD*, Lee Kneer, MD

KEYWORDS

- Tendinopathy • Platelet-rich plasma (PRP) • Biologics • Tendons

KEY POINTS

- Pain and dysfunction related to tendinopathy are often refractory to traditionally available treatments and offer a unique challenge to physicians as there is no current gold standard treatment.
- Injectable biologics including platelet-rich plasma (PRP) may represent a new modality in conjunction with a multifaceted treatment approach.
- PRP injections are not associated with the systemic or tendon degradation risks of corticosteroids or the inherent risks of surgery.
- Basic science studies are promising but have not been replicated with high-powered evidence at the clinical level.
- Given this promise and the lack of a definitive treatment, further evidence to expand understanding of the role of PRP in the treatment of tendinopathy is needed.

CAUSES OF TENDINOPATHY

Tendons serve as the interface between muscles and the skeletal structures on which energy is transferred, ultimately leading to motion. They typically function at 30% to 40% of their maximum tensile strength and are injured when exposed to supramaximal loading.[1] A low metabolic rate allows tendons to function under prolonged stress but can also lead to delayed healing when injury occurs.[2,3] Common terms used in the past to describe tendon disorders include tendinitis, tendinopathy, and tendinosis. Tendinitis, which implies an inflammatory cause, has largely been abandoned as a term because of multiple studies showing a degenerative rather than inflammatory milieu in affected tendons.[4–6] Tendinopathy is an often-used term that implies a painful subacute functional loss that may or may not involve an inflammatory component. Tendinosis refers to the degenerative structural changes that occur in tendons that

Departments of Physical Medicine and Rehabilitation and Orthopaedics, Emory Orthopaedics and Spine Center, 59 Executive Park Dr South, Suite 1000, Atlanta, GA 30329
* Corresponding author.
E-mail address: kmautne@emory.edu

Phys Med Rehabil Clin N Am 25 (2014) 865–880
http://dx.doi.org/10.1016/j.pmr.2014.06.008
1047-9651/14/$ – see front matter © 2014 Elsevier Inc. All rights reserved.

fail to heal after injury. Once thought to represent a persistent inflammatory process, tendinosis is now understood to be characterized by a scarcity of clinical or histologic signs of inflammation and instead shows fibrotic replacement of collagen, poor organization of remaining collagen fibers, increased neovascularity, and a lack of inflammatory mediators.[7–12]

Although the end result is more clear, the pathophysiology of tendinosis is still being debated, because multiple factors likely contribute to the hallmark pain and dysfunction of incomplete tendon healing.[11,12] Structures that are commonly involved include the rotator cuff tendons of the shoulder, the wrist flexor and extensor tendons, and the patellar and Achilles tendons of the knee and ankle, respectively. Like many other types of musculoskeletal disorder, both intrinsic and extrinsic risk factors are associated with the tendinopathy. Common intrinsic factors identified include altered biomechanics, decreased strength, both hypoflexibility and hyperflexibility, increasing age, female gender, certain medication use, and diabetes.[5,13–16] Extrinsic factors including load amount, duration, frequency, and direction of movement also contribute to the risk of developing tendinopathy.[17,18] In addition to pain and dysfunction, studies have shown a profound increase in risk for tendon rupture in degenerated tendons, highlighting the importance of developing effective treatment strategies not only for pain relief but also for tendon healing.[19]

HISTORY OF TENDINOPATHY MANAGEMENT

The classic tendinopathy treatment algorithm focused initially on palliation via arrest of a presumed inflammatory process. Nonsteroidal antiinflammatory drugs (NSAIDs), relative immobilization, topical modalities, compression, and corticosteroid injections are all common interventions used to quell pain and allow participation in a rehabilitation program focusing on stretching and eccentric strengthening. Although pain relief is an important goal in treating the patient with tendinopathy, modalities that are intended to decrease pain in the short term do not address the underlying tissue disorder. The inflammatory cascade that was previously targeted as a means of treating tendinopathy is now understood to be integral in the wound healing process, and blunting its effects may lead to delayed healing and slower functional recovery.[20–23]

It has been theorized that resetting the healing process via the introduction of concentrated growth factors, proteins, and many other bioactive substances, all of which are plentiful in platelet-rich plasma (PRP), may be an effective means of treating recalcitrant tendinopathies. PRP preparations have been used with proven efficacy for years to augment tissue healing in surgical wound closure as well as fat, skin, and bone grafting, and more recently have been used with success in treating tendinopathy as well.[24–28]

What is PRP?

PRP has been defined as an autologous concentration of platelets obtained after gentle centrifugation of whole blood.[29,30] The resultant supernatant contains a high concentration of platelets and the 7 fundamental protein growth factors secreted by the alpha granules of platelets to promote wound healing, including platelet-derived growth factors (PDGF) alpha, beta, and alpha/beta, transforming growth factors (TGF) beta 1 and beta 2, vascular endothelial growth factor (VEGF), and epithelial growth factor (EGF).[31,32] A summary of the functions of these and other bioactive components of PRP is presented in **Table 1**.

The plasma component of the centrifuged supernatant also contains 3 important proteins for tissue regeneration: fibrin, fibronectin, and vitronectin. Fibrin polymerizes

Table 1
Bioactive components of PRP

Factor	Origin	Function
PDGF αα	Alpha granule of platelets	Cell differentiation, neovascularization[33,34]
PDGF αβ	Alpha granule of platelets	Cell differentiation, fibroblast migration, ECM synthesis[34,35]
PDGF ββ	Alpha granule of platelets	Cell proliferation and differentiation, collagen remodeling[34,36–38]
TGF β1	Alpha granule of platelets	Stimulation of collagen formation[34,39]
TGF β2	Alpha granule of platelets	Tendon differentiation[34,40]
VEGF	Alpha granule of platelets	Neovascularization, prevention of apoptosis[34,41,42]
EGF	Alpha granule of platelets	Fibroblast proliferation[41]
Stromal-derived factor 1α	Alpha granule of platelets	Promotes catabolism of degenerative tissue; recruitment of mesenchymal stem cells and fibroblasts[43,44]
Fibrin	Plasma	Component of ECM; stimulation of phagocytosis[47]
Fibronectin	Plasma	Component of ECM; stimulation of phagocytosis[47]
Vitronectin	Plasma	Coordination of cell migration[40]
Interleukin-1β	Macrophage	Increases leukocyte maturation and FGF activity[43]
FGF	Alpha granule of platelets	Neovascularization, stimulation of ECM production and cell migration[34,37,45,46]
IGF-1	Alpha granule of platelets	ECM synthesis, fibroblast proliferation[34,47]
IGF-2	Alpha granule of platelets	ECM synthesis, protein cell proliferation[47]

Abbreviations: ECM, extracellular matrix; FGF, fibroblast growth factor; IGF, insulinlike growth factor.

and cross-links with fibronectin to form the proper substratum for the development of new tissue, and both are also involved in signal transduction to stimulate phagocytosis of designated tissue.[47] Vitronectin coordinates cell migration via proteolysis and cell adhesion[48]

PRP Preparations

Multiple variables can influence the efficacy of PRP, including platelet and leukocyte concentrations, the use of activators, and pH of the injectant. Attempts to determine the optimum platelet product for soft tissue healing are discussed later.

Platelet concentration
Normal platelet concentrations range from 150,000 to 300,000/μL in the healthy adult. Early studies promoted an optimal platelet concentration of 2.5 to 3 times the baseline platelet count and suggested that concentrations higher than this might have an inhibitory effect on healing.[49,50] However, recent research has challenged the use of lower platelet concentrations, suggesting instead the use of preparations of 1.5 million/μL, or 5 to 7 times the typical baseline concentration. Higher platelet concentrations o induce greater angiogenesis and are not inhibitory up to 2 million to 3 million per

microliter, or 10 times the baseline platelet count.[51,52] In addition, Haynesworth and colleagues[53] showed an exponential increase in mesenchymal stem cell proliferation as platelet concentration increased from 2.5 to 10 times that contained in whole blood. The current body of literature suggests greater tissue healing with the use of higher platelet concentrations, although additional well-designed studies are needed to further answer this question.

Leukocyte concentrations

The use of leukocytes in PRP preparations is a topic of continuing debate. There are commercially available platelet-concentrating systems that remove leukocytes from the preparation, which is then termed leukocyte poor. However, other units centrifuge whole blood to yield a leukocyte-rich supernatant that has been shown to contain primarily monocytes and leukocytes, and few neutrophils. The presence of leukocytes has been associated with prolonged soft tissue healing. Enzymatic activation of matrix metalloproteinases (MMPs) by granules released from neutrophils present in leukocyte-rich PRP has been shown to injure soft tissues and delay healing in vitro.[54–56] In contrast, monocytes and lymphocytes have been shown to recruit and promote the differentiation of stem cells in vitro, and it has been theorized that their presence may result in higher stem cell counts and promotion of the wound healing cascade in vivo.[52,57,58] Furthermore, El-Sharkawy and colleagues[59] compared the stimulation of cytokine release (a marker of inflammation) in tissues treated with whole blood, leukocyte-rich PRP, and platelet-poor plasma and exposure to PRP with leukocytes was associated with a decrease in cytokine release. Again, there are not enough well-designed in vivo clinical studies to determine optimum amount and distribution of leukocytes in PRP preparations.

Use of activators

Some clinicians have theorized that activating platelets via the use of thrombin or other activating agents may lead to improved concentrations of growth factors at the site of injection because of concerns for migration of the PRP away from the intended region.[60] Scherer and colleagues[61] examined the effects of platelet activation on wound healing in vivo and in vitro and found that wounds treated with nonactivated PRP healed more quickly, and other studies have yielded similar results.[62] One theory for this finding is the concept of a healing cascade schedule, whereby growth factors may have an optimal effect when present on demand rather than being released immediately at the time of injection. The cells effecting change at the site of healing require different growth factors at different times because their concentrations follow a temporal schedule during the wound repair cascade, as shown in (**Fig. 1**).

pH of injectant

Regarding pH, commercially available PRP preparation systems typically use citrate dextrose for its anticoagulant properties. By binding to free calcium in the blood it arrests the coagulation cascade, stabilizing the blood in a liquid state to allow centrifugation. However, the presence of citrate dextrose in the PRP preparation creates a slightly more acidic injectate, which initially raised concern for impairment of tissue regeneration. The wound healing process is known to involve an acidic environment initially followed by a transition to a neutral and then slightly alkaline pH later.[63,64] The timing of pH variations stimulates the release of growth factors at the appropriate time, as shown by Wahlström and colleagues,[65] who exposed platelets to media of differing acidity and found that, at the lowest pH, PDGFs were more prevalent. PDGFs are important in all stages of wound healing, but are particularly active early.[66] Given the acidic milieu of the targeted tissue, buffering PRP to counteract the acidity of

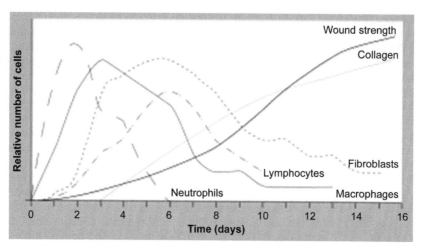

Fig. 1. Leukocytes and Wound Healing. (*From* Mautner A, Malanga G, Colberg R. Optimization of ingredients, procedures, and rehabilitation for platelet-rich plasma injections for chronic tendinopathy. Pain Manag 2011;1(6):527; with permission.)

citrate dextrose is generally viewed as unnecessary, and may even delay soft tissue healing.

Local anesthetics

Given the volume of fluid injected and the sensitive soft tissues targeted with PRP injections, many practitioners use local anesthetic for the procedure. Previous studies have yielded conflicting results on the effects of local anesthetics on wound healing, tenocytes, and platelets. Kevy and colleagues[52] showed noninferiority of platelets when mixed with local anesthetics, but multiple studies have shown decreased tenocyte cell proliferation and decreased cell viability.[67,68] Studies have also associated the concomitant use of methylprednisolone, a corticosteroid sometimes used for relief of the expected postprocedure pain, with decreased tenocyte proliferation and cell viability.[67,69] The authors prefer to use only minimal, diluted anesthetics and no corticosteroids with PRP injections.

Basic Science Studies on PRP

Injectable biologics represent a promising, novel means of treating tendinopathy, a common diagnosis with few overwhelmingly efficacious treatments to date. Although PRP is a proven treatment of surgical wound closure and graft incorporation, as stated earlier, its use has increased in musculoskeletal medicine despite a paucity of prospective, large-scale, randomized controlled clinical trials of high methodologic quality to support its use. However, numerous preliminary proof of concept studies have shown a beneficial effect of PRP on tenocyte healing, and several of these are discussed here.

Many basic science studies have examined the association between treatment with PRP and an increase in mediators that are known to contribute to tissue healing and regeneration. Baksh and colleagues[70] conducted a review of the available literature evaluating the effects of PRP at the cellular level and described multiple studies showing initial increased angiogenesis, improved tenocyte formation, and tendon healing. PRP has been shown to have a positive effect on the expression of several growth factors, including the various PDGFs, TGFs, insulinlike growth factors, hepatocyte growth factor, and VEGF.[31,32,34,71-76]

In theory, the upregulation of growth factors leads to increased formation of tenocytes and the structures that support them, and the current body of literature supports this. Zhang and Wang[77] exposed tendon stem cells to PRP in vitro and found an increased rate of differentiation into tenocytes, increased tenocyte-related gene and protein expression, as well as the production of collagen, and others have shown similar increases in collagen formation.[76–80] Increased vascularity at the site of PRP injection indirectly promotes tendon healing via recruitment of additional platelets, leukocytes, and their associated growth factors, and multiple studies have shown increased angiogenesis in vivo compared with controls with the use of PRP.[81–84] Kajikawa and colleagues[85] showed that this increase was functional, with improved recruitment of native circulation–derived cells with a resultant increase in type I and III collagen levels at the site of PRP application. This finding was confirmed by Bosch and colleagues,[84] who showed not only quantitative changes in collagen but qualitative improvements in the collagen network and increased metabolic activity as well. The improved collagen matrix size and quality has been shown to improve the tensile strength of tendons treated with PRP.[79] In this way the effects of PRP probably extend beyond the mediators in the injectate alone, and this lends support to the longer-term expected recovery compared with the brief time in which PRP is present at the site of injection.

Human Clinical Studies on PRP

For PRP to be clinically relevant, the promising results seen in basic science studies need to translate into improved patient outcomes. Although there is a dearth of well-designed clinical studies of significant power this body of research is expanding understanding of the effects of PRP on tendon healing. Taylor and colleagues[86] reviewed the available literature regarding outcomes following PRP treatment of tendon injury. Thirteen studies met criteria, including 3 randomized controlled trials. Of those, nearly all showed benefit with PRP except for the treatment of chronic Achilles tendinopathy, which yielded conflicting results.

Lateral epicondyle extensor tendinopathy

PRP use in the treatment of chronic lateral elbow pain has been associated with long-term efficacy in multiple studies examining both pain and function,[87–90] including a recent well-powered multicenter double-blind randomized controlled trial by Mishra and colleagues[90] showing statistically significant improvement in pain at 6 months after the procedure compared with percutaneous needling of the tendon. Peerbooms and colleagues[87] also showed in a double-blind, randomized control trial at 2 years' follow-up that individuals receiving a single injection of PRP fared significantly better than individuals receiving a corticosteroid injection for chronic lateral epicondylitis.[91] Ultrasonographic examinations of extensor tendons treated with PRP have also shown promising results for tendon healing, suggesting that preclinical study findings may translate into clinical benefit. A pilot study by Chaudhury and colleagues[92] found morphologic improvements, defined as an increase in vascularity, at the myotendinous junction in all 5 patients evaluated at 6 months after PRP injection (1 subject was lost to follow-up). In contrast, other studies have failed to replicate these results, including a randomized, double-blind, placebo-controlled trial by Krogh and colleagues.[93,94] This study examined the association of either PRP, glucocorticoid, or saline (placebo) injections with pain relief, vascularity, and tendon thickness at 1 and 3 months. Injection of glucocorticoid was associated with superior pain relief at 1 but not 3 months, and decreased vascularity and tendon diameter at 3 months. Neither glucocorticoid nor PRP was superior to saline injection by any measured variable at 3 months. The merits of saline as a true placebo have not been established, and longer-term follow-up may have revealed different outcomes because the full benefits of PRP cannot be measured at 3 months after injection.[87–92]

Patellar tendinopathy

Chronic patellar tendinopathy causes great pain and functional limitations, and conservative means of treatment including eccentric training have only been estimated to be 50% to 70% effective at restoring pain and function to allow participation in sports.[95,96] As such, it is a potential target for PRP therapy. Clinical studies have shown significant pain reduction, even in patients who had failed other treatments. Gosens and colleagues[97] evaluated improvements in pain prospectively and found significant improvements both in patients who had never sought interventional treatment as well as in those that had been treated surgically or received prolotherapy or corticosteroid injections. Other studies found similar results with augmented pain relief and improved tendinous echotexture under ultrasonography when PRP and physical therapy were both used and injections were performed with ultrasonography guidance.[98–100] Medium-term follow-up found statistically significant improvements in pain and return to sports activity up to 4 years following injection.[101] Unilateral pain and shorter duration of symptoms predicted a positive response, whereas BMI and previous surgical treatment did not significantly affect outcome, all of which are important considerations for appropriate patient selection. A multicenter retrospective review of outcomes after PRP in multiple tendons by Mautner and colleagues[102] showed the least improvement in pain, function, and patient satisfaction with patellar tendon injections (59% vs 81%–100% at other sites).

Achilles tendinopathy

Achilles tendinopathy is a common target of PRP therapy, although its efficacy is a source of continuing debate. Several small studies have shown postinjection improvements in pain, tendon structure, return to activities, and quality of life.[100,102–107] In addition to decreased pain, Ferrero and colleagues[100] found statistically significant structural changes in Achilles tendons 6 months after PRP combined with dry needling treatment including decreased tendon size, decreased echogenicity, and increased power Doppler signal indicating an induced vascular response. Other studies have supported these results, with subjective and objective positive benefits as much as 18 months after PRP.[106] Deans and colleagues[107] used a comprehensive program including PRP followed by 6 weeks of immobilization with therapeutic ultrasonography before beginning an eccentric exercise program. This protocol led to excellent pain relief, improved quality of life, and return to sport at 6 months after the procedure and represents a multimodal treatment approach that may be more effective at relieving chronic Achilles tendinopathic pain and restoring function than PRP treatment alone.

There have been studies that have failed to replicate these positive results and that call into question the role of PRP in treating chronic midportion Achilles tendinopathy. De Jonge and colleagues[108] designed a double-blind, randomized controlled trial evaluating the effect of PRP injection versus a saline injection (deemed a placebo) combined with an eccentric strengthening program on pain, tendon size, and neovascularity. Both groups improved significantly regarding pain and sonographic outcomes at 12 months without a significant difference between treatment groups.[109,110] A review of the literature conducted by Sadoghi and colleagues[111] found no well-designed in vivo evidence to support the use of platelet therapy in chronic Achilles tendinopathy among the 4 studies meeting criteria. A subsequent review by Kaux and Crielaard[112] highlighted the conflicting results found in several studies examining the clinical effects of PRP injection to the Achilles and other tendon targets, as well as the challenges of controlling variables such as preinjection and postinjection rehabilitation, timing of follow-up, injectate quality, and design of a proper control. Overall, these mixed results highlight the complex nature of tendon healing and the need for further research.

Rehabilitation Following PRP

The use of PRP in the treatment of musculotendinous injuries involves a postprocedure rehabilitation plan that is specific to the treated structure. In general, the affected area is treated as though a new tissue injury has occurred and rehabilitation follows a stepwise progression that follows the stages of wound healing as shown in **Table 2**.[102,108,113,114]

Table 2
After PRP rehabilitation

Phase	Length of Time	Restrictions	Rehabilitation
Phase I: tissue protection	Days 0–3	Consider NWB or protected WB for lower extremity procedures, especially if in pain No weight training Avoid NSAIDS Limited ice	Relative rest Activities as tolerated; avoiding excess loading or stress to treated area Gentle AROM
Phase II: early tissue healing; facilitation of collagen deposition	Days 4–14	Progress to FWB without protective device Avoid NSAIDs Limited ice	Light activities to provide motion to tendon; aerobic exercise that avoids loading of the treated tendon Gentle prolonged stretching Begin treatment on kinetic chain/adjacent regions
	Weeks 2–6	Avoid eccentric exercises Limited NSAIDs Limited ice	Progress weight-bearing activities Low-weight, high-repetition isometrics (pain scale <3/10) Open kinetic chain activities Soft tissue work to tendon with CFM, IASTM Dynamic stretching
Phase III: collagen strengthening	Weeks 6–12	—	Eccentric exercises (keep pain scale <3/10) 2 sets of 15 repetitions 2/d then increase to 3/d Closed kinetic chain activities Plyometrics; proprioceptive training and other sport-specific exercises Progress weight-bearing activities and consider return to sport if pain <3/10
	Months 3+	Reassess improvement; if not >75% improved consider repeat injection and return to phase I	Progress back to functional sport-specific activities with increasing load on tendon as pain allows

Abbreviations: AROM, active range of motion; CFM, cross-friction massage; FWB, full weight bearing; IASTM, instrument-assisted soft tissue massage; NWB, non–weight bearing; WB, weight bearing.

In the immediate postinjection period the inflammatory cascade is activated. Mediators from the injected PRP as well as the body's inherent immunologic response result in a milieu rich in cytokines and growth factors necessary for tissue healing. This phase typically lasts up to 72 hours, during which time patients are advised to use acetaminophen and other oral agents that do not affect the inflammatory cascade for subjective pain relief. There is a theoretic risk of disruption of the fibrin plug that develops during the initial healing response, and, as a result, a degree of immobility of the affected tissue is typically recommended for the first few days, although there is little evidence to refute or support this practice.

Over the following six weeks, the secondary immune response consisting of the sustained recruitment of lymphocytes, polymorphic neutrophils, and macrophages results in proteolytic degradation of injured tissue. Fibroblasts also begin to secrete precursors of the extracellular matrix during this, the proliferative phase. Initial rehabilitation during this phase prepares the tissue for remodeling. After the period of immobilization described earlier, controlled passive range of motion exercises are recommended and evidence exists to suggest that motion and mild stretching guide nascent tendinogenesis and remodeling.[115] At two weeks after injection the patient can begin to undergo soft tissue massage to the affected tendon and can begin low-intensity strengthening exercises, both under the guidance of a physical therapist.

The third and final postinjection phase involves the synthesis, accumulation, and organization of the type I collagen fibers that will make up the nascent healthy tendon.[116] This maturation phase is expected to last several months and the patient should be counseled to allow adequate time for tissue healing. The timing of initiating eccentric strengthening exercise has been debated and positive outcomes have been documented after as early as one week and as late as six weeks.[87,89,117–119] There is some evidence that eccentric loading may subject the injured tendon to excessive force and hinder early angiogenesis. In theory, if performed too early, this could negatively affect the healing cascade.[118] The authors recommend waiting until six weeks after the procedure to initiate eccentric exercise. Return to preinjection athletic pursuits should follow symptomatic improvement, because linear improvements in pain and function are expected during the first six months after the procedure. Over time, continued tendon healing and symptomatic improvement are expected with evidence to support minimal risk of rupture.[91]

Patients typically require no more than one PRP injection in the setting of adequate rest followed by gradually progressive rehabilitation. However, in certain cases, especially in patients who experienced a partial response to the first injection, a second or even a third injection can be considered for continued improvement. Postprocedure evaluation at six to eight weeks commonly finds the patient with only partial benefit, and there is no clear evidence-based protocol regarding reinjection. It has been the author's experience that subjective improvement of greater than 50% at eight weeks and 75% at twelve weeks has been associated with long-term pain relief and functional improvement without the need for additional injections. Further objective sonographic tendon improvements often cannot be visualized at the time of initial follow-up and are generally not used to determine the need for additional injections.[100,103,106] Complete tendon remodeling may take up to two years to occur, leaving the clinician with few objective data to guide the decision to repeat the procedure, which highlights the need for well-designed and well-powered studies to establish injection criteria that leave both physician and patient confident in the expected outcome.

SUMMARY

Pain and dysfunction related to tendinopathy are often refractory to traditionally available treatments and offer a unique challenge to physicians, because no current gold standard treatment exists. Injectable biologics, including PRP, may represent a new modality in conjunction with a multifaceted treatment approach. PRP injections are not associated with the systemic or tendon degradation risks of corticosteroids or the inherent risks of surgery. Basic science studies are promising but have not been replicated with high-powered evidence at the clinical level. Given this promise and the lack of a definitive treatment, further evidence to expand understanding of the role of PRP in the treatment of tendinopathy is needed.

REFERENCES

1. Butler DL, Dressler M, Awad H. Functional tissue engineering: assessment of function in tendon and ligament repair. In: Guilak F, Butler DL, Goldstein SA, et al, editors. Functional tissue engineering. New York: Springer; 2003. p. 213–26.
2. Vailas AC, Tipton CM, Laughlin HL, et al. Physical activity and hypophysectomy on the aerobic capacity of ligaments and tendons. J Appl Physiol Respir Environ Exerc Physiol 1978;44:542–6.
3. Williams JG. Achilles tendon lesions in sport. Sports Med 1986;3:114–35.
4. Puddu G, Ippolito E, Postacchini F. A classification of Achilles tendon disease. Am J Sports Med 1976;4(4):145–50.
5. Khan KM, Cook JL, Bonar F, et al. Histopathology of common tendinopathies. Update and implications for clinical management. Sports Med 1999;27(6): 393–408.
6. Aström M, Rausing A. Chronic Achilles tendinopathy. A survey of surgical and histopathologic findings. Clin Orthop Relat Res 1995;(316):151–64.
7. Pingel J, Fredberg U, Qvortrup K, et al. Local biochemical and morphological differences in human Achilles tendinopathy: a case control study. BMC Musculoskelet Disord 2012;13:53.
8. de Mos M, van El B, DeGroot J, et al. Achilles tendinosis: changes in biochemical composition and collagen turnover rate. Am J Sports Med 2007; 35(9):1549–56.
9. Khan K, Cook J. The painful nonruptured tendon: clinical aspects. Clin Sports Med 2003;22(4):711–25.
10. Hart DA, Frank CB, Bray RC. Inflammatory processes in repetitive motion and overuse syndromes: potential role of neurogenic mechanisms in tendons and ligaments. In: Gordon SL, Blair SJ, Fine LJ, editors. Repetitive motion disorders of the upper extremity. Rosemont (IL): American Academy of Orthopaedic Surgeons; 1995. p. 247–62.
11. Rees JD, Wilson AM, Wolman RL. Current concepts in the management of tendon disorders. Rheumatology 2006;45(5):508–21.
12. Adler SC, Kent KJ. Enhancing healing with growth factors. Facial Plast Surg Clin North Am 2002;10:129.
13. Maffulli N, Khan K, Puddu G. Overuse tendon conditions: time to change a confusing terminology. Arthroscopy 1998;14(8):840–3.
14. Viikari-Juntura E, Shiri R, Solovieva S, et al. Risk factors of atherosclerosis and shoulder pain–is there an association? A systematic review. Eur J Pain 2008; 12(4):412–26.
15. Stephenson AL, Wu W, Cortes D, et al. Tendon injury and fluoroquinolone use: a systematic review. Drug Saf 2013;36:709–21.

16. Janssen I, Steele JR, Munro BJ, et al. The relationship between patellar tendinopathy risk factors and ground reaction forces during cross-over block jump landings. Br J Sports Med 2011;45(5):545.
17. Witvrouw E, Bellemans J, Lysens R, et al. Intrinsic risk factors for the development of patellar tendinitis in an athletic population: a two-year prospective study. Am J Sports Med 2001;29(2):190–5.
18. Steinberg N, Siev-Ner I, Peleg S, et al. Extrinsic and intrinsic risk factors associated with injuries in young dancers aged 8-16 years. J Sports Sci 2012; 30(5):485–95.
19. Butler DL, Grood ES, Noyes FR, et al. Biomechanics of ligaments and tendons. Exerc Sport Sci Rev 1978;6:125–81.
20. Braun S, Millett PJ, Yongpravat C, et al. Biomechanical evaluation of shear force vectors leading to injury of the biceps reflection pulley: a biplane fluoroscopy study on cadaveric shoulders. Am J Sports Med 2010;38: 1015–24.
21. Kannus P, Jozsa L. Histopathological changes preceding spontaneous rupture of a tendon. A controlled study of 891 patients. J Bone Joint Surg Am 1991; 73(10):1507–25.
22. Jones MK, Wang H, Peskar BM, et al. Inhibition of angiogenesis by nonsteroidal anti-inflammatory drugs: insight into mechanisms and implications for cancer growth and ulcer healing. Nat Med 1999;5(12):1418–23.
23. Diegelmann RF, Evans MC. Wound healing: an overview of acute, fibrotic and delayed healing. Front Biosci 2004;9:283–9.
24. Abuzeni P, Alexander RW. Enhancement of autologous fat transplantation with platelet rich plasma. Am J Cosmetic Surg 2001;18:59–70.
25. Crovetti G, Martinellia G, Issia M, et al. Platelet gel for healing cutaneous chronic wounds. Transfus Apher Sci 2004;30(2):145–51.
26. Berghoff W, Pietrzak W, Rhodes R. Platelet-rich plasma application during closure following total knee arthroplasty. Orthopedics 2006;29(7):590–8.
27. DelRossi AJ, Cernaianu AC, Vertrees RA, et al. Platelet-rich plasma reduces postoperative blood loss after cardiopulmonary bypass. J Thorac Cardiovasc Surg 1990;100:281–6.
28. Roback J, Combs M, Grossman B, et al. Technical manual of the American Association of Blood Banks. 16th edition. Bethesda (MD): American Association of Blood Banks; 2008.
29. Marx RE. Platelet-rich plasma: evidence to support its use. J Oral Maxillofac Surg 2004;62:489–96.
30. Marx RE, Carlson ER, Eichstaedt R. Platelet rich plasma: growth factor enhancement for bone grafts. Oral Surg Oral Med Oral Pathol Oral Radiol Endod 1998; 85:638.
31. Eppley BL, Woodell JE, Higgins J. Platelet quantification and growth factor analysis from platelet-rich plasma: implications for wound healing. Plast Reconstr Surg 2004;114(6):1502–8.
32. Heldin C, Westermark B. Mechanism of action and in vivo role of platelet-derived growth factor. Physiol Rev 1999;79(4):1284–301.
33. Molloy T, Wang Y, Murrell G. The roles of growth factors in tendon and ligament healing. Sports Med 2003;33:381–94.
34. Kirchberg K, Lange TS, Klein EC, et al. Induction of β1 integrin synthesis by recombinant platelet derived growth factor (PDGF-AB) correlates with an enhanced migratory response of human dermal fibroblasts to various extracellular matrix proteins. Exp Cell Res 1995;220:29–35.

35. Thomopoulos S, Zaegel M, Das R, et al. PDGF-BB released in tendon repair using a novel delivery system promotes cell proliferation and collagen remodeling. J Orthop Res 2007;25(10):1358–68.

36. Sarkissian M, Lafyatis R. Transforming growth factor and platelet derived growth factor regulation of fibrillar fibronectin matrix formation by synovial fibroblasts. J Rheumatol 1998;25:613–22.

37. De Mos M, van der Windt AE, Jahr H, et al. Can platelet rich plasma enhance tendon repair? A cell culture study. Am J Sports Med 2008;36:1171–8.

38. Kashiwagi K, Mochizuki Y, Yasunaga Y, et al. Effects of transforming growth factor-beta 1 on the early stages of healing of the Achilles tendon in a rat model. Scand J Plast Reconstr Surg Hand Surg 2004;38(4):193–7.

39. Guerguin MJ, Charvet B, Nourissat G, et al. Transcription factor EGR1 directs tendon differentiation and promotes tendon repair. J Clin Invest 2013;123(8):3564–76.

40. Zhang F, Liu H, Stile F, et al. Effect of vascular endothelial growth factor on rat Achilles tendon healing. Plast Reconstr Surg 2003;112(6):1613–9.

41. Fong G, Backman LJ, Andersson G, et al. Human tenocytes are stimulated to proliferate by acetylcholine through an EGFR signaling pathway. Cell Tissue Res 2013;351(3):465–75.

42. Kanbe K, Takagishi K, Chen Q. Stimulation of matrix metalloprotease 3 release from human chondrocytes by the interaction of stromal cell-derived factor 1 and CXC chemokine receptor 4. Arthritis Rheum 2002;46:130–7.

43. Mobasheri A, Shakibaei M. Is tendinitis an inflammatory disease initiated and driven by pro-inflammatory cytokines such as interleukin 1β? Histol Histopathol 2013;28(8):955–64.

44. Harwood FL, Goomer RS, Gelberman RH, et al. Regulation of alpha (v) beta3 and alpha5beta1 integrin receptors by basic fibroblast growth factor and platelet-derived growth factor-BB in intrasynovial flexor tendon cells. Wound Repair Regen 1999;7(5):381–8.

45. Hoying JB, Williams SK. Effects of basic fibroblast growth factor human on microvessel endothelial cell migration on collagen I correlates inversely with adhesion and is cell density dependent. J Cell Physiol 1996;168:294–304.

46. Abrahamsson SO. Similar effects of recombinant human insulin-like growth factor-I and II on cellular activities in flexor tendons of young rabbits: experimental studies in vitro. J Orthop Res 1997;15(2):256–62.

47. Nagy JA, Dvorak AM, Dvorak HF. Vascular hyperpermeability, angiogenesis, and stroma generation. Cold Spring Harb Perspect Med 2012;2(2):a006544.

48. Preissner KT, Reuning U. Vitronectin in vascular context: facets of a multitalented matricellular protein. Semin Thromb Hemost 2011;37(4):408–24.

49. Graziani F, Ivanovski S, Cei S, et al. The in vitro effect of different PRP concentrations on osteoblasts and fibroblasts. Clin Oral Implants Res 2006;17(2):212–9.

50. Weibrich G, Hansen T, Kleis W, et al. Effect of platelet concentration in platelet-rich plasma on peri-implant bone regeneration. Bone 2004;34(4):665–71.

51. Giusti I, Rughetti A, D'Ascenzo S. Identification of an optimal concentration of platelet gel for promoting angiogenesis in human endothelial cells. Transfusion 2009;49(4):771–8.

52. Kevy S, Jacobson M, Mandle R. Defining the composition and healing effect of platelet-rich plasma. Presented at: platelet rich plasma symposium. Hospital for special surgery. NY, USA, August 5, 2010.

53. Haynesworth SE, Kadiyala S, Liang LN. Mitogenic stimulation of human mesenchymal stem cells by platelet release suggest a mechanism for enhancement of

bone repair by platelet concentrates. Presented at the 48th Meeting of the Orthopedic Research Society. Dallas, TX, February 10–13, 2002.

54. Tidball JG. Inflammatory processes in muscle injury and repair. Am J Physiol Regul Integr Comp Physiol 2005;288(2):345–53.

55. Pizza FX, McLoughlin TJ, McGregor SJ, et al. Neutrophils injure cultured skeletal myotubes. Am J Physiol Cell Physiol 2001;281(1):335–41.

56. Pizza FX, Peterson JM, Baas JH, et al. Neutrophils contribute to muscle injury and impair its resolution after lengthening contractions in mice. J Physiol 2005;562(3):899–913.

57. Dainiak N, Cohen CM. Surface membrane vesicles from mononuclear cells stimulate erythroid stem cells to proliferate in culture. Blood 1982;60:583–94.

58. Kapacee Z, Yeung CY, Lu Y, et al. Synthesis of embryonic tendon-like tissue by human marrow stromal/mesenchymal stem cells requires a three-dimensional environment and transforming growth factor β3. Matrix Biol 2010;29(8):668–77.

59. El-Sharkawy H, Kantarci A, Deady J, et al. Platelet-rich plasma: growth factors and pro- and anti-inflammatory properties. J Periodontol 2007;78(4):661–9.

60. Fufa D, Shealy B, Jacobson M, et al. Activation of platelet-rich plasma using soluble type I collagen. J Oral Maxillofac Surg 2008;66(4):684–90.

61. Scherer SS, Tobalem M, Vigato E, et al. Nonactivated versus thrombin-activated platelets on wound healing and fibroblast-to-myofibroblast differentiation in vivo and in vitro. Plast Reconstr Surg 2012;129(1):46e–54e.

62. Han B, Woodell-May J, Ponticiello M, et al. The effect of thrombin activation of platelet-rich plasma on demineralized bone matrix osteoinductivity. J Bone Joint Surg Am 2009;91(6):1459–70.

63. Edlow DW, Sheldon WH. The pH of inflammatory exudates. Proc Soc Exp Biol Med 1971;137(4):1328–32.

64. Leveen HH, Falk G, Borek B, et al. Chemical acidification of wounds: an adjuvant to healing and the unfavorable action of alkalinity and ammonia. Ann Surg 1973;178(6):745–53.

65. Wahlström O, Linder C, Kalén A, et al. Variation of pH in lysed platelet concentrates influence proliferation and alkaline phosphatase activity in human osteoblast-like cells. Platelets 2007;18(2):113–8.

66. Kaltalioglu K, Coskun-Cevher S, Tugcu-Demiroz F, et al. PDGF supplementation alters oxidative events in wound healing process: a time course study. Arch Dermatol Res 2013;305(5):415–22.

67. Carofino B, Chowaniec DM, McCarthy MB, et al. Corticosteroids and local anesthetics decrease positive effects of platelet-rich plasma: an in vitro study on human tendon cells. Arthroscopy 2012;28(5):711–9.

68. Scherb MB, Han SH, Courneya JP, et al. Effect of bupivacaine on cultured tenocytes. Orthopedics 2009;32(1):26.

69. Beitzel K, McCarthy MB, Cote MP, et al. The effect of ketorolac tromethamine, methylprednisolone, and platelet-rich plasma on human chondrocyte and tenocyte viability. Arthroscopy 2013;29(7):1164–74.

70. Baksh N, Hannon CP, Murawski CD, et al. Platelet-rich plasma in tendon models: a systematic review of basic science literature. Arthroscopy 2013;29(3):596–607.

71. Anitua E, Sánchez M, Zalduendo MM, et al. Fibroblastic response to treatment with different preparations rich in growth factors. Cell Prolif 2009;42:162–70.

72. Lyras DN, Kazakos K, Tryfonidis M, et al. Temporal and spatial expression of TGF-beta1 in an Achilles tendon section model after application of platelet-rich plasma. Foot Ankle Surg 2010;16:137–41.

73. McCarrel T, Fortier L. Temporal growth factor release from platelet-rich plasma, trehalose lyophilized platelets, and bone marrow aspirate and their effect on tendon and ligament gene expression. J Orthop Res 2009;27(8):1033–42.

74. Lyras DN, Kazakos K, Georgiadis G, et al. Does a single application of PRP alter the expression of IGF-I in the early phase of tendon healing? J Foot Ankle Surg 2011;50(3):276–82.

75. Zhang J, Middleton KK, Fu FH, et al. HGF mediates the anti-inflammatory effects of PRP on injured tendons. PLoS One 2013;8(6):e67303.

76. Sánchez-Ilárduya MB, Trouche E, Tejero R, et al. Time-dependent release of growth factors from implant surfaces treated with plasma rich in growth factors. J Biomed Mater Res A 2013;101(5):1478–88.

77. Zhang J, Wang JH. Platelet-rich plasma releasate promotes differentiation of tendon stem cells into active tenocytes. Am J Sports Med 2010;38(12):2477–86.

78. Chen L, Dong SW, Liu JP, et al. Synergy of tendon stem cells and platelet-rich plasma in tendon healing. J Orthop Res 2012;30(6):991–7.

79. Kaux JF, Drion PV, Colige A, et al. Effects of platelet-rich plasma (PRP) on the healing of Achilles tendons of rats. Wound Repair Regen 2012;20(5):748–56.

80. Jo CH, Kim JE, Yoon KS, et al. Platelet-rich plasma stimulates cell proliferation and enhances matrix gene expression and synthesis in tenocytes from human rotator cuff tendons with degenerative tears. Am J Sports Med 2012;40(5):1035–45.

81. Bosch G, Moleman M, Barneveld A, et al. The effect of platelet-rich plasma on the neovascularization of surgically created equine superficial digital flexor tendon lesions. Scand J Med Sci Sports 2011;21:554–61.

82. Lyras DN, Kazakos K, Verettas D, et al. The influence of platelet-rich plasma on angiogenesis during the early phase of tendon healing. Foot Ankle Int 2009;30(11):1101–6.

83. Dong Z, Li B, Liu B, et al. Platelet-rich plasma promotes angiogenesis of prefabricated vascularized bone graft. J Oral Maxillofac Surg 2012;70(9):2191–7.

84. Bosch G, van Schie HT, de Groot MW, et al. Effects of platelet-rich plasma on the quality of repair of mechanically induced core lesions in equine superficial digital flexor tendons: a placebo-controlled experimental study. J Orthop Res 2010;28(2):211–7.

85. Kajikawa Y, Morihara T, Sakamoto H, et al. Platelet-rich plasma enhances the initial mobilization of circulation-derived cells for tendon healing. J Cell Physiol 2008;215(3):837–45.

86. Taylor DW, Petrera M, Hendry M, et al. A systematic review of the use of platelet-rich plasma in sports medicine as a new treatment for tendon and ligament injuries. Clin J Sport Med 2011;21(4):344–52.

87. Peerbooms JC, Sluimer J, Bruijn DJ, et al. Positive effect of an autologous platelet concentrate in lateral epicondylitis in a double-blind randomized controlled trial: platelet-rich plasma versus corticosteroid injection with a 1-year follow-up. Am J Sports Med 2010;38(2):255–62.

88. Mishra A, Pavelko T. Treatment of chronic elbow tendinosis with buffered platelet-rich plasma. Am J Sports Med 2006;34(11):1774–8.

89. Thanasas C, Papadimitriou G, Charalambidis C, et al. Platelet-rich plasma versus autologous whole blood for the treatment of chronic lateral elbow epicondylitis: a randomized controlled clinical trial. Am J Sports Med 2011;39(10):2130–4.

90. Mishra AK, Skrepnik NV, Edwards SG, et al. Platelet-rich plasma significantly improves clinical outcomes in patients with chronic tennis elbow: a double-blind,

prospective, multicenter, controlled trial of 230 patients. Am J Sports Med 2014; 42(2):463–71.

91. Gosens T, Peerbooms JC, van Laar W, et al. Ongoing positive effect of platelet-rich plasma versus corticosteroid injection in lateral epicondylitis: a double-blind randomized controlled trial with 2-year follow-up. Am J Sports Med 2011;39(6): 1200–8.

92. Chaudhury S, de La Lama M, Adler RS, et al. Platelet-rich plasma for the treatment of lateral epicondylitis: sonographic assessment of tendon morphology and vascularity (pilot study). Skeletal Radiol 2013;42(1):91–7.

93. Krogh TP, Fredberg U, Stengaard-Pedersen K, et al. Treatment of lateral epicondylitis with platelet-rich plasma, glucocorticoid, or saline: a randomized, double-blind, placebo-controlled trial. Am J Sports Med 2013;41(3):625–35.

94. Behrens SB, Deren ME, Blaine TA. Lateral epicondylitis: an internal comparison in the same patient. Orthopedics 2011;34(4).

95. Malliaras P, Barton CJ, Reeves ND, et al. Achilles and patellar tendinopathy loading programmes: a systematic review comparing clinical outcomes and identifying potential mechanisms for effectiveness. Sports Med 2013;43(4):267–86.

96. Visnes H, Bahr R. The evolution of eccentric training as treatment for patellar tendinopathy (jumper's knee): a critical review of exercise programmes. Br J Sports Med 2007;41(4):217–23.

97. Gosens T, Den Oudsten BL, Fievez E, et al. Pain and activity levels before and after platelet-rich plasma injection treatment of patellar tendinopathy: a prospective cohort study and the influence of previous treatments. Int Orthop 2012;36(9):1941–6.

98. Filardo G, Kon E, Della Villa S, et al. Use of platelet-rich plasma for the treatment of refractory jumper's knee. Int Orthop 2010;34:909–15.

99. Kon E, Filardo G, Delcogliano M, et al. Platelet-rich plasma: new clinical application: a pilot study for treatment of jumper's knee. Injury 2009;40:598–603.

100. Ferrero G, Fabbro E, Orlandi D, et al. Ultrasound-guided injection of platelet-rich plasma in chronic Achilles and patellar tendinopathy. J Ultrasound 2012;15(4): 260–6.

101. Filardo G, Kon E, Di Matteo B, et al. Platelet-rich plasma for the treatment of patellar tendinopathy: clinical and imaging findings at medium-term follow-up. Int Orthop 2013;37(8):1583–9.

102. Mautner K, Colberg RE, Malanga G, et al. Outcomes after ultrasound-guided platelet-rich plasma injections for chronic tendinopathy: a multicenter, retrospective review. PM R 2013;5(3):169–75.

103. Finnoff JT, Fowler SP, Lai JK, et al. Treatment of chronic tendinopathy with ultrasound-guided needle tenotomy and platelet-rich plasma injection. PM R 2011;3(10):900–11.

104. Monto RR. Platelet rich plasma treatment for chronic Achilles tendinosis. Foot Ankle Int 2012;33(5):379–85.

105. Owens RF Jr, Ginnetti J, Conti SF, et al. Clinical and magnetic resonance imaging outcomes following platelet rich plasma injection for chronic midsubstance Achilles tendinopathy. Foot Ankle Int 2011;32(11):1032–9.

106. Gaweda K, Tarczynska M, Krzyzanowski W. Treatment of Achilles tendinopathy with platelet-rich plasma. Int J Sports Med 2010;31(8):577–83.

107. Deans VM, Miller A, Ramos J. A prospective series of patients with chronic Achilles tendinopathy treated with autologous-conditioned plasma injections combined with exercise and therapeutic ultrasonography. J Foot Ankle Surg 2012;51(6):706–10.

108. de Jonge S, de Vos RJ, Weir A, et al. One-year follow-up of platelet-rich plasma treatment in chronic Achilles tendinopathy: a double-blind randomized placebo-controlled trial. Am J Sports Med 2011;39(8):1623–9.

109. de Vos RJ, Weir A, Tol JL, et al. No effects of PRP on ultrasonographic tendon structure and neovascularisation in chronic midportion Achilles tendinopathy. Br J Sports Med 2011;45(5):387–92.

110. de Vos RJ, Weir A, van Schie HT, et al. Platelet-rich plasma injection for chronic Achilles tendinopathy: a randomized controlled trial. JAMA 2010;303(2):144–9.

111. Sadoghi P, Rosso C, Valderrabano V, et al. The role of platelets in the treatment of Achilles tendon injuries. J Orthop Res 2013;31(1):111–8.

112. Kaux JF, Crielaard JM. Platelet-rich plasma application in the management of chronic tendinopathies. Acta Orthop Belg 2013;79(1):10–5.

113. Mautner K, Malanga G, Colberg R. Optimization of ingredients, procedures, and rehabilitation for platelet-rich plasma injections for chronic tendinopathy. Pain Manag 2011;1(6):523–32.

114. Filardo G, Kon E, Buda R, et al. Platelet-rich plasma intra-articular knee injections for the treatment of degenerative cartilage lesions and osteoarthritis. Knee Surg Sports Traumatol Arthrosc 2011;19:528–35.

115. Virchenko O, Aspenberg P. How can one platelet injection after tendon injury lead to a stronger tendon after four weeks? Interplay between early regeneration and mechanical stimulation. Acta Orthop 2006;77(5):806–12.

116. Ohberg L, Alfredson H. Effects on neovascularisation behind the good results with eccentric training in chronic mid-portion Achilles tendinosis? Knee Surg Sports Traumatol Arthrosc 2004;12(5):465–70.

117. Nguyen RT, Borg-Stein J, McInnis K. Applications of platelet-rich plasma in musculoskeletal and sports medicine: an evidence-based approach. PM R 2011;3(3):226–50.

118. Yu J, Park D, Lee G. Effect of eccentric strengthening on pain, muscle strength, endurance, and functional fitness factors in male patients with Achilles tendinopathy. Am J Phys Med Rehabil 2013;92(1):68–76.

119. Murtaugh B, Ihm JM. Eccentric training for the treatment of tendinopathies. Curr Sports Med Rep 2013;12(3):175–82.

The Role of Regenerative Medicine in the Treatment of Sports Injuries

Gerard Malanga, MD[a,b,]*, Reina Nakamurra, MD[a]

KEYWORDS

- Regenerative medicine • Stem cell therapy • Platelet-rich plasma • Biological agents
- Sports injuries • Tendon • Ligament • Cartilage

KEY POINTS

- Regenerative medicine is of particular interest in the treatment of sports injuries, as historical and recent evidence increasingly refute the commonly used treatments of anti-inflammatory medications and corticosteroid injections.
- The use of biological treatments using a patient's own stem cells and growth factors to heal damaged tissues is an attractive option.
- Use of these treatments in conjunction with aggressive/comprehensive rehabilitation may maximize nonsurgical treatments of these various sports injuries.
- More rigorous studies using these biological agents to treat such injuries could potentially change the way most sports injuries are managed.
- The true utility of regenerative medicine for sports injuries will become clearer as more high-quality research is published.

INTRODUCTION

The treatment of sports injuries historically has included the use of the PRICE principle (Protection, Rest, Ice/cold, Compression, and Elevation), analgesics/nonsteroidal anti-inflammatory drugs (NSAIDs), and, commonly, corticosteroids. The PRICE principle, widely used in the initial treatment of soft-tissue sports injury, is thought to generally reduce hemorrhage into the injured area and thereby reduce pain and swelling.[1] Rest is recommended to minimize additional stress or strain to promote healing, while cooling decreases bleeding and ultimately serves as a counterirritant to reduce pain.[2] Both compression and elevation work to control swelling.[2] The clinical basis for the

[a] Department of Physical Medicine & Rehabilitation, Rutgers University-New Jersey Medical School, Newark, NJ 07103, USA; [b] New Jersey Regenerative Institute, 197 Ridgedale Avenue, Cedar Knolls, NJ 07927, USA
* Corresponding author. New Jersey Regenerative Institute, 197 Ridgedale Avenue, Cedar Knolls, NJ 07927.
E-mail address: gmalangamd@hotmail.com

Phys Med Rehabil Clin N Am 25 (2014) 881–895
http://dx.doi.org/10.1016/j.pmr.2014.06.007
1047-9651/14/$ – see front matter © 2014 Elsevier Inc. All rights reserved.

application of the PRICE principle is well supported in experimental studies, though not by randomized controlled clinical trials.[1]

NSAIDs are often used during and after acute injuries, and in chronic overuse injuries to control pain and inflammation.[3] As a class of medications, they have varying effects on inflammation, analgesia, and fever. NSAIDs work to inhibit the cyclooxygenase enzymes from which prostaglandins, prostacyclins, and thromboxanes are produced from arachidonic acid.[4] Cyclooxygenase has 2 isoforms, COX-1 and COX-2.[4] Whereas COX-1 is physiologic and is present in numerous tissues in the body, COX-2 is released in response to injury.[4] This isoform produces compounds that increase temperature, sensitize pain receptors, and play a role in inflammation.[4] NSAIDs are used in sports injuries for their capabilities to inhibit COX-2, and are available as general cyclooxygenase inhibitors or COX-2–specific inhibitors.[4]

NSAIDs have significant side effects, most notably in the upper gastrointestinal tract,[5] which include gastrointestinal perforation/hemorrhage, peptic ulcer disease, abdominal pain, diarrhea, nausea/vomiting, and stricture formation.[5] Other effects such as hypertension, congestive heart failure, renal insufficiency, and hyperkalemia have been reported.[5] Furthermore, ibuprofen may potentially inhibit aspirin's antiplatelet activity.[5] A review of NSAIDs on various acute sports soft-tissue injuries showed that NSAIDs have a modest role in the treatment of acute injuries, without harmful effects when used for a short period.[3] Ibuprofen, celecoxib, and diclofenac decreased synovial fluid levels of tumor necrosis factor α, interleukin-6, and vascular endothelial growth factor (VEGF), which in turn significantly improved patient Western Ontario and McMaster scores in a dose-dependent fashion after 14 days of treatment.[6]

Injectable corticosteroids are another class of medications frequently used to treat sports injuries because of their anti-inflammatory effects. Corticosteroids inhibit cyclooxygenase enzyme isoforms and lipoxygenase, which converts arachidonic acid to leukotrienes.[7] These compounds play a key role in chemotaxis and inflammation, which is the rationale for their ubiquitous use in sports injuries. Side effects include corticosteroid-induced cutaneous atrophy, hyperglucocorticoidism, temporary deterioration of diabetes mellitus, facial flushing, and anaphylaxis.[5]

Historical and recent evidence increasingly refute the commonly used treatments of anti-inflammatory medications and corticosteroid injections for most sports injuries. This view holds particularly true for tendinopathies. Cohen and colleagues[8] revealed that indomethacin and celecoxib had a negative effect on rotator cuff tendon-to-bone healing, and organization of collagen fibrils in a murine model. Coombes and colleagues[9] conducted a meta-analysis on the effect of corticosteroids in various tendons in comparison with other nonsurgical interventions. Although corticosteroids provided short-term (0–12 weeks) benefit, there was a decline in function and increased pain from intermediate (13–26 weeks) to long term (>1 year) for lateral epicondylalgia.[10] Short-term effectiveness for rotator cuff tendon was inconclusive, and no significant difference was noted regarding intermediate and long-term results.[10] There was a short-term decrease in pain for patellar tendon, but not for Achilles tendon.[10] In a randomized placebo-controlled trial of unilateral epicondylalgia, the same group reported that patients treated with corticosteroid injection had poorer outcome and higher recurrence after 1 year.[10] The corticosteroid group had better outcomes than the placebo group at 4 weeks, although this difference was not significant when physical therapy was taken into account. At 26 weeks and 1 year, patients who received corticosteroid had poorer outcomes in comparison with placebo.

Tendinopathy, also referred to as tendinosis, is a very common injury presenting to sports medicine physicians. These injuries have previously been improperly named tendonitis, implying the presence of an inflammatory process.[11] It is now well recognized that chronic tendon complaints are an overuse injury that is degenerative in nature.[8] Contributing factors to tendinopathy pain include excessive load or frequent microtrauma, in addition to intrinsic biomechanical changes predisposing to injury.[8]

The pain accompanying tendinosis was previously thought to be due to inflammation; however, it is now known that tendinosis is histologically characterized by random and disorganized structure, hypercellularity, and neovascularization, and is devoid of inflammatory cells.[8] Although the exact mediators of pain are uncertain, irritants and neurotransmitters seem to play a role; these include lactic acid, glutamate, and substance P.[8]

Healing and repair of a tendon occurs in 3 stages.[8] The inflammatory phase in the first few days is characterized by inflammation and migration of erythrocytes and polymorphonuclear leukocytes.[8] Monocytes and macrophages are also present for phagocytosis of necrotic tissue.[8] Chemokines are released, leading to chemotaxis of tenocytes, which lay down collagen III.[8] This process is followed by the proliferative phase, which is characterized by more collagen III and increased ground substance, lasting several weeks.[8] From week 6 up to 1 year, remodeling takes place.[8] Collagen I is synthesized along the path of stress,[8] followed by scar formation.[8] Ligament and muscle injuries undergo basic stages of healing similar to those of tendons.

Based on the current literature, it is the opinion of the author that NSAIDs play a minor role, if any, in most postacute sports injuries, and may even truncate the healing response by interfering with physiology. A short course, (ie, 7–10 days) may be of benefit during the initial acute inflammatory phase of treatment. Similarly, although corticosteroids may offer short-term relief of symptoms, it is likely more harmful in the long term, for the same reasons.

The key to the successful treatment of most sports injuries, following the control of the initial pain and inflammation phase, is a functional rehabilitation program stressing restoration of normal range of motion, strength, and proprioceptive training, with a gradual return-to-sport program.

REGENERATIVE BIOLOGICAL TREATMENTS

The application of regenerative biological treatments for ailments of the musculoskeletal system emerged in the 1930s.[12] The purpose of regenerative medicine is to heal a pathologic process by augmenting the body's physiology by nature or by means of bioengineering.[12] The current practice of regenerative medicine encompasses prolotherapy, platelet-rich plasma (PRP), and mesenchymal stem cell therapy (**Table 1**).[12]

Table 1	
Various regenerative treatments and their mechanism of action	
Treatment	**Mechanism of Action**
Prolotherapy	Introduce irritating agent Trigger inflammatory cascade Proliferation of fibroblasts, deposition of collagen Healing
Platelet-rich plasma	Degranulation of activated platelets Increased vascular permeability leading to chemotaxis of inflammatory cells Cellular proliferation and formation of extrafibrillar matrix Formation of collagen
Stem cell therapy	Cells differentiate into various cells in the mesenchymal lineage including bone, cartilage, adipose, and other soft tissues

Prolotherapy

Prolotherapy introduces an irritating agent to pathologic tissue to obtain a healing response.[12] It first emerged in the musculoskeletal literature in the 1950s, although the concept has been around since the 1930s and possibly dates back to the time of Ancient Greek and Egyptian medicine.[12] Although the exact mechanism of prolotherapy is uncertain, it is postulated that proliferant solutions increase collagen synthesis and cause transient neurolysis,[12] which is accomplished by cytokines that mediate chemomodulation and chemoneuromodulation.[12] The irritating vehicles, which include hyperosmolar dextrose, zinc sulfate, glycerin, phenol, guaiacol, pumic acid, and sodium morrhuate, are theorized to trigger the inflammatory cascade that ultimately leads to proliferation of fibroblasts and deposition of collagen.[12] Although animal studies on tendons show benefit, the results on ligaments are inconclusive.[12]

In humans, prolotherapy has been shown to be an effective treatment for the symptoms of pain in various sports injuries including groin pain, Achilles tendinosis, and plantar fasciitis.[13–16] In a pilot study including 24 patients with chronic lateral epicondylar pain, Scarpone and colleagues[17] found that an injection of a 10.7% dextrose/14.7% sodium morrhuate solution given every 4 weeks at baseline, 4, and 8 weeks, offered significant improvement in pain and isometric contraction strength 16 weeks after treatment when compared with baseline and controls.

In a randomized study, Yelland and colleagues[14] compared prolotherapy with eccentric loading exercises for Achilles tendinosis. Although there was improved pain in favor of prolotherapy at 6 months, and prolotherapy combined with eccentric loading exercises at 12 months, the differences were not significant in the long term.[14] Despite encouraging results, there are few quality trials with rigorous medical evidence from which to build a general consensus regarding prolotherapy and its use in sports injuries.

Platelet-Rich Plasma

PRP is broadly defined as plasma with platelet concentration higher than baseline.[18,19] However, the concentration of platelets necessary to induce a healing response is thought to require a minimum of 1 million platelets per microliter in 5 mL of plasma.[19–21] This burden necessitates centrifugation of whole blood to separate the various components, which include red blood cells, platelet-poor plasma, and a layer of PRP. Platelets have been well known to participate in blood-clot formation and in modulation of inflammation and healing, achieved through release of various growth factors, cytokines, and chemokines contained in mitochondria, dense granules, α granules, and lysosomal granules.[22] Eicosanoids are also newly synthesized from arachidonic acid, partaking in the process of inflammation.[22] Degranulation of 70% to 95% of growth factors occurs within 10 minutes of activation, with the remainder slowly released over a few days.[19,21] Various methods of processing autologous venous blood exist with the goal of platelet concentration, activation, and release of bioactive proteins.[23]

PRP is typically made in a 2-step centrifugation process.[23] The first cycle separates venous blood into red blood cells, platelet-poor plasma, and a buffy coat.[23] The platelets and leukocytes separate into the buffy coat.[23] The second step isolates the buffy coat from the other 2 layers for application.[23] Because the layers are separated by pipette, this process is subject to human error and therefore is imprecise.

Multiple devices are now available to process PRP, each yielding various concentrations of platelets, white blood cells, and red blood cells. The clinical significance of differing concentrations of cells is uncertain. Mazzocca and colleagues[24] studied the effect of various PRP preparations and concentrations on cells of bone, muscle, and tendon. The investigators were unable to conclude which preparation was best suited to treat the various cell types in vitro, and also noted that a higher concentration of platelets did not necessarily result in better outcomes.

Dense granules contain serotonin, histamine, dopamine, calcium, and adenosine.[20] Serotonin and histamine increase vascular permeability, allowing movement of cells that participate in inflammation to the area.[20] This process results in activation of macrophages and chemotaxis of polymorphonuclear cells.[20] Cellular proliferation and formation of extrafibrillar matrix follows, which leads to formation of collagen.[20] This process works in synergy with other growth factors and cytokines released from platelets.

The α granules in platelets are mostly composed of transforming growth factor β (TGFβ), platelet-derived growth factor (PDGF), insulin-like growth factor (IGF I and II), β fibroblast growth factor (βFGF), epidermal growth factor, VEGF, and endothelial cell growth factor.[20] These various growth factors stimulate angiogenesis, epithelialization, granule tissue formation, extracellular matrix formation, and differentiation of cells.[25]

The main function of IGF-I in inflammation and healing is thought to be in migration and multiplication of fibroblasts, which leads to collagen and extracellular matrix protein synthesis.[26] Although IGF-I is present in all phases of healing and repair, it is most prominent during inflammation and proliferation.[26] Molly and colleagues[26] referenced a study by Sciore and colleagues, who demonstrated an increase of IGF-I and its receptor in rabbit medial collateral ligaments 3 weeks after injury. In transected Achilles tendon of rats, exposure to recombinant IGF-I resulted in improved healing starting 24 hours after injury/exposure to IGF-I, which lasted for 15 days.[27]

The widespread effects of TGF-β include mitosis control, activation and differentiation of mesenchymal stem cells, production and secretion of collagen, migration of endothelial cells, and angiogenesis.[21] TGF-β appears to have a large presence immediately following injury.[26] A study of flexor tendon cells showed that lactic acid, a substance that builds in early response to tissue hypoxia, stimulates TGF-β.[28] Research shows increased levels of TGF-β in the patellar ligament of rats up to 8 weeks after injury.[26] As cited in Molly and colleagues,[26] murine Achilles tendons exposed to cartilage-derived morphogenic protein 2, a growth factor in the TGF-β superfamily, had increased thickness and density in comparison with controls.

Another function of TGF-β1 is in fibrotic differentiation of skeletal muscle.[29] In vitro stimulation of myoblasts with TGF-β1 resulted in a further increase of the cytokine, production of proteins that regulate fibrosis, and formation of scar tissue in murine skeletal muscle.[30]

PDGF is found early in inflammation and stimulates production of growth factors such as IGF-I, in addition to remodeling of tissue.[26] Molly and colleagues[26] reviewed an in vivo study of rat medial collateral ligaments which showed that exposure to PDGF increased the strength, stiffness, and energy required to break the ligament.

The main function of VEGF is angiogenesis.[26] Contrary to previously discussed growth factors, which are most active during the inflammatory phase of healing and repair, VEGF levels are highest in the later phases.[26] As reviewed in Molly and colleagues,[26] VEGF was shown to increase the length and density of vessels in the flexor tendons of canines, from days 3 to 21 after injury.

βFGF plays a key role in angiogenesis, cell proliferation, and migration.[26] An article by Chan and colleagues, reviewed by Molly and colleagues,[26] showed an increase in type III collagen and cellular proliferation with varying doses of βFGF injected into damaged patellar tendons of rats (**Table 2**).

Table 2
Growth factors released from α granules of platelets, and their mechanism of action

Growth Factors Released from α Granules of Platelets	Action
Transforming growth factor β	Mitosis control, activation and differentiation of mesenchymal stem cells, production and secretion of collagen, migration of endothelial cells, angiogenesis, and fibrotic differentiation of skeletal muscle
Platelet-derived growth factor	Stimulates production of growth factors such as IGF-I, in addition to remodeling of tissue
Insulin-like growth factor I (IGF-I)	Migration and multiplication of fibroblasts, which leads to collagen and extracellular matrix protein synthesis
β Fibroblast growth factor	Angiogenesis, cell proliferation, and migration
Vascular endothelial growth factor	Angiogenesis

PRP and muscle

Some animal studies support the use of PRP in muscle strain. Hammond and colleagues[31] looked at the effect of PRP versus platelet-poor plasma on 2 different types of muscle strain, and found that the strain injuries from multiple light strains, previously shown to heal by myogenesis,[30] had better progress and faster return to full function compared with single heavy strain, which repairs by different means.[31] Myogenesis in those treated with PRP was also demonstrated by a significant increase in the number of central nucleated muscle fibers.[31] These central nucleated fibers are generally recognized as an indicator of muscle regeneration.[31] A potential obstacle in achieving healing of muscle tissue with PRP is the presence of TGF-β1, a profibrotic cytokine. Terada and colleagues[32] discovered that PRP and losartan, a TGF-β1 antagonist, provided skeletal muscle healing with minimal fibrosis in a murine model. Despite such promising findings, evidence regarding the clinical utility of PRP on muscle strain is mostly limited to case reports. Therefore, the clinical usefulness of PRP remains uncertain until more high-quality trials with adequate power are performed.

PRP and tendons

The utility of PRP for tendinosis at various anatomic locations has been examined in recent years, with varying results. Finnoff and colleagues[33] conducted a retrospective study on the effect of ultrasound-guided needle tenotomy followed by PRP on chronic tendinosis. The postprocedure ultrasound characteristics were evaluated prospectively. There was a 68% benefit in overall function and 58% improvement in worst-pain an average of 14 months after treatment. Follow-up ultrasonography showed improved echotexture in addition to fewer calcifications and neovessels. In a multicenter, retrospective survey study of PRP, Mautner and colleagues[34] examined patient satisfaction and perceived improvement for various chronic tendinopathies (most commonly lateral epicondyle Achilles and patella tendon). In this study population, there was an average reduction in visual analog scale (VAS) for pain of 74% (7.0 ± 1.8 to 1.8 ± 2). Eighty-five percent of patients were satisfied with their PRP treatment, with 82% reporting "moderate (>50%) to complete" improvement of symptoms at an average of 15 months after the injection. In general, PRP appears to be of benefit for tendinosis, although specific individual tendons achieve a better response (see later discussion).

Rotator cuff In recent years, multiple investigators have evaluated the efficacy of PRP for rotator cuff disorder. Some have studied the ability of PRP to augment the healing of operative rotator cuff repairs,[35–37] whereas others have looked at PRP as a direct treatment for rotator cuff injuries.[38,39] In a prospective, randomized, double-blind study, Weber and colleagues[35] compared recovery from arthroscopic rotator cuff repair with and without application of a platelet-rich fibrin matrix. There were no differences in range of motion, pain, and rate of retear at multiple time points up to 12 weeks postoperatively. In a prospective cohort study, Jo and colleagues[36] found that PRP did not enhance healing from arthroscopic rotator cuff repair in terms of discomfort, strength, movement, function, and satisfaction after 16 months. Similarly, Bergeson and colleagues[37] were unable to show the benefits of a platelet-rich fibrin matrix for arthroscopic rotator cuff repair in comparison with controls. Kesikburun and colleagues[38] compared PRP with saline for the treatment of chronic rotator cuff tendinopathy. There was significant improvement in both groups, with sizeable improvements in both pain and function. All patients underwent a 3-week therapy program 2 days following the injection. There was no difference in discomfort, mobility, quality of life, and disability between the 2 groups.[38] Rha and colleagues[39] compared ultrasound-guided PRP injection with dry needling. Dry needling or 2 PRP injections were performed 4 weeks apart. In contrast to the other studies, there was significant improvement in the Shoulder Pain and Disability Index scores, passive internal rotation, and flexion of patients treated with PRP as early as 6 weeks, which continued until 6 months postinjection. Although the utility of PRP for augmenting postoperative healing may be dubious, there seems to be a role for nonoperative management of rotator cuff tendinopathy.

PRP and the knee

Patellar tendon In a case series of 20 athletes with patellar tendinosis, Kon and colleagues[40] evaluated the effects of a series of 3 PRP injections, each given 15 days apart. The subjects had significantly improved overall function, pain, perception of physical and emotional health, vitality, and a sense of limitation at 6 months.[40] James and colleagues[41] looked at the utility of 2 injections of autologous blood at 4-week intervals, in combination with dry needling. The procedure resulted in significant improvement in the Victorian Institute of Sports Assessment score at follow-up, which averaged approximately 15 months.

Meniscus Ishida and colleagues[42] showed the regenerative properties of PRP on meniscal cells in vitro. The same study demonstrated that in vivo PRP combined with a hydrogel significantly improved healing of surgically produced meniscal lesions in a rabbit model.

Anterior cruciate ligament Murray and colleagues[43] showed that placement of a collagen-PRP framework after central anterior cruciate ligament (ACL) transection and suture repair stimulated healing of ACL as evidenced by histology and biomechanics in pigs.

PRP and Achilles tendon

A randomized, placebo-controlled trial by de Vos and colleagues[44] comparing PRP with saline injection failed to show the benefits of PRP for chronic Achilles tendinopathy after 24 weeks. Both interventions provided statistically significant improvement compared with baseline in terms of pain and level of activity, based on Victorian Institute of Sports Assessment Score A. All patients participated in a standardized therapy program consisting of eccentric loading exercises. However, the difference between the PRP and control groups was not meaningful. On the other hand, Sanchez and colleagues[45] looked at the ability of platelet-rich fibrin to enhance healing of surgically repaired Achilles tendon ruptures. Patients who received the platelet-rich fibrin had improved ankle motion, with faster return to gentle running and sport. Moreover, subjects treated with platelet-rich fibrin returned to preinjury activity levels at a mean interval of 14 weeks, an average of 8 weeks earlier than controls.

PRP and the elbow complex

Ulnar collateral ligament Podesta and colleagues[46] reported the efficacy of PRP for partial ulnar collateral ligament tears in a case series of 34 athletes. Athletes returned to sport after a mean of 12 weeks. In addition, there was a statistically significant improvement in the mean Kerlan-Jobe Orthopedic Clinic Shoulder and Elbow score, and Disabilities of the Arm, Shoulder, and Hand score (DASH) at an average of 70 weeks after treatment. The mean elbow joint-space laxity on valgus stress also improved at follow-up.

Medial and lateral epicondylosis Creaney and colleagues[47] compared PRP and autologous blood injection for tennis elbow resistant to conservative management. Both methods offered significant benefit for pain and function; however, the differences between the interventions were negligible. A similar study of tennis elbow showed statistically significant improvement of the VAS pain score in favor of PRP, compared with autologous blood injection 6 weeks after treatment.[48] Mishra and Pavelko[49] reported the efficacy of PRP 8 weeks after treatment, in comparison with bupivacaine and epinephrine, for chronic elbow tendinosis. The Mayo elbow score and VAS pain score was used to assess outcome. In a randomized controlled trial, Krogh and colleagues[50] compared the effects of saline, glucocorticoid, and PRP on chronic lateral epicondylitis. No significant differences were observed between the groups 3 months after treatment, although patients who received steroid injection reported improved pain compared with saline and PRP 4 weeks following treatment. The investigators concluded that PRP and steroid injections did not result in better recovery when compared with saline injections, although steroid offered benefit in the short term. The potential long-term clinical benefits of PRP were elucidated by a randomized controlled trial by Peerbooms and colleagues.[51] PRP was compared with a corticosteroid injection using VAS pain score and DASH as primary outcomes. A 25% improvement in either score was defined as treatment success. At 4 weeks, patients treated with corticosteroids did better than those with PRP. As time passed, patients treated with PRP started to improve more than those who received steroids. By the time 6 months had passed, there was a meaningful improvement in PRP patients in comparison with those on steroids. This trend continued for up to 1 year. An interesting point is that those treated with corticosteroids, although showing improvement in the short term, started to decline, with minimal improvement at 6-month and 1-year follow-up. The benefits were sustained up to 2 years after treatment, which was shown in a continuation study by Gosens and colleagues.[52]

PRP and osteoarthritis

Osteoarthritis is degenerative in nature, and results from wear of articular cartilage and fibrocartilagenous structures. Growth factors play a role in monitoring the development and maintaining stability of articular cartilage, resulting in a growing interest in PRP as a potential treatment modality. Recent research regarding the utility of PRP in osteoarthritis has been promising. In the laboratory, PRP releasate was shown to reduce the numerous inflammatory effects of interleukin-1β in human chondrocytes.[53] Moreover, Akeda and colleagues[54] demonstrated a statistically significant increase in chondrocyte DNA and collagen synthesis of chondrocytes treated with PRP in comparison with platelet-poor plasma or fetal bovine serum in a porcine model.

In human trials, several case series and cohort studies have shown favorable outcomes of PRP in the treatment of osteoarthritis of the knee.[55] In a prospective case series, Harpern and colleagues[56] found that a cohort of patients with grade I to III osteoarthritis (Kellgren-Lawrence radiographic classification) had better pain, function, and stiffness 6 months and 1 year following PRP.[56] Similar results were obtained in mild to severe osteoarthritis with 2 injections of PRP, 4 weeks apart, at 6 months and 1 year in terms of pain, function, and activity level. A prospective cohort study found that an intra-articular injection of PRP reduced VAS pain scores 6 months following the injection.[57] Increasing age, disease severity, and patellofemoral disease was associated with poorer outcomes. Sampson and colleagues[58] found an upward trend in the relief of pain and symptoms over 1 year in patients treated with a series of PRP injections every 4 months.

The benefits of PRP are also shown in multiple studies comparing PRP with hyaluronic acid (HA) injections. Cerza and colleagues[59] conducted a randomized controlled trial of 4 weekly injections of PRP with HA for grade I to III osteoarthritis (Kellgren-Lawrence radiographic classification). Although overall data showed a superior clinical outcome measured by the Western Ontario and McMaster (WOMAC) score at 4, 12, and 24 weeks, patients with grade III disease did not obtain significant benefit until 12 weeks after treatment. Similarly, in a prospective cohort study by Spakova and colleagues,[60] a series of 3 intra-articular PRP injections significantly improved WOMAC scores after 3 and 6 months in comparison with HA. A retrospective cohort study comparing PRP with HA found a statistically significant improvement in PRP 5 weeks after treatment.[61] Lastly, a prospective cohort study comparing a series of 3 intra-articular injections of PRP, low molecular weight HA, and high molecular weight HA discovered no difference between low molecular weight HA and PRP 2 months after treatment.[62] However, after 6 months, patients treated with PRP were meaningfully improved compared with both types of HA. The investigators observed that outcomes from PRP were similar to those after low molecular weight HA in older patients and worse disease, but were improved in younger subjects with milder disease.[62]

Stem Cells

The most recent and, perhaps, most exciting area of regenerative biological treatments is the use of mesenchymal stem cells in the treatment of various orthopedic conditions. There are various sources of stem cells that have been used for a variety of medical conditions, ranging from embryonic stem cells to human adult stem cells. Embryonic stem cell therapy is subject to significant regulatory and religious issues with potential adverse effects, with no studies supporting its use for orthopedic conditions. Human adult stem cells are available from various tissues including blood, adipose, bone marrow, and synovial tissue. The literature would support bone marrow as the main source and having most published research for orthopedic conditions. Harvesting mesenchymal stem cells (MSCs) from bone marrow is also associated with a lower complication rate in comparison with adipose-derived stem cell extraction. The multipotent nature of MSCs allows them to differentiate into various cells in the mesenchymal lineage, including bone, cartilage, adipose, and other soft tissues.[63]

At present, the literature supporting stem cell therapies for orthopedic conditions consists of some basic science and animal studies along with case reports, case series, and cohort studies in humans.[64]

Kuroda and colleagues[65] described the ability of MSCs to repair a 20 × 30 mm lesion of the medial femoral condyle in a Judo player. Seven months after treatment, the defect was filled with smooth tissue on arthroscopic evaluation. Biopsy of the tissue consisted of layers of fibrous tissue, hyaline-like cartilage, and chondral bone. Imaging studies also displayed filling of the defect, although a minor flaw was still detectable. Symptoms improved dramatically, and the patient resumed the previous level of athleticism. Similar findings were reported by Centeno and colleagues[66] for knee and hip osteoarthritis.[67] The investigators reported that magnetic resonance imaging (MRI) confirmed thickening of cartilage within the hip joint, in addition to resolving bone spur in severe hip osteoarthritis 4 weeks after injection of MSCs in a PRP scaffold.[67] The same group showed thickening of the meniscus and cartilage in a case of knee osteoarthritis at 24 weeks.[68] The patient reported significantly better pain and range of motion.

In addition, there have been case reports from the Regenexx Center regarding the effectiveness of stem cell treatments for patients who have suffered nonretracted ACL tears, with improvement noted clinically and on posttreatment MRI.

A case series of 6 female patients with severe knee osteoarthritis who received intra-articular mesenchymal stem cell injections showed improvement at 6 months and 1 year.[68] The VAS pain score, WOMAC index, and walking distance showed steady improvement until 6 months, followed by a slight decline at 1 year. Repeat MRI evaluation at 6 months showed thicker cartilage and smoother chondral surfaces. A cohort of 30 patients (≥65 years) with knee osteoarthritis underwent arthroscopic lavage and injection of adipose-derived stem cells under arthroscopic guidance.[69] Subjects were followed for 2 years. There was a significant decrease in VAS score at 2 years, and an increase in the Knee Injury and Osteoarthritis Outcome Score at all points of follow-up (3 months, 1 year, and 2 years). Long-term healing was demonstrated by significant improvement in clinical parameters from 1 to 2 years of follow-up. After 2 years, 16 subjects underwent repeat arthroscopy. Compared with baseline, 87.5% had preservation or improvement of the appearance of cartilage. At present there are no prospective, randomized controlled trials with adequate power to elucidate the true clinical value of stem cell therapy. Regenexx has now collected registry data from its multiple centers throughout the United States using a standardized approach to extraction and delivery of bone marrow stem cell therapy for a variety of orthopedic conditions, which includes: osteoarthritis of the shoulder, hip, and knee; meniscal tears of the knee; avascular necrosis of the hip; rotator cuff tears; Achilles tendon tears; and ACL tears. A stratification of patients was performed at the time of these procedures with patients classified as being good, fair, or poor candidates based on a variety of factors including the patient's age, comorbidities, body mass index, activity level, severity of the condition, and so forth, to better determine which patient type best responds to stem cell therapy. The data from this registry have demonstrated that more than 90% of these patients had at least some level of improvement, with those rated good candidates showing 55% to 60 % improvement in pain and function; fair candidates improving on average 45% to 50%, and poor candidates improving by approximately 35%. Recent results from this registry have demonstrated a durability of up to 3 years for these improvements. In addition, in case reports of fluoroscopically placed bone marrow stem cells, there is evidence of healing of partial ACL tears and nonretracted rotator cuff tears on serial MRI (see Regenexx.com.)

Although this area of treatment remains exciting and with great potential, more rigorous research is necessary before any reliable conclusions can be made regarding the role of stem cell therapy in the treatment of severe tendon and cartilage pathologies.

SUMMARY

Regenerative medicine is of particular interest in the treatment of sports injuries, as historical and recent evidence increasingly refute the commonly used treatments of anti-inflammatory medications and corticosteroid injections. The use of biological treatments using a patient's own stem cells and growth factors to heal damaged tissues is an attractive option. These treatments, in conjunction with aggressive/comprehensive rehabilitation, may maximize the nonsurgical treatment of these various sports injuries. This review is by no means a complete review of the literature. There is currently level-1 evidence to support the use of PRP for tendinopathies of the elbow complex and osteoarthritis of the knee. Additional studies appear to demonstrate efficacy in other tendons and ligaments. Although some reports have shown effectiveness, stringent medical evidence is lacking for the use of prolotherapy and stem cell therapy, in addition to PRP for muscle strain, most ligamentous sprains, patellar tendinosis, Achilles tendinosis, and rotator cuff injuries to a certain extent. More rigorous studies using these biological agents to treat such injuries could potentially change the way most sports injuries are managed. The true utility of regenerative medicine for sports injuries will become clearer as more high-quality research is published.

REFERENCES

1. Jarvinen TA, Jarvinen TL, Minna Kaariainen M, et al. Muscle injuries: biology and treatment. Am J Sports Med 2005;33(5):745–62.
2. van den Bekerom MP, Struijs PA, Blankevoort L, et al. What is the evidence for rest, ice, compression, and elevation therapy in the treatment of ankle sprains in adults? J Athl Train 2012;47(4):435–43.
3. Weiler JM. Medical modifiers of sports injury: the use of nonsteroidal anti-inflammatory drugs (NSAIDs) in sports-soft tissue injuries. Clin Sports Med 1992;11(3):625–44.
4. Mehallo CJ, Drezner JA, Bytomski JR. Practical management: nonsteroidal anti-inflammatory drug (NSAID) use in athletic injuries. Clin J Sport Med 2006;16(2): 170–4.
5. Brandt KD. Non selective NSAIDS in diagnosis and nonsurgical management of osteoarthritis. 5th edition. West Islip (NY): Professional Communications Inc; 2010. p. 171–211.
6. Gallelli L, Galasso O, Falcone D, et al. The effects of nonsteroidal anti-inflammatory drugs on clinical outcomes, synovial fluid cytokine concentration and signal transduction pathways in knee osteoarthritis: a randomized open label trial. Osteoarthritis Cartilage 2013;21:1400–8.
7. Katzung and Trevor's pharmacology: examination and board review. 7th edition. New York: McGraw-Hill; 1998. p. 163.
8. Cohen DB, Kawamura S, Ehteshami JR, et al. Indomethacin and celecoxib impair rotator cuff tendon-to-bone healing. Am J Sports Med 2006;34(3):362–9.
9. Coombes BK, Bisset L, Vicenzino B. Efficacy and safety of corticosteroid injections and other injections for management of tendinopathy: a systematic review of randomized controlled trials. Lancet 2010;376:1751–67.
10. Coombes BK, Bisset L, Brooks P, et al. Effect of corticosteroid injection, physiotherapy, or both on clinical outcomes in patients with unilateral lateral epicondalgia: a randomized controlled trial. JAMA 2013;309(5):461–9.
11. Sharma P, Maffulli N. Tendon injury and tendinopathy: healing and repair. J Bone Joint Surg 2005;87(1):187–202.

12. DeChellis DM, Cortazzo MH. Regenerative medicine in the field of pain medicine: prolotherapy, platelet-rich plasma therapy, and stem cell therapy-theory and evidence. Tech Reg Anesth Pain Manag 2011;15(2):74–80.

13. Topol GA, Reeves KD, Hassanein KM. Efficacy of dextrose prolotherapy in elite male kicking-sport athletes with chronic groin pain. Arch Phys Med Rehabil 2005;86:697–702.

14. Yelland MJ, Sweeting KR, Lyftogt JA, et al. Prolotherapy injections for painful Achilles tendinosis: a randomized trial. Br J Sports Med 2011;45:421–8.

15. Topol GA, Reeves DK. Regenerative injection of elite athletes with career-altering chronic groin pain who fail conservative treatment: a consecutive case series. Am J Phys Med Rehabil 2008;87(11):890–902.

16. Ryan MB, Wong AD, Gillies JH. Sonographically guided intratendinous injections of hyperosmolar dextrose/lidocaine: a pilot study for the treatment of chronic plantar fasciitis. Br J Sports Med 2009;43:303–6.

17. Scarpone M, Rabago DP, Zgierska A, et al. The efficacy of prolotherapy for lateral epicondylosis: a pilot study. Clin J Sport Med 2008;18:248–54.

18. Alsousou J, Thompson M, Hulley P, et al. The biology of platelet-rich plasma and its application in trauma and orthopaedic surgery: a review of the literature. J Bone Joint Surg 2009;91(8):987–96.

19. Marx RE. Platelet-rich plasma (PRP): what is PRP and what is not PRP? Implant Dent 2001;10(4):225–8.

20. Foster TE, Pukas BL, Mandelbaum BR, et al. Platelet-rich plasma: from basic science to clinical applications. Am J Sports Med 2009;37(11):2259–72.

21. Lee KS, Wilson JJ, Rabago DP, et al. Musculoskeletal applications of platelet-rich plasma: fad or future? Am J Roentgenol 2011;196:628–36.

22. Anitua E, Andia I, Ardanza B, et al. Autologous platelets as a source of proteins for healing and tissue regeneration. Thromb Haemost 2004;91:4–15.

23. Dohan Ehrenfest DM, Rasmusson L, Albrektsson T. Classification of platelet concentrates: from pure platelet-rich plasma (P-PRP) to leucocyte-and platelet-rich fibrin (L-PRF). Trends Biotechnol 2008;27(3):158–67.

24. Mazzocca AD, McCarthy MB, Chowaniec DM, et al. The positive effects of different platelet-rich plasma methods on human muscle, bone, and tendon cells. Am J Sports Med 2012;40:1742–9.

25. Sampson S, Gerhardt M, Mandelbaum B. Platelet rich plasma injection for musculoskeletal injuries: a review. Curr Rev Musculoskelet Med 2008;1:165–74.

26. Molly T, Wang Y, Murrell GA. The roles of growth factors in tendon and ligament healing. Sports Med 2003;33(5):381–94.

27. Kurtz CA, Loebig T, Anderson DD, et al. Insulin-like growth factor 1 accelerates functional recovery from Achilles tendon injury in a rat model. Am J Sports Med 1999;27(3):363–9.

28. Klein MB, Pham H, Yalamanchi N, et al. Flexor tendon wound healing in vitro: the effect of lactate on tendon cell proliferation and collagen production. J Hand Surg Am 2001;26A:847–54.

29. Li Y, Foster W, Deasy BM, et al. Transforming growth factor-β1 induces the differentiation of myogenic cells into fibrotic cells in injured skeletal muscle: a key event in muscle fibrogenesis. Am J Pathol 2004;164(3):1007–19.

30. Lovering RM, Roche JA, Block RJ, et al. Recovery of function in skeletal muscle following 2 different contraction inducted injuries. Arch Phys Med Rehabil 2007;88:617–25.

31. Hammond JW, Hinton RY, Curl LA, et al. Use of autologous platelet-rich plasma to treat muscle strain injuries. Am J Sports Med 2009;37(6):1135–42.

32. Terada S, Ota S, Kobayashi M, et al. Use of an antifibrotic agent improves the effect of platelet-rich plasma on muscle healing after injury. J Bone Joint Surg Am 2013;95:980–8.

33. Finnoff JT, Fowler SP, Lai JK, et al. Treatment of chronic tendinopathy with ultrasound-guided needle tenotomy and platelet-rich plasma injection. PM R 2011;3:900–11.

34. Mautner K, Colberg RE, Malanga G, et al. Outcomes after ultrasound-guided platelet-rich-plasma injections for chronic tendinopathy: a multicenter, retrospective review. PM R 2013;5:169–75.

35. Weber SC, Kauffman NJ, Parise C, et al. Platelet-rich plasma matrix in the management of arthroscopic repair of the rotator cuff. Am J Sports Med 2012;41(2):263–70.

36. Jo CH, Kim JE, Yoon KS, et al. Does platelet-rich plasma accelerate recovery after rotator cuff repair? Am J Sports Med 2011;39(10):2082–90.

37. Bergeson AG, Tashjian RZ, Greis PE, et al. Effects of platelet-rich fibrin matrix on repair integrity of at-risk rotator cuff tears. Am J Sports Med 2012;40(2):286–93.

38. Kesikburun S, Tan AK, Yilmaz B, et al. Platelet-rich plasma injections in the treatment of chronic rotator cuff tendinopathy: a randomized controlled trial with 1-year follow-up. Am J Sports Med 2013;41(11):2609–16. http://dx.doi.org/10.1177/0363546513496542.

39. Rha DW, Park GY, Kim YK, et al. Comparison of the therapeutic effects of ultrasound-guided platelet-rich plasma injection and dry needling in rotator cuff disease: a randomized controlled trial. Clin Rehabil 2012;27(2):113–22.

40. Kon E, Filardo G, Delcogliano M, et al. Platelet-rich plasma: new clinical application a pilot study for treatment of jumper's knee. Injury 2009;40(6):598–603.

41. James SL, Ali K, Pocock C, et al. Ultrasound guided dry needling and autologous blood injection for patellar tendinosis. Br J Sports Med 2007;41:518–22.

42. Ishida K, Kuroda R, Miwa M, et al. The regenerative effects of platelet-rich plasma on meniscal cells in vitro and its in vivo application with biodegradable gelatin hydrogel. Tissue Eng 2007;13(5):1103–12.

43. Murray MM, Spindler KP, Abreu E, et al. Collagen-platelet rich plasma hydrogel enhances primary repair of the porcine anterior cruciate ligament. J Orthop Res 2007;25(1):81–91.

44. de Vos RJ, Weir A, van Schie HT, et al. Platelet-rich plasma injection for chronic Achilles tendinopathy: a randomized controlled trial. JAMA 2010;303(2):144–9.

45. Sanchez M, Anitua E, Azofra J, et al. Comparison of surgically repaired Achilles tendon tears using platelet-rich fibrin matrices. Am J Sports Med 2007;35(2):245–51.

46. Podesta L, Crow SA, Volkmer D, et al. Treatment of partial ulnar collateral ligament tears in the elbow with platelet-rich plasma. Am J Sports Med 2013;41(7):1687–94.

47. Creaney L, Wallace A, Curtis M, et al. Growth factor-based therapies provide additional benefit beyond physical therapy in resistant elbow tendinopathy: a prospective, single-blind, randomized trial of autologous blood injections versus platelet-rich plasma. Br J Sports Med 2011;45:966–91.

48. Thanasas C, Papadimitriou G, Charalambidis C, et al. Platelet-rich plasma versus autologous whole blood for the treatment of chronic lateral epicondylitis: a randomized controlled clinical trial. Am J Sports Med 2011;39(10):2130–4.

49. Mishra A, Pavelko T. Treatment of chronic elbow tendinosis with buffered platelet-rich plasma. Am J Sports Med 2006;34(11):1774048.

50. Krogh TP, Fredberg U, Stengaard-Pedersen K, et al. Treatment of lateral epicondylitis with platelet-rich plasma, glucocorticoid, or saline. Am J Sports Med 2013;41(3):625–35.

51. Peerbooms JC, Sluimer J, Brujn DJ, et al. Positive effect of an autologous platelet concentrate in lateral epicondylitis in a double-blind randomized controlled trial: platelet-rich plasma versus corticosteroid injection with a 1-year follow-up. Am J Sports Med 2010;38(2):255–62.

52. Gosens T, Peerbooms JC, vanLaar W, et al. Ongoing positive effect of platelet-rich plasma versus corticosteroid injection in lateral epicondylitis. Am J Sports Med 2011;39(6):1200–8.

53. van Buul G, Koevoet WL, Kops N, et al. Platelet-rich plasma releasate inhibits inflammatory processes in osteoarthritic chondrocytes. Am J Sports Med 2011;39(11):2362–73.

54. Akeda K, An HS, Okuma M, et al. Platelet-rich plasma stimulates porcine articular chondrocyte proliferation and matrix biosynthesis. Osteoarthritis Cartilage 2006;14:1272–80.

55. Gobbi A, Karnatzikos G, Mahajan V, et al. Platelet-rich plasma treatment in symptomatic patients with knee osteoarthritis: preliminary results in a group of active patients. Sports Health 2012;4(2):162–72.

56. Harpern B, Chaudhry S, Rodeo SA, et al. Clinical and MRI outcomes after platelet-rich plasma treatment of knee osteoarthritis. Clin J Sport Med 2013; 23(3):238–9.

57. Jang SJ, Kim JD, Cha SS. Platelet-rich plasma (PRP) injections as an effective treatment for early osteoarthritis. Eur J Orthop Surg Traumatol 2013;23:572–80.

58. Sampson S, Reed M, Silvers H, et al. Injection of platelet-rich plasma in patients with primary and secondary knee osteoarthritis: a pilot study. Am J Phys Med Rehabil 2010;89:961–9.

59. Cerza F, Carni S, Carcangiu A, et al. Comparison between hyaluronic acid and platelet-rich plasma, intra-articular infiltration in the treatment of gonarthrosis. Am J Sports Med 2012;40:2822–7.

60. Spakova T, Rosocha J, Lacko M, et al. Treatment of knee joint osteoarthritis with autologous platelet-rich plasma in comparison to hyaluronic acid. Am J Phys Med Rehabil 2012;91(4):1–7.

61. Sanchez M, Anitua E, Azofra J, et al. Intra-articular injection of an autologous preparation rich in growth factors for the treatment of knee OA: a retrospective cohort study. Clin Exp Rheumatol 2008;26:910–3.

62. Kon E, Mandelbaum B, Buda R, et al. Platelet-rich plasma intra-articular injection versus hyaluronic acid viscosupplementations as treatments for cartilage pathology: from early degeneration to osteoarthritis. Arthroscopy 2011;27(11): 1490–501.

63. Steinert AF, Noth U, Tuan RS. Concepts in gene therapy for cartilage repair. Injury 2008;39(Suppl 1):S97–113.

64. Pastides P, Chimutengwende-Gordon M, Maffulli N, et al. Stem cell therapy for human cartilage defects: a systematic review. OsteoArthritis Cartilage 2013;21: 646–54.

65. Kuroda R, Ishida K, Matsumoto T, et al. Brief report: treatment of a full-thickness articular cartilage defect in the femoral condyle of an athlete with autologous bone-marrow stromal cells. OsteoArthritis Cartilage 2007;15:226–31.

66. Centeno CJ, Kisiday J, Freeman M, et al. Partial regeneration of the human hip via autologous bone marrow nucleated cell transfer: a case study. Pain Physician 2006;9:135–7.

67. Centeno CJ, Busse D, Kisiday J, et al. Increased knee cartilage volume in degenerative joint disease using percutaneously implanted, autologous mesenchymal stem cells. Pain Physician 2008;11:343–53.

68. Emadedin M, Aghdami N, Taghiyar L, et al. Intra-articular injection of autologous mesenchymal stem cells in six patients with knee osteoarthritis. Arch Iran Med 2012;15(7):422–8.

69. Koh YG, Choi YJ, Kon SK. Clinical results and second-look arthroscopic findings after treatment with adipose-derived stem cells for knee osteoarthritis. Knee Surg Sports Traumatol Arthrosc 2013. [Epub ahead of print].

Performance-Enhancing Drugs: Understanding the Risks

Caroline K. Hatton, PhD[a],*, Gary A. Green, MD[b], Peter J. Ambrose, PharmD[c]

KEYWORDS

- Anabolic steroids • Blood doping • Dietary supplements • Growth hormone
- Nonanalytical positive doping cases • Sports doping • Stimulants
- Therapeutic use exemptions

KEY POINTS

- The risks associated with taking performance-enhancing drugs concern users other than athletes because the general public, including youth, also takes them.
- The risks go beyond textbook side effects because adverse reactions can be triggered by megadoses, polypharmacy practices, drugs unapproved for human use, and exercise.
- Athletes who need a prohibited substance for legitimate medical reasons can request a Therapeutic Use Exemption with their physician's help.
- A positive anti-doping test is only 1 of 10 ways to commit an anti-doping rule violation.
- Athletes are not the only ones at risk for violating anti-doping rules. Physicians and other entourage members can do so even inadvertently.

INTRODUCTION

Risk in sport takes many shapes, and doping issues add many ways for athletes and their health care professionals to violate the rules. In addition to the adverse effects of misused pharmaceuticals, dopers are at risk for toxicity with black market products unapproved for human use, and clean athletes are at risk for inadvertent doping offenses because of dietary supplement contamination or failure to respect administrative procedures, to give only a few examples. Some unethical physicians deliberately engage in doping activities, as highlighted by occasional sports headlines.

Disclosure Statement: C.K. Hatton and G.A. Green have received payments from Major League Baseball for consultation on anti-doping matters. P.J. Ambrose has received payments from the National Center for Drug Free Sport for drug-testing collections.
[a] Sports Antidoping Science Consultant, PO Box 4795, Culver City, CA 90231, USA; [b] Division of Sports Medicine, Pacific Palisades Medical Group, University of California, Los Angeles, 15200 Sunset Boulevard, Suite 107, Pacific Palisades, CA 90272, USA; [c] Department of Clinical Pharmacy, School of Pharmacy, University of California at San Francisco, 450 Parnassus Avenue, San Francisco, CA 94143, USA
* Corresponding author.
E-mail address: ckhatton@aol.com

Phys Med Rehabil Clin N Am 25 (2014) 897–913
http://dx.doi.org/10.1016/j.pmr.2014.06.013
1047-9651/14/$ – see front matter © 2014 Elsevier Inc. All rights reserved.

However, in this article the case examples were selected to illustrate how even honest physicians and athletes have also had to cope with doping problems.

OVERVIEW
Anti-Doping Programs

Doping is prohibited in most sports. Anti-doping programs should include the following:

- A written drug-testing protocol
- A list of prohibited substances and methods
- A consent form
- A process for athletes to request permission to use a banned substance for legitimate medical treatment (Therapeutic Use Exemption [TUE])
- Sanctions
- An appeal process

Athletes in Olympic sports are subject to the rules of their sports federations, which are signatories to the World Anti-Doping Code.[1] The National Collegiate Athletic Association (NCAA)[2] and professional sports organizations, such as Major League Baseball (MLB)[3] or the National Football League (NFL), also conduct anti-doping programs.

Prohibited Lists

For a given athlete, the relevant prohibited list depends on which sport authority has jurisdiction over the athlete, which may depend on the event. For example, it would be the NCAA Banned Drugs list[4] when competing at the NCAA Championships, but the World Anti-Doping Agency (WADA) Prohibited List[5] at the Olympics.

WADA's harmonization efforts have led sports and national anti-doping organizations (eg, the United States Anti-Doping Agency [USADA]) to accept and implement the Code, including by adopting the WADA Prohibited List. To reflect trends in drug use, WADA updates the list annually as one of its responsibilities for monitoring anti-doping worldwide.

Substances or methods are considered for inclusion on the list if they meet any 2 of the following 3 criteria:

- Scientific evidence of (potential) sport performance enhancement
- Scientific evidence of (potential) health risk
- Violation of the spirit of sport

Alternatively, a single criterion is that the substance or method could mask doping.[1]

One skeleton athlete paid a high price for missing an update. He was using finasteride to treat alopecia and did not notice when WADA banned the drug as a masking agent in 2005. After a positive test and appeal procedures, he was barred from the 2006 Turin Olympics.[6] By 2009, testing advances made it possible to remove finasteride from the banned list.[7]

To help athletes and their entourage stay up to date, WADA makes its list available as an App, USADA helps to manage a global drug reference online database (www. globaldro.org), and the National Center for Drug Free Sport, which manages the NCAA drug testing program, operates the Resource Exchange Center, a drug information service to which anti-doping programs (eg, NCAA, MLB) can subscribe so that their athletes can consult it.[8]

Table 1
World Anti-Doping Agency 2014 prohibited list

Prohibited Substances	Examples
Substances and methods prohibited at all times (in competition and out of competition)	
S0. Nonapproved substances[a]	Rycals (eg, S107, a Ca^{2+} channel stabilizer that improves impaired contractility, such as in heart and skeletal muscle),[9] LH receptor agonists[10]
S1. Anabolic agents	
1. Anabolic androgenic steroids	
a. Exogenous	Stanozolol, nandrolone, methandienone, boldenone, dehydrochloromethyltestosterone[b,c]
b. Endogenous	Testosterone, dehydroepiandrosterone[b]
2. Other anabolic agents	Clenbuterol, tibolone, selective androgen receptor modulators (SARMs)
S2. Peptide hormones, growth factors, and related substances	
1. Erythropoiesis-stimulating agents	Erythropoietin (EPO), darbepoetin[b]
2. Chorionic gonadotropin (CG) and luteinizing hormone (LH) in males	CG, LH[b]
3. Corticotropins	Tetracosactide hexaacetate (Synacthen)
4. Growth hormone (GH) Insulin-like growth factor 1 (IGF-1) Fibroblast growth factors (FGFs) Hepatocyte growth factor (HGF) Mechano growth factors (MGFs) Platelet-derived growth factor (PDGF) Vascular-endothelial growth factor (VEGF)	
S3. β2-Agonists	Terbutaline, salbutamol, fenoterol, salmeterol[b]
S4. Hormone and metabolic modulators	
1. Aromatase inhibitors	Letrozole, androstatrienedione, anastrozole, formestane, androstene-3,6,17-trione (6-oxo)
2. Selective estrogen receptor modulators	Tamoxifen
3. Other antiestrogenic substances	Clomiphene
4. Agents modifying myostatin function(s)	Myostatin inhibitors
5. Metabolic modulators a. Insulins b. Peroxisome proliferator activated receptor δ (PPARδ) agonists (eg, GW 1516), PPARδ-AMP-activated protein kinase (AMPK) axis agonists (eg, AICAR)	PPARδ agonists
S5. Diuretics and other masking agents	Furosemide, hydrochlorothiazide, chlorothiazide, canrenone, acetazolamide, indapamide[b–d]

(continued on next page)

Table 1 (continued)	
Prohibited Substances	**Examples**
Substances and methods prohibited in competition	
S6. Stimulants	Methylhexaneamine (dimethylpentylamine), cocaine, amphetamine, methylphenidate, methamphetamine (D-)[b,c] for some stimulants
S7. Narcotics	Morphine, oxycodone, fentanyl and derivatives, methadone[b]
S8. Cannabinoids	Carboxy-THC, JWH-018, JWH-073[b]
S9. Glucocorticosteroids	Budesonide, prednisolone, prednisone, betamethasone, dexamethasone[b]
M1. Manipulation of blood and blood components	1. Autologous, homologous, or heterologous blood transfusion or red blood cell products administration 2. Enhancement of oxygen transfer: perfluorochemicals, efaproxiral (RSR13) and modified hemoglobin products (eg, hemoglobin-based blood substitutes, microencapsulated hemoglobin products), excluding supplemental oxygen 3. Intravascular blood manipulation
M2. Chemical and physical manipulation	Tampering by urine substitution or adulteration (eg, proteases)
M3. Gene doping	Using polymers of nucleic acids or genetically modified cells
Substances prohibited in particular sports	
P1. Alcohol	
P2. β-Blockers	Metoprolol, atenolol, labetalol, acebutolol, bisoprolol, propranolol, sotalol[b]

[a] Any pharmacologic substance not addressed by any of the other sections of the List and with no current approval for human use by any governmental regulatory health authority.
[b] Examples listed in order of decreasing frequency of identification by laboratories in 2012.[11]
[c] And other substances with a similar chemical structure or similar biological effect(s).
[d] And other substances with similar biological effect(s).
Adapted from WADA. The World Anti-Doping Code. The 2014 prohibited list international standard. Montreal: World Anti-Doping Agency; 2014.

The WADA list[5] (**Table 1**) includes 14 classes of substances and methods. The substances are banned with no threshold (ie, at any urinary concentration), with few exceptions. To cover drugs not named as examples, several classes (eg, steroids, stimulants), include "other substances with a similar chemical structure or similar biological effect(s)."

The 2013-2014 NCAA Banned Drugs list also includes any chemically related substance. As an example of a difference between different organizations' lists, caffeine is banned by the NCAA (if >15 μg/mL urine), but not by WADA, although it is included in WADA's 2014 Monitoring Program to detect abuse patterns.[4,5,12] There is thus a risk for athletes being misinformed about which list applies in competition or at all times, and testing positive.

Therapeutic Use Exemptions

For athletes who need a prohibited drug for legitimate medical reasons, comprehensive anti-doping programs offer a way to request a TUE. WADA rules may allow athletes to possess or use a prohibited substance or method without violating anti-doping rules if the conditions in **Box 1** are satisfied.[13]

Such athletes must provide a statement by an appropriate physician, attesting to the need to use the prohibited substance or method, to treat a documented medical condition. TUE applications must specify dosage, frequency, route, and duration of administration.

TUEs must be obtained before possessing the substance, using it, and potentially testing positive for it at a time when it is banned, whether in competition or during training, so it is best to allow ample time by applying as soon as the need is known. A common reason for delays is that incomplete or illegible applications are returned for resubmission. The TUE committee reviewing the application may need extra time to request additional information or consult other experts. Any change in dosage, frequency, route, or dates of administration requires obtaining a new TUE first. Retroactive TUE approval is possible after emergency treatment or in exceptional circumstances where there has been insufficient time to obtain a TUE first (eg, short-term use of narcotic analgesics).

If possession of a substance or its presence in urine or blood is not consistent with the terms of a TUE, the athlete may be charged with an anti-doping rule violation.[13] Athletes risk committing such violations owing to the inadvertent lack of a TUE, because it was not requested, was requested too late, was requested for the wrong drug, dose, frequency, or duration (start and end date), or was not renewed in time.

What Happens to a Positive Test?

Following a laboratory report of an "adverse analytical finding" (eg, the presence of a prohibited substance in an athlete's sample), the anti-doping organization may impose individual or team sanctions. Appeals are typically subject to arbitration (eg, before the Court of Arbitration for Sport [CAS] in cases involving WADA signatories).[1]

If a prohibited drug is present, a sanction is imposed, regardless of how the drug got there and whether the athlete was aware of it. Strict liability has consistently been upheld by CAS beginning even before the unfortunate case of a gymnast at the 2000 Sydney Olympics. She tested positive for pseudoephedrine, which her team physician had given her for a cold. She lost her gold medal and her appeal to CAS. Her physician was expelled from the Games and barred from the next 2 Olympics.[14,15] In 2004 WADA removed pseudoephedrine from the prohibited list, but global monitoring showed increasing urinary concentrations as evidence of abuse, so in 2010 WADA banned pseudoephedrine again.[16,17]

Box 1
WADA TUE conditions

- The prohibited substance or method is needed to treat a medical condition and withholding such treatment would result in a significant impairment to the athlete's health

- The therapeutic use of the substance or method is highly unlikely to enhance performance beyond returning the athlete to a normal state of health

- That there is no reasonable, permitted alternative must be clinically justified

- The need to use the substance or method is not a consequence of prior doping

Adapted from WADA. World Anti-Doping Program. Therapeutic use exemption guidelines. Montreal: World Anti-Doping Agency; 2012.

SELECTED DRUG CLASSES

The most problematic classes of substances prohibited by WADA are covered here. Stimulants,[18–20] anabolic androgenic steroids,[21] and drugs that enhance oxygen transfer[22] are substantially misused for doping because they enhance performance. Growth hormone is a hotly debated issue.[23] The WADA 2012 statistics[11] list the substances identified in 267,645 samples from more than 90 sports tested by the 34 WADA-accredited laboratories worldwide. The substances most often reported within each class are discussed.

Stimulants

Legitimate medical indications

Among the 5 prohibited stimulants most often identified in athletes' urine samples by WADA-accredited laboratories worldwide are amphetamine, d-methamphetamine, and methylphenidate.[11] Amphetamine and combinations of its derivatives are indicated for the treatment of attention-deficit/hyperactivity disorder (ADHD) and narcolepsy. Methamphetamine is approved for use in weight-loss treatments for simple obesity and for the treatment of ADHD. Methylphenidate indications include the treatment of ADHD, autistic disorder, bipolar disorder, and narcolepsy.[24]

Misuse

Stimulants have enjoyed popularity in a variety of sports owing to their purported ability to increase energy and concentration, and because they enhance performance.[18–20] In the NFL, the "Sunday syndrome" referred to amphetamine highs and lows.[25] In Major League Baseball, "greenies" were the green clobenzorex capsules used in the 1980s and 1990s.

The latest NCAA study of substance abuse by athletes revealed that 5% of athletes across all sports had used amphetamines, ephedrine, or both in the preceding year. Interestingly most of the amphetamine users stated that athletic performance was not their main reason for use. Perhaps it was to improve studying, which may explain why 6% had taken Adderall or Ritalin without a prescription. Almost 8% of male wrestlers had used amphetamines,[26] and clinicians should be aware that athletes use stimulants to lose weight in sports with weight classes.

Adverse effects

The side effects of stimulants are associated with central nervous system[24] and cardiovascular[24,27] stimulation. With amphetamine-like compounds, beyond tremor, tachycardia, insomnia, and other well-known adverse effects, severe effects include myocardial infarction, stroke, and death. Adverse effects of methylphenidate also include Raynaud phenomenon, diaphoresis, and decreased appetite.[24]

The demands of sports can increase the thermogenic effects of stimulants and cause heat illness, perhaps because of increased muscle mass in athletes or because stimulants can reduce skin blood flow and limit cooling. Indeed, ephedrine was a contributing factor in several heat-related deaths of American football players.[28] Exercise can also trigger cardiac arrhythmias, and stimulants, which are arrhythmogenic, heighten such risk.[29] It is imperative for sports medicine professionals to be aware of these complications when assessing athletes, and to know which athletes have TUEs for stimulants.

The stimulant most often reported in athletes' samples by WADA laboratories in 2012 was methylhexaneamine (1,3-dimethylamylamine [DMAA]) in 320 samples.[11] Although DMAA was once marketed as a nasal decongestant,[30] it no longer has any Food and Drug Administration (FDA)-approved medical indication in the United States. Nonetheless, it is sold as a dietary supplement promising weight loss, muscle building, and performance enhancement. In 2012, the FDA began warning supplement manufacturers that products containing DMAA are illegal.[31] By 2013, the FDA had received 86 reports of illnesses and deaths associated with DMAA-containing supplements.[32] The illnesses consisted of cardiac complications and nervous system or psychiatric disorders. One study noted significant blood pressure increases following DMAA consumption.[33] There is also a case report of a young man suffering a cerebral hemorrhage after ingesting DMAA with caffeine and alcohol.[34]

Anabolic Androgenic Steroids

Legitimate indications

The primary therapeutic use of anabolic androgenic steroids (AAS) is to treat testosterone (T) deficiency. T is indicated for the treatment of hypogonadism in males and delayed puberty in adolescent males,[24] and also used to treat symptoms of T deficiency.

Stanozolol, the exogenous AAS most often reported by WADA laboratories in 2012,[11] is approved in the United States for the treatment of hereditary angioedema.[24] It is less androgenic than T.[35] Veterinary stanozolol has been used to treat debilitated horses and to help horses recover from surgery or injuries.[36]

Nandrolone was approved by the FDA for the treatment of anemia in chronic renal failure, and has been used as an off-label treatment for inoperable metastatic breast cancer in women, but it has not been legally available in the United States since 2007.[24] It is less androgenic than T.[35]

Misuse

AAS studies in the 1960s, using replacement or therapeutic doses, found no evidence of an anabolic effect. Not until 1996 did Bhasin and colleagues[21] demonstrate that supraphysiologic doses are required for muscle building. However, athletes knew this well before 1996, as did the government officials running the former German Democratic Republic's systematic sports doping program.[37] Users combine multiple AAS ("stacking"), increase then decrease doses ("pyramiding") during each cycle of use, and cycle on and off to let their hormonal systems recover[38]; take human growth hormone (hGH)[37]; and add drugs to counteract AAS side effects (eg, human chorionic gonadotropin,[37] tamoxifen, and isotretinoin, to limit testicular atrophy, gynecomastia, and acne, respectively).[27]

Because of constant improvements in drug testing in recent decades, athlete AAS use has shifted from pharmaceutical xenobiotics to T, to prohormones, to designer steroids (developed only to elude anti-doping tests).[35,37] Meanwhile, AAS use has spread to the general population. Although legitimate uses are mostly limited to treating hypogonadal men (age >50 years) with T, and AAS are controlled substances, they are widely available through antiaging clinics and the Internet. An online search for "buy anabolic steroids" yielded 2.8 million hits in 2013. A 2007 study of 7500 high school girls found a 5% AAS usage rate.[39] Therefore, clinicians need to maintain suspicion for AAS use by a variety of patients in terms of activity, age, and gender.

AAS have been used in cases of severe burns.[35] However, although athletes often claim that they used AAS to assist in injury recovery, there are no human studies to support this, and it is not a legitimate use of AAS.

Adverse effects

Adverse effects of AAS are well described.[37,38] Physiologic T doses for T replacement are relatively safe, but AAS abusers consume megadoses, risking dose-dependent complications (eg, psychiatric[40]) and the additive effects of multiple AAS and other doping agents.

Although AAS can affect every bodily system, cardiovascular risks are a major concern.[27,41] High-dose AAS can increase total cholesterol[42]; they increase low-density lipoprotein cholesterol and markedly suppress high-density lipoprotein (HDL) cholesterol.[18,27] One author (G.A.G.) has seen an HDL level of less than 10 mg/dL in users of multiple AAS, especially nandrolone. This level represents a major risk factor for coronary artery disease, and there are case reports of myocardial infarctions even in young bodybuilders.[43] AAS have also been used for anemia. One author (G.A.G.) has seen AAS users with a hemoglobin level greater than 18 g/dL to the point that phlebotomies were required to reduce red cell mass.

Liver damage, particularly with the water-soluble, 17-alkylated oral AAS, is due to first-pass metabolism, and can cause elevated liver function test results,[35] peliosis hepatis, and hepatomas.[18] Therefore, liver function tests and hepatic ultrasonography should be part of the evaluation of an AAS user.

Diffuse acne, especially on the chest and back, occurs so often[37] that AAS users combat it by taking oral isotretinoin. Unusual tendon ruptures (eg, triceps,[44] pectoralis major[45]) are generally ascribed to muscle strength exceeding tendon tensile strength.

Men who use large AAS doses may overload the liver and aromatize the excess to estrogens, causing gynecomastia. To counteract it, many AAS users also take antiestrogens (eg, clomiphene)[37] or aromatase inhibitors (eg, anastrozole),[27] ie, drugs never used in the treatment of hypogonadism with replacement doses of T. Estrogen may actually play a prominent role in male libido.[46]

Women can suffer loss or alteration of menses[18,37,38] and virilization.[18,37] Deepening of the voice,[37] male pattern alopecia,[38] and clitoromegaly are often irreversible.[35]

Youth can suffer accelerated puberty and stunted growth from epiphyseal closure.[37,38] Some young men have committed suicide while cycling off AAS.[47,48]

Risks are heightened when users take AAS never approved for human use, such as boldenone, used in veterinary medicine to treat debilitated horses to increase weight and appetite, and to improve performance.[49,50] This agent was identified by WADA laboratories in 63 samples in 2012.[11] The risks are most unpredictable with designer steroids (eg, BALCO's tetrahydrogestrinone).[35]

Enhancement of Oxygen Transfer

Legitimate indications

Recombinant epoetin-α (rHuEPO) is structurally very similar to endogenous erythropoietin (EPO).[24] Darbepoetin-α is a genetically modified EPO with a longer duration of action than epoetin-α.[51] Both are used to treat anemia secondary to chemotherapy, neoplastic disease, and chronic renal failure.[24] Epoetin-α is also approved for use in anemic patients at high risk of blood loss from surgery. It has been used for other conditions associated with anemia. Methoxy polyethylene glycol-epoetin β is a continuous EPO receptor activator (CERA),[24] which can be given once a month and is indicated for the treatment of the anemia of chronic renal failure.

Misuse

Whereas most doping agents have a ceiling effect with respect to performance enhancement, endurance activity is highly dependent on peak oxygen uptake (Vo_{2max}), which depends on hemoglobin mass.[22,52] When winners are determined by small percentages of overall race time, a clinically insignificant difference can have significant sports implications.

Before 1987, "blood doping" by transfusion was the mainstay for athletes attempting to increase red cell mass. Risks involved storage issues, transfusion reactions, and infection. The introduction of rHuEPO in 1987 ushered in a new era of doping.[22]

Because rHuEPO is so similar to natural EPO, it took years to develop a urine test. Meanwhile, athletes had unfettered use of rHuEPO, and this led to an "arms race" of elevated hemoglobins. A cluster of up to 20 deaths among Dutch and Belgian cyclists in the late 1980s led to speculation that rHuEPO may have been involved.[22] By 1997, the International Cycling Federation had adopted a health requirement of a hematocrit less than 50% for males (47% for females), a harm-reduction strategy while awaiting a test for rHuEPO,[53] which took until 2000. In 2001, darbepoetin-α was released and a few competitors were caught using it. In 2003, the BALCO scandal showed that rHuEPO was no longer the province of endurance athletes, as it was also given to sprinters.[54] Athletes also turned to some of the proliferating (foreign pharmaceutical or rogue), nearly identical biosimilar EPOs, and got away with it until WADA adapted identification criteria.[22] Next came very-long-acting CERA.[55] Not surprisingly, athletes had also moved back to the use of blood transfusions, and some were caught.[56]

Adverse effects
Serious adverse effects from the therapeutic use of rHuEPO include myocardial infarction and thromboembolic events.[24] This possibility makes the athlete mentality of "if a little is good, then more is better" particularly dangerous when applied to erythropoietic agents, as suggested by the 1980s cluster of cyclist deaths. Although dopers do not publish their findings, one case report on an athlete seems to link rHuEPO to cerebral thrombosis, and athletes using rHuEPO are at risk for iron disorders and exercise-induced elevated systolic pressure.[22]

Growth Hormone

Legitimate indications
By law, recombinant human growth hormone (rhGH), or somatropin, can be prescribed in the United States only for a few conditions including short stature, Turner syndrome, and Prader-Willi syndrome in children, and in adults, growth hormone (GH) deficiency and wasting in AIDS patients.[57–59]

Misuse
In the United States, the use of rhGH to improve athletic performance, to help with injury recovery, for bodybuilding purposes, and as an antiaging agent are illegal; GH is one of the few drugs that cannot be given legally for off-label indications.[59] Current evidence is vastly insufficient to warrant rhGH use to promote injury healing.[23] However, rhGH is rarely used by itself by antiaging doctors. One author (G.A.G.) has reviewed antiaging clinics cases and has yet to find a case whereby rhGH was not used in combination with AAS. Indeed, 25% of AAS users surveyed admitted to also using rhGH, often in combination with insulin.[60] This finding is consistent with the physiology of hGH, which can become catabolic if not combined with AAS or insulin.[61]

There are no studies demonstrating that hGH alone can increase physical performance in healthy subjects. Reasons for this include underpowered sample sizes, inadequate dosing regimens, and inappropriate subject populations, reminiscent of 1960s AAS research.[23] However, athletes apparently use hGH with AAS, even in low doses of the latter.

Although athletes have been using hGH for many years, its use in the general population far exceeds that of the sports group. United States congressional testimony in 2008 revealed 276 antiaging, rejuvenation, or wellness clinics in the United States that advertised online that they provided hGH,[62] none of which provided legitimate prescriptions. Nevertheless, such clinics have since proliferated. An Internet search for "buy hGH" yielded more than 5 million hits in 2013. In addition, GH-releasing peptides are on the increase.[23]

Adverse effects

Adverse effects of the therapeutic use of hGH include edema, arthralgia, myalgia, anti-social behavior, and depression.[57] Studies of hGH administration in older subjects have documented glucose intolerance, diabetes, and, commonly, carpal tunnel syndrome (caused by median nerve edema).[63] Acromegalics develop a classic coarsening of the bones of the face, hands, and feet. However, acromegalics typically produce slightly increased amounts of GH over many years and may not represent an apt comparison with an athlete on ill-documented high doses over a shorter time,[24,57] which no ethics committee would approve. Thus, the adverse effects of hGH doping remain difficult to ascertain.

Drug Detection in Doping Control

The periods of detectability by current laboratory tests are shown in **Table 2**.

At the Olympics, sample storage for 8 years (to increase to 10 years as of 2015) helps as a deterrent.[1] Retrospective analysis of stored blood samples from the Beijing 2008 Olympics detected CERA use by 5 athletes.[52]

EXTRA RISKS
Dietary Supplements

Most athletes, in their quest for peak performance, use multiple supplements. Many supplements marketed to athletes as "ergogenic" are popular among them.[64] Therefore, dietary supplements may represent the greatest risk of a positive test for any athlete because of their lack of regulation, possible contamination (perhaps resulting from unclean mixing vats, questionable ingredients, or intentional spiking), and mislabeling.[65,66]

Indeed, since the 1990s numerous prohibited substances have been found in a variety of dietary supplements, but not on their labels, including stimulants (eg, DMAA, ephedrines, fenfluramine, methylenedioxymethamphetamine, sibutramine)[31,65,67,68]; AAS (eg, androstenedione, boldenone, dehydrochlormethyltestosterone, dehydroepiandrosterone, methandienone, 19-norandrost-4-enedione, oxandrolone, stanozolol, T); designer AAS (dimethazine, methasterone, prostanozol)[65,67,69–71]; an aromatase inhibitor (androstatrienedione)[65]; and GH-releasing peptide 2.[72] Pharmaceutical human insulin-like growth factor 1, a prohibited GH action mediator, was identified in deer antler velvet supplements, typically marketed as growth promoting.[73]

To protect athletes, USADA[74] and the NCAA[4] emphasize the risks inherent to supplements. The only way to get a 100% guarantee that a supplement will not cause a positive test or adverse effects is to avoid using any supplement at all. The NFL and

---

Table 2
Approximate periods of detectability after last dose

Prohibited Drug Class	Sample Type	Period of Detectability
Stimulants	Urine	A few hours to a few days
Anabolic steroids	Urine	A few hours to a few months
Erythropoiesis-stimulating agents	Urine (blood for CERA)	A day to a few weeks
Growth hormone	Blood	A day to several days

Abbreviation: CERA, continuous EPO receptor activator (methoxy polyethylene glycol-epoetin β).

MLB have partnered with a supplement certification company, NSF International, which conducts manufacturing audits and product testing before certifying that no banned substances from the relevant prohibited list were detected, but does not provide a 100% guarantee against positives nor assesses efficacy.

A swimmer tested positive for clenbuterol, which was found in the supplement she had taken. She withdrew from the 2008 US Olympic Team, and was suspended for 1 year and barred from the 2012 Olympics. She had studied the manufacturer's Web site, which promoted "natural," not "steroidal" bodybuilding, talked to the manufacturer about purity, was told that products were tested by an independent company, consulted her team nutritionist, the US Olympic Committee psychologist, and her coach, obtained the supplements directly from the manufacturer and not from an unknown source, checked for no red flags (eg, no "steroidal" label), and had been taking the supplement for months before testing positive. This course of action may approximate extreme caution, but because she took the supplements despite her hesitation, CAS found her negligent.[75] CAS has acknowledged in more cases that prohibited drugs have come from contaminated supplements.[76]

Meat in Mexico or China

Contamination with clenbuterol, an anabolic agent prohibited in cattle in the United States and Europe, and prohibited by WADA, has caused athletes to test positive after eating meat in Mexico[77,78] or China.[79]

Whereabouts Requirements

Elite athletes are tested in competition (on crossing the finish line) and out of competition (any day at any time, with no advance notice). Together, the 2 types of testing deter doping at all times. To be able to locate athletes with no advance notice, international sports federations and national anti-doping agencies require them to declare their whereabouts in advance of each trimester.[80]

Reactions to whereabouts requirements have ranged from star athletes welcoming them as no big deal[81] to legal challenges to WADA for breaking European Union privacy laws.[82,83] Related risks are the failure to meet requirements (3 missed tests or failures to file acceptable information in 12 months = one anti-doping rule violation) and target testing in case of suspicious whereabouts filings (eg, pattern of last-minute changes).[1,80]

More Ways to Break Anti-Doping Rules

A positive test is far from the only way to break anti-doping rules. The 2015 World Anti-Doping Code[1] defines 10 types of violations (**Box 2**).

One infamous cyclist was stripped of 7 Tour de France titles and banned for life in the absence of any positive test.[84] The risks for athletes who commit anti-doping rule violations also include embarrassment and shame for teammates, coaches, family, and fans.

Physicians and anyone else may be sanctioned for their role in doping or insufficient role in anti-doping. Recall how the team doctor who gave pseudoephedrine to a gymnast was barred from the Olympics.[15]

Another example is that of a national Olympic team physician in the 2002 Salt Lake City Winter Olympics "blood bag affair." Heaps of used blood transfusion paraphernalia found in the cross-country ski and biathlon teams' trash led the International Olympic Committee to throw the book at them, including a strong warning to the physician, whose blissful ignorance of athletes' blood withdrawal and infusion by nonmedical personnel was deemed to have facilitated doping. At the 2006 Torino

---

Box 2
World Anti-Doping Code anti-doping rule violations

- Presence of a prohibited substance or its metabolites or markers in an athlete's sample
- (Attempted) use by an athlete of a prohibited substance or method
- Evading, refusing, or failing to submit to sample collection
- Whereabouts failures
- (Attempted) tampering with any part of doping control
- Possession of a prohibited substance or method
- (Attempted) trafficking in any prohibited substance or method
- (Attempted) administration to any athlete of any prohibited substance or method
- Complicity
- Prohibited association

Adapted from WADA. World Anti-Doping Code 2015—final draft. Montreal: World Anti-Doping Agency; 2014.

Winter Olympics, the same physician left the Games when the Italian police showed up and found more paraphernalia and more people involved than in 2002.[85]

Physicians also risk professional or criminal sanctions when applicable to doping activities, and financial penalties have been imposed on athletes and sport organizations.[86,87]

SUMMARY

The risks associated with deliberate or inadvertent performance-enhancing drug use are an unfortunate reality for physicians and their patients. Physicians need to avoid prescribing errors that might cause competitive patients to test positive, help patients apply for TUEs if they need to take prohibited substances, and caution patients against the dangers of supplements. Physicians must understand doping by athletes and nonathletes, because physicians are in a position of power to help fight doping, a growing public health issue.

Sports doping control is a difficult process involving administrators, physicians, scientists, lawyers, and athletes. It will never catch every doper, yet it is worth the effort so as to maintain an ethical framework for the clean athletes' sake. If doping were allowed, athletes would face 3 choices: (1) take drugs, (2) compete at a disadvantage, or (3) quit the sport. Competitions would not be between athletes, but between their pharmacologists. One only has to look at the German Democratic Republic in the 1970s-1980s to see what sport could become. In fact, most athletes compete cleanly and want strict anti-doping rules. In 2013, several MLB players were suspended for doping offenses and the active players clamored for harsher penalties. Performance-enhancing drugs corrupt the essence of sport, whereas preserving it is at the root of the anti-doping movement.

REFERENCES

1. WADA. World Anti-Doping Code 2015 – Draft - Version 3.0. Available at: http://www.wada-ama.org/Documents/World_Anti-Doping_Program/WADP-The-Code/Code_Review/Code%20Review%202015/WADC-2015-draft-version-3.0.pdf. Accessed January 30, 2014.

2. NCAA. Drug testing. Indianapolis, IN: National Collegiate Athletic Association (NCAA); 2013. Available at: http://www.ncaa.org/health-and-safety/policy/drug-testing. Accessed January 30, 2014.

3. MLB. Major league baseball's joint drug prevention and treatment program. New York, NY: Major League Baseball (MLB); 2016. Available at: http://www.mlb.com/pa/pdf/jda.pdf. Accessed January 30, 2014.

4. NCAA. 2013-14 NCAA banned drugs. 2013. Available at: http://www.ncaa.org/health-and-safety/policy/2013-14-ncaa-banned-drugs. Accessed July 13, 2014.

5. WADA. The World Anti-Doping Code. The 2014 prohibited list international standard. Available at: http://www.wada-ama.org/en/World-Anti-Doping-Program/Sports-and-Anti-Doping-Organizations/International-Standards/Prohibited-List/. Accessed January 30, 2014.

6. CAS. CAS arbitration No. CAS OG 06/001. 2006. Available at: http://www.usada.org/wp-content/uploads/CAS-Decision_Zach-Lund_Feb-20061.pdf. Accessed January 30, 2014.

7. WADA. The World Anti-Doping Code. The 2009 prohibited list international standard. Available at: http://www.wada-ama.org/Documents/World_Anti-Doping_Program/WADP-Prohibited-list/WADA_Prohibited_List_2009_EN.pdf. Accessed January 30, 2014.

8. NCDFS. Resource exchange center. Available at: http://www.drugfreesport.com/rec/. Accessed January 30, 2014.

9. Thevis M, Kuuranne T, Geyer H, et al. Annual banned-substance review: analytical approaches in human sports drug testing. Drug Test Anal 2012;4:2–16.

10. Thevis M, Kuuranne T, Geyer H, et al. Annual banned-substance review: analytical approaches in human sports drug testing. Drug Test Anal 2013;5:1–19.

11. WADA. 2012 anti-doping testing figures report. Available at: http://www.wada-ama.org/Documents/Resources/Testing-Figures/WADA-2012-Anti-Doping-Testing-Figures-Report-EN.pdf. Accessed January 30, 2014.

12. WADA. The 2014 monitoring program. Available at: http://www.wada-ama.org/Documents/World_Anti-Doping_Program/WADP-Prohibited-list/2014/WADA-Monitoring-Program-2014-EN.pdf. Accessed January 30, 2014.

13. WADA. International standard for therapeutic use exemptions. Montreal, Canada: World Anti-Doping Agency (WADA); 2011. Available at: http://www.wada-ama.org/Documents/World_Anti-Doping_Program/WADP-IS-TUE/2011/WADA_ISTUE_2011_revJanuary-2012_EN.pdf. Accessed January 30, 2014.

14. CAS. Arbitration CAS ad hoc division (O.G. Sydney) 00/011 Andreea Raducan/International Olympic Committee (IOC), award of 28 September 2000. Available at: http://arbitrationlaw.com/files/free_pdfs/CAS%2000-011%20AR%20v%20IOC%20Award.pdf. Accessed January 30, 2014.

15. Birchard K. Olympic committee bans doctor after doping case. Lancet 2000;356:1171.

16. WADA. 2010 prohibited list summary of major modifications. Available at: http://www.wada-ama.org/Documents/World_Anti-Doping_Program/WADP-Prohibited-list/WADA_Summary_of_Modifications_2010_EN.pdf. Accessed January 30, 2014.

17. WADA. Additional information in regards to the reintroduction of pseudoephedrine to the 2010 prohibited list. Available at: http://www.wada-ama.org/Documents/World_Anti-Doping_Program/WADP-Prohibited-list/WADA_Additional_Info_Pseudoephedrine_2010_EN.pdf. Accessed January 30, 2014.

18. Catlin DH, Hatton CK. Use and abuse of anabolic and other drugs for athletic enhancement. Adv Intern Med 1991;36:399–424.

19. Gill ND, Shield A, Blazevich AJ, et al. Muscular and cardiorespiratory effects of pseudoephedrine in human athletes. Br J Clin Pharmacol 2000;50:205–13.

20. Hodges K, Hancock S, Currell K, et al. Pseudoephedrine enhances performance in 1500-m runners. Med Sci Sports Exerc 2006;38:329–33.

21. Bhasin S, Storer TW, Berman N, et al. The effects of supraphysiologic doses of testosterone on muscle size and strength in normal men. N Engl J Med 1996; 335:1–7.

22. Catlin DH, Hatton CK. Abuse of recombinant erythropoietins and blood products by athletes. In: Elliott SG, Foote MA, Molineux G, editors. Erythropoietins, erythropoietic factors, and erythropoiesis. Molecular, cellular, preclinical, and clinical biology. 2nd edition. Basel (Switzerland): Birkhäuser; 2009. p. 249–78.

23. Baumann GP. Growth hormone doping in sports: a critical review of use and detection strategies. Endocr Rev 2012;33:155–86.

24. Micromedex healthcare series. DRUGDEX System. Greenwood Village (CO): Truven Health Analytics; 2013. Available at: http://www.micromedexsolutions.com/. Accessed January 30, 2014.

25. Mandell AJ, Stewart KD, Russo PV. The Sunday syndrome: from kinetics to altered consciousness. Fed Proc 1981;40:2693–8.

26. NCAA. National study of substance use trends among NCAA college student-athletes. 2012. Available at: http://www.ncaapublications.com/productdownloads/SAHS09.pdf. Accessed January 30, 2014.

27. Angell PJ, Chester N, Sculthorpe N, et al. Performance enhancing drug abuse and cardiovascular risk in athletes: implications for the clinician. Br J Sports Med 2012;46(Suppl I):i78–84.

28. George AJ. Central nervous system stimulants. Baillieres Best Pract Res Clin Endocrinol Metab 2000;14:79–88.

29. Furlanello F, Bentivegna S, Cappato R, et al. Arrhythmogenic effects of illicit drugs in athletes. Ital Heart J 2003;4:829–37.

30. Cohen PA. DMAA as a Dietary Supplement Ingredient. Arch Intern Med 2012; 172:1038–9.

31. FDA. DMAA in dietary supplements. 2013. Available at: http://www.fda.gov/Food/DietarySupplements/QADietarySupplements/ucm346576.htm. Accessed January 30, 2014.

32. FDA. Stimulant potentially dangerous to health, FDA warns. 2013. Available at: http://www.fda.gov/ForConsumers/ConsumerUpdates/ucm347270.htm. Accessed January 30, 2014.

33. Bloomer RJ, Harvey IC, Farney TM, et al. Effects of 1,3-dimethylamylamine and caffeine alone in combination on heart rate and blood pressure in healthy men and women. Phys Sportsmed 2011;39:111–20.

34. Gee P, Jackson S, Easton J. Another bitter pill: a case of toxicity from DMAA party pills. N Z Med J 2010;123:124–7.

35. Kicman AT. Pharmacology of anabolic steroids. Br J Pharmacol 2008;154: 502–21.

36. Soma LR, Uboh CE, Guan F, et al. Pharmacokinetics of boldenone and stanozolol and the results of quantification of anabolic and androgenic steroids in race horses and nonrace horses. J Vet Pharmacol Ther 2007;30:101–8.

37. Franke WW, Berendonk B. Hormonal doping and androgenization of athletes: a secret program of the GDR. Clin Chem 1997;15:141–6.

38. van Amsterdam J, Opperhuizen A, Hartgens F. Adverse health effects of anabolic-androgenic steroids. Regul Toxicol Pharmacol 2010;57:117–23.

39. Elliot DL, Cheong J, Moe EL, et al. Cross-sectional study of female students reporting anabolic steroid use. Arch Pediatr Adolesc Med 2007;16:572–7.
40. Pagonis TA, Angelopoulos NV, Koukoulis GN, et al. Psychiatric side effects induced by supraphysiological doses of combinations of anabolic steroids correlate to the severity of abuse. Eur Psychiatry 2006;21:551–62.
41. Montisci M, El Mazloum R, Cecchetto G, et al. Anabolic androgenic steroids abuse and cardiac death in athletes: morphological and toxicological findings in four fatal cases. Forensic Sci Int 2012;217:e13–8.
42. Gårevik N, Skogastierna C, Rane A, et al. Single dose testosterone increases total cholesterol levels and induces the expression of HMG CoA Reductase. Subst Abuse Treat Prev Policy 2012;7:12.
43. Wysoczanski M, Rachko M, Bergman SR. Acute myocardial infarction in a young man using anabolic steroids. Angiology 2008;59:376–8.
44. Sollender JL, Rayan GM, Barden GA. Triceps tendon rupture in weight lifters. J Shoulder Elbow Surg 1998;7:151–3.
45. März J, Novotný P. Pectoralis major tendon rupture and anabolic steroids in anamnesis–a case review. Rozhl Chir 2008;87:380–3.
46. Finkelstein JS, Lee H, Burnett-Bowie SA, et al. Gonadal steroids and body composition strength and sexual function in men. N Engl J Med 2013;369:1011–22.
47. Taylor Hooton Foundation. Taylor Hooton. Available at: http://taylorhooton.org/taylor-hooton/. Accessed January 30, 2014.
48. Taylor Hooton Foundation. Efrain Marrero. Available at: http://taylorhooton.org/efrain-marrero/. Accessed January 30, 2014.
49. Houghton E, Maynard S. Chapter 17 - Some aspects of doping and medication control in equine sports. In: Thieme D, Hemmersbach P, editors; In: Hoffmann FB, editor. Doping in Sports. Handbook of experimental pharmacology, vol. 195. Heidelberg (Germany): 2010. p. 369–410.
50. O'Connor JJ, Stillions MC, Reynolds WA, et al. Evaluation of boldenone undecylenate as an anabolic agent in horses. Can Vet J 1973;14:154–8.
51. Kaushansky K, Kipps TJ. Hematopoietic agents: growth factors, minerals, and vitamins. In: Brunton LL, Chabner BA, Knollman BC, editors. Goodman and Gilman's the pharmacologic basis of therapeutics. 12th edition. New York: McGraw-Hill; 2011. p. 1067–99.
52. Stray-Gundersen J, Viderman T, Penttilä I, et al. Abnormal hematologic profiles in elite cross country skiers: blood doping or ? Clin J Sport Med 2003;13:132–7.
53. Union Cycliste Internationale. 40 years of fighting against doping. Aigle, Switzerland: Union Cycliste Internationale; 2001. Available at: http://www.uci.ch/Modules/BUILTIN/getObject.asp?MenuId=&ObjTypeCode=FILE&type=FILE&id=MzIyNjM&LangId=1. Accessed January 30, 2014.
54. USADA. Kelli White – losing to win, vol. 5. Colorado Springs, CO: True Sport; 2005. Issue 2. Available at: http://www.usada.org/wp-content/uploads/spirit_of_sport_q2_2005.pdf. Accessed July 13, 2014.
55. International Olympic Committee. IOC sanctions five athletes who competed in Beijing. 2009. Available at: http://www.olympic.org/content/news/media-resources/manual-news/1999-2009/20091/11/16/ioc-sanctions-five-athletes-who-competed-in-beijing-/. Accessed January 30, 2014.
56. CAS. CAS 2005/A/884 Tyler Hamilton V/USADA & UCI. 2006. Available at: http://www.usada.org/wp-content/uploads/CAS-Decision-Tyler-Hamilton_Feb2006.pdf. Accessed January 30, 2014.

57. Facts & Comparisons eAnswers. Drug facts and comparisons. Indianapolis (IN): Wolters Kluwer Health; 2013. Available at: http://www.factsandcomparisons.com/facts-comparisons-online/. Accessed January 30, 2014.

58. United States Code Title 21 U.S.C. § 333(e)(1). Available at: http://uscode.regstoday.com/21USC_CHAPTER9.aspx#21USC333. Accessed July 14, 2014.

59. DEA. Human growth hormone. 2013. Available at http://www.deadiversion.usdoj.gov/drug_chem_info/hgh.pdf. Accessed January 30, 2014.

60. Parkinson AB, Evans NA. Anabolic androgenic steroids: a survey of 500 users. Med Sci Sports Exerc 2006;38:644–51.

61. Sonksen PH. Insulin, growth hormone and sport. J Endocrinol 2001;170:13–25.

62. Perls T. The growth hormone craze. 2008. Available at: http://oversight-archive.waxman.house.gov/documents/20080212150143.pdf. Accessed January 30, 2014.

63. Blackman MR, Sorkin JD, Münzer T, et al. Growth hormone and sex steroid administration in healthy aged women and men: a randomized controlled trial. JAMA 2002;288:2282–92.

64. Ambrose PJ. Drug use in sports: a veritable arena for pharmacists. J Am Pharm Assoc 2004;44:501–16.

65. Geyer H, Parr MK, Koehler K, et al. Nutritional supplements cross-contaminated and faked with doping substances. J Mass Spectrom 2008;43:892–902.

66. Judkins C, Prock P. Supplements and inadvertent doping - how big is the risk to athletes. Med Sport Sci 2012;59:143–52.

67. De Hon O, Coumans B. The continuing story of nutritional supplements and doping infractions. Br J Sports Med 2007;41:800–5.

68. Wang J, Chen B, Yao S. Analysis of six synthetic adulterants in herbal weight-reducing dietary supplements by LC electrospray ionization-MS. Food Addit Contam Part A Chem Anal Control Expo Risk Assess 2008;25:822–30.

69. van der Merwe PJ, Grobbelaar E. Unintentional doping through the use of contaminated nutritional supplements. S Afr Med J 2005;95:510–1.

70. Geyer H, Parr MK, Mareck U, et al. Analysis of non-hormonal nutritional supplements for anabolic-androgenic steroids - results of an international study. Int J Sports Med 2004;25:124–9.

71. FDA. FDA warns consumers about health risks with healthy life chemistry dietary supplement. Silver Spring, MD: Food and Drug Administration (FDA); 2013. Available at: http://www.fda.gov/newsevents/newsroom/pressannouncements/ucm362799.htm. Accessed January 30, 2014.

72. Kohler A, Thomas A, Geyer H, et al. Non-approved ingredients analyzed in the Cologne Doping Control Laboratory 2009. Drug Test Anal 2010;2:533–7.

73. Cox HD, Eichner D. Detection of human insulin-like growth factor-1 in deer antler velvet supplements. Rapid Commun Mass Spectrom 2013;27:2170–8.

74. USADA. Supplement 411. Available at: http://www.usada.org/supplement411. Accessed January 30, 2014.

75. CAS. Arbitration CAS 2009/A/1870 World Anti-Doping Agency (WADA) v. Jessica Hardy & United States Anti-Doping Agency (USADA), award of 21 May 2010. Available at: http://www.tas-cas.org/d2wfiles/document/4218/5048/0/Award20187020FINAL.pdf. Accessed January 30, 2014.

76. CAS. CAS 2011/A/2384 UCI v. Alberto Contador Velasco & RFEC ad CAS 2011/A/2386 WADA v. Alberto Contador Velasco & RFEC. 2012. and references therein. Available at: http://www.tas-cas.org/d2wfiles/document/5648/5048/0/FINAL20AWARD202012.02.06.pdf. Accessed January 30, 2014.

77. USADA. US cycling athlete, Godby, accepts loss of results. 2013. Available at: http://www.usada.org/us-cycling-athlete-godby-accepts-loss-of-results/. Accessed July 13, 2014.
78. FIFA. Dvorak: an excellent and unique collaboration. 2011. Available at: http://www.fifa.com/aboutfifa/footballdevelopment/medical/news/newsid=1528706/index.html. Accessed January 30, 2014.
79. Guddat S, Fusshöller G, Geyer H, et al. Clenbuterol – regional food contamination a possible source for inadvertent doping in sports. Drug Test Anal 2012;4:534.
80. WADA. International standard for testing. Available at: http://www.wada-ama.org/Documents/World_Anti-Doping_Program/WADP-IS-Testing/2012/WADA_IST_2012_EN.pdf. Accessed January 30, 2014.
81. WADA. Athlete testimonies on whereabouts system. 2009. Available at: http://www.wada-ama.org/Documents/World_Anti-Doping_Program/WADP-IS-Testing/WADA_Athlete_Testimonies_Whereabouts_EN.pdf. Accessed January 30, 2014.
82. FIFpro World Players' Union. WADA "whereabouts" rule breaks EU laws. 2010. Available at: http://www.fifpro.org/news/news_details/1181. Accessed January 30, 2014.
83. ESPN. Belgian group challenges WADA rule. 2009. Available at: http://sports.espn.go.com/oly/news/story?id=3863905. Accessed January 30, 2014.
84. USADA. US Postal Service pro cycling team investigation. 2012. Available at: http://cyclinginvestigation.usada.org/. Accessed January 30, 2014.
85. International Olympic Committee. IOC disciplinary commission recommendations regarding the National Olympic Committee of Austria. Available at: http://www.olympic.org/Documents/Reports/EN/en_report_1182.pdf. Accessed January 30, 2014. http://www.olympic.org/Documents/Reports/EN/en_report_1183.pdf. Accessed July 13, 2014.
86. Fédération Équestre Internationale. FEI tribunal takes a final decision in the prohibited substance case involving the horse CAMIRO. 2008. Available at: http://www.fei.org/news/fei-tribunal-takes-final-decision-prohibited-substance-case-involving-horse-camiro. Accessed January 30, 2014.
87. Yahoo Sports. Kazakhstan fined for multiple doping cases. 2013. Available at: http://sports.yahoo.com/news/kazakhstan-fined-multiple-doping-cases-173846856-spt.html. Accessed January 30, 2014.

Psychosocial Factors in Sports Injury Rehabilitation and Return to Play

CrossMark

Leslie Podlog, PhD[a],*, John Heil, DA[b], Stefanie Schulte, PhD[a]

KEYWORDS

- Cognitions • Social support • Intervention plan • Fear of injury • Denial • Distress
- Pain

KEY POINTS

- Research on psychological factors has found that cognitive appraisals, emotional reactions, and behavioral responses to injury influence the quality and nature of athletes' rehabilitation.
- The 2 most influential social factors influencing athletes' injury rehabilitation are the nature of patient-practitioner interactions and the effectiveness of social support provisions.
- Taking into account the psychological nature of rehabilitation as well as the plethora of demands confronting returning athletes, the need for evaluation of psychological readiness to return is imperative.
- Injury is an emotionally disruptive experience for anyone, but perhaps more so for athletes, especially those for whom sport is central to lifestyle and personal identity.
- There is an extensive array of psychological factors, positive and negative, that play into the recovery process for better or worse.

PART 1: THE RESEARCH LITERATURE
Impact of Psychological Factors on Rehabilitation

Research on psychological factors has found that cognitive appraisals, emotional reactions, and behavioral responses to injury influence the quality and nature of athletes' rehabilitation. Cognitive, emotional, and behavioral factors influencing athletes' rehabilitation are discussed separately in this article.

Cognitions

A range of cognitions has been identified that influence athletes' emotions and behaviors in rehabilitation settings, including attributions for injury occurrence,

---

[a] Department of Exercise and Sport Science, University of Utah, 250 South 1850 East, Room 200, Salt Lake City, UT 84112, USA; [b] Psychological Health Roanoke, 2840 Electric Road, Suite 200, Roanoke, VA 24018, USA
* Corresponding author.
E-mail address: les.podlog@utah.edu

Phys Med Rehabil Clin N Am 25 (2014) 915–930
http://dx.doi.org/10.1016/j.pmr.2014.06.011
1047-9651/14/$ – see front matter © 2014 Elsevier Inc. All rights reserved.
pmr.theclinics.com

self-perceptions following injury, cognitively based coping strategies, and perceived injury benefits. Self-perceptions of esteem and worth have also been shown to diminish following injury in some studies (eg, Leddy and colleagues,[1] 1994) but not in others (eg, Smith and colleagues,[2] 1993). Cognitive appraisals of the potential benefits of injury have been described, including opportunities to develop nonsport interests, viewing injury as a test of character, enhanced appreciation for sport, greater resilience, and enhanced knowledge of the body and technical mastery.[3,4] Quinn and Fallon[5] (1999) found differences in sport self-confidence over the course of rehabilitation, with confidence levels high at the onset of injury, declining during rehabilitation, and increasing with recovery. However, there is little other study of change in appraisal over time and how this is related to recovery.

Emotions

Athletes' emotional reactions to injury include feelings of loss, denial, frustration, anger, and depression (eg, Tracey,[6] 2003). Positive emotions such as happiness, relief, and excitement have been reported as well.[7] The attainment of rehabilitation goals and the prospect of recovery may engender a host of positive emotional responses throughout the course of rehabilitation. It seems that these responses are influenced by a wide array of personal factors (eg, athletic identity, previous injury experience, injury severity, injury type, current injury status) and situational factors (eg, life stress, social support satisfaction, timing of the injury).[2,8–16]

Emotions typically fluctuate in response to rehabilitation progress and/or setbacks (see Brewer,[17] 2007, for a review). Emotional states typically move from negative to positive as athletes progress through their rehabilitation and a return to competition draws nearer. Studies have shown an increase in negative affect as the return to sport approaches, possibly because of anxieties over reinjury, the uncertainty of what lies ahead, as well as concerns that postinjury goals may be unrealized.[18] Return to sport may alternatively be viewed as a functional reality check challenging denial that may have falsely bolstered athlete expectation. In summary, individual differences in emotional response over the course of rehabilitation are varied, complex, and fluctuate with rehabilitation progress and setbacks.

Behaviors

The extent to which athletes use various coping skills (eg, goal setting, imagery, seeking out social support) and adhere to rehabilitation have received the greatest amount of research attention. Personal factors linked to adherence including pain tolerance,[19] self-motivation,[20] tough-mindedness,[21] perceived injury severity,[22] internal health locus of control,[23] self-efficacy,[24,25] and self-esteem[26] have all been positively associated with rehabilitation adherence, whereas mood disturbance[9] and fear of reinjury[27] are negatively associated. Demographic factors such as age have also been found to influence rehabilitation adherence. For example, Brewer and colleagues[28] found that age moderated the relationship between psychological factors and 2 kinds of adherence: home exercise completion and home cryotherapy completion. Older patients were more adherent when they were self-motivated and perceived high levels of social support, whereas younger patients were more adherent when they were highly invested in the athlete role as a source of self-worth.[28]

Adherence has been positively associated with enhanced clinical outcomes such as proprioception, range of motion, joint/ligament stability, muscular strength and endurance, as well as reductions in the subsequent risk of reinjury.[9,17,29–31] However, nonsignificant[32] and negative relationships[31,32] have also been found. The negative relationship in particular is likely a function of methodological problems. Although it is a simple matter to get measures of compliance such as attendance, assessing the more subtle elements such as motivation and psychological coping behaviors is more difficult. Active coping responses such as use of positive self-talk,[33] imagery,[24] goal setting,[34] and seeking out additional information about injury[35] are also associated with adherence. In addition, situational factors, mostly related to perception of treatment, also predict adherence, including a belief in the efficacy of the treatment,[28] information about rehabilitation,[36] the clinical environment,[36] value of rehabilitation to the athlete,[22] and hours a week of sport involvement.[37]

Psychological interventions that have shown efficacy in enhancing the rate or quality of sport injury rehabilitation include goal setting,[34] imagery and relaxation,[38] and stress inoculation.[39] The use of self-directed cognitive coping strategies similarly predict favorable psychosocial outcomes such as accepting injury, focusing on getting better, thinking positively, and using imagery.[10] There is also speculation that psychological factors may expedite the recovery process through neurochemical or physiologic changes such as increased blood flow and enhanced proprioception, muscular endurance and strength, and coordination. However, empirical support for such contentions is lacking.[40]

Social Factors Affecting Injury Rehabilitation

The 2 most influential social factors influencing athletes' injury rehabilitation are the nature of patient-practitioner interactions and the effectiveness of social support provisions.

Patient-practitioner interactions
Patient-practitioner interactions, specifically those between the athlete and athletic trainer/sport physiotherapist, have been found to be crucial factors influencing athletes' psychological state, the quality of their rehabilitation experiences, and eventual treatment outcomes.[41] Given the close proximity and regularity of contact, sport medicine professionals are uniquely positioned to play an influential role in the psychological well-being of injured athletes through behavioral intervention as well as through effective psychological triage and referral.[42,43] Positive behaviors shown by rehabilitation specialists include building patient alliances based on acceptance, genuineness, and empathy[44]; effective communication[45]; counseling[46]; and the provision of social support (discussed in greater detail later).[40] The delineation of athletes' roles (eg, motivation, compliance, communication of concerns) and the establishment of clear expectations also seem to be crucial in optimizing athletes' rehabilitation motivation and adherence.[47] Practitioners may also facilitate rehabilitation by clarifying their own role in the treatment process; specifically, providing clear information about treatment, adequate pain control, and participation in key decisions.[48]

Social support
A wealth of evidence highlights the benefit of social support in coping with difficult life events and facilitating rehabilitation from a variety of ailments (eg, cardiac rehabilitation).[49] The value of social support in a sport injury context is no exception. Social support and assistance from a variety of sources, including sport medicine practitioners, coaches, teammates, and family, may be vital in enhancing injured athletes' resilience and facilitating adaptive coping (eg, Bianco and Eklund,[40] 2001). The athlete may benefit from support expressed by listening to the athlete, acknowledging advances in rehabilitation progress (eg, greater range of motion), providing emotional support, encouraging the achievement of physical-rehabilitation goals, encouraging positive coping, and the personal sharing of practitioners' own experiences and opinions.[50]

Initial research suggests that gender differences may exist with regard to perceptions of available social support. Using a sample of 207 injured athletes (male, 111; female, 96), Mitchell and colleagues[51] found that women reported significantly higher scores than men on the availability of emotional and esteem support, whereas no significant differences were reported for the information and tangible forms of support. The investigators suggested that their findings enhance understanding of the moderating role of gender within the social support process and potential coping actions of male and female athletes during rehabilitation. Further research is needed to examine the moderating influence of other variables influencing perceived social support availability and preferences, including type of sport (team vs individual), level of competition, and cultural differences.

Highlighting the value of social support, Canadian national team skiers reported that social support from coaches and rehabilitation practitioners was important in providing reassurance about getting better, keeping things in perspective, focusing on future opportunities, and encouragement to adhere to the rehabilitation program.[52] US alpine and freestyle skiers in Gould and colleagues'[53] (1997) study similarly thought that their injury recovery was facilitated by coach interest and assistance. Johnston and Carroll[54] (1998) also found that social support from several sources, including coaches and rehabilitation specialists, was beneficial in assisting athletes throughout the injury rehabilitation period. Athletes reported that they needed various forms of social support from the coach and sport medicine practitioner (ie, informational, emotional, and practical) at different points in the recovery period. For example, emotional support was particularly important at the beginning of rehabilitation when athletes were trying to adjust to the severity of their injuries. At the end of rehabilitation, the need for informational support was most salient in ensuring that athletes did not return to sport prematurely. One athlete stated: "At this stage you are raring to go and just want to get back into playing your sport competitively, but you need someone to monitor your re-entry into sport and your training and to make sure you ease back into it and don't re-injure yourself."[54(p277)] It was at this time that some athletes indicated a lack of sport-specific advice, encouragement, and feedback, especially from physiotherapists and coaches.[54,55] For example, athletes indicated that they perceived their coaches to be distant and insensitive to injury, did not provide sufficient or appropriate rehabilitation guidance, and did not show a belief in them.[56] Athletes in a later investigation similarly indicated a lack of (informational) support from coaches and physiotherapists as they were returning to play.[54] Athletes reported receiving insufficient advice, guidance, and information from their coaches about how to train as they reentered the competitive arena.[54] These findings are supported by more recent work[57] that reveals that injured athletes in National Collegiate Athletic Association division II to III were significantly more satisfied with the social support provided by certified athletic trainers (ATCs) than that provided by coaches and teammates. In addition, injured athletes reported that social support provided by ATCs contributed significantly more to their overall well-being.

A lack of social support from relevant individuals such as coaches contradicts the substantial evidence of the benefits discussed earlier.[40] Social support from coaches, family members, and medical practitioners may be essential in assisting athletes in dealing with the demands of injury recovery and complying with the rigors of their rehabilitation regimens.[54] Coaches and sport medicine practitioners are encouraged to stay involved and to provide alternative activities (such as developing special practice routines) so athletes can achieve appropriate clinical outcomes and sport-specific skills as they transition back into training and competition. This ongoing involvement diminishes feelings of isolation from the team, allows athletes to continue to develop in their sports, reduces feelings that athletes are falling behind, and helps maintain confidence in their capabilities when they are returning to their sports.[58]

Performance Concerns Facing Returning Athletes

As the completion of rehabilitation draws near and the prospect of a return to sport approaches, a range of performance concerns may develop. The degree to which athletes experience apprehension regarding the return to sport may be a reflection of the success of the preceding rehabilitation.[59,60] However, psychological recovery from injury does not inevitably ensue following medical clearance to return to sport.[61] A range of psychosocial issues has been documented during the return-to-sport transition including anxieties associated with reinjury, concerns about achieving preinjury levels of athletic proficiency, perceptions of being disconnected from relevant others (eg, coaches, teammates), a lack of athletic identity, and insufficient social support.[3,27] External and internal pressures to return to sport may compound the challenges inherent in this transitional period and further test athletes' coping resources.[62] In addition, athletes may experience self-presentational concerns about the prospect of appearing unfit, incompetent, or lacking in skill.

Methods for Assessing Psychological Readiness to Return

Taking into account the psychological nature of rehabilitation as well as the plethora of demands confronting returning athletes, evaluation of psychological readiness to return is imperative. Several user-friendly assessments exist in the literature that can help guide return-to-sport decisions. These assessments include Creighton and colleagues'[63] 3-step return-to-competition decision-making model, the Injury Psychological Readiness to Return to Sport Scale (I-PRRS) 2009,[64] and the Reinjury Anxiety Inventory.[27] Creighton and colleagues'[63] 3-step return-to-competition decision-making model is a useful heuristic for conceptualizing the various stages of athletes' return to sport as well as key considerations for each step. In step 1 of the model, the health status of the athlete is assessed through the evaluation of medical factors (eg, medical history of the patient, laboratory tests such as radiographs or magnetic resonance imaging, severity of the injury, functional ability, and psychological state). Step 2 involves consideration of the risks associated with participation by assessing variables such as the type of sport played (eg, collision, noncontact), the position played (eg, goalie, forward), the competitive level (eg, recreational, professional), the ability to protect (eg, bracing, taping, padding), and the limb dominance of the patient. Step 3 in the decision-making process includes consideration of nonmedical factors that can influence return-to-competition decisions. Relevant considerations here include the timing in the season (eg, playoffs), pressure from the athlete or others (eg, coach, athlete's family), ability to mask the injury (eg, pain medications), conflict of interest (eg, potential financial gain or loss to the patient or clinician), and fear of litigation (eg, if participation is restricted or permitted). The model provides a framework outlining the complex interaction of factors ultimately contributing to return-to-competition decisions. Using the 3-step process outlined (and the associated considerations of each step) can help guide practitioner decisions regarding athletes' return to play.

The I-PRRS consists of 6 items that ask athletes to rate dimensions of confidence on a scale from 0 to 100. Initial validation of the instrument suggests that it is a reliable and valid measure. Given its concise nature, the I-PRRS can be easily administered by health practitioners in the rehabilitation setting. The 6 items are (1) "My overall confidence to play is...," (2) "My confidence to play without pain is...," (3) "My confidence to give 100% effort is...," (4) "My confidence to not concentrate on the injury is…" (5) "My confidence in the injured body part to handle the demands of the situation is …," and (6) "My confidence in my skill level/ability is…."

The Reinjury Anxiety Inventory is a 28-item measure of 2 factors: anxieties regarding rehabilitation (RIA-R: 15 items; eg, "I am worried about becoming reinjured during rehabilitation," "I feel nervous about becoming reinjured during rehabilitation) and on reentry into competitive sport (RIA-RE: 13 items, eg, "I am worried about becoming reinjured during reentry into competition," "I feel nervous about becoming reinjured during reentry into competition"). Walker and colleagues,[27] (2010) differentiated fear (a flight-or-fight response to danger) from anxiety (uncertainty, worry, or concern), suggesting that anxiety more precisely captures the athlete's state of mind. Reliability measures, as well as face, content, and factorial validity, provide strong preliminary evidence for the psychometric utility of this inventory, rendering it a useful tool in the identification of at-risk athletes.

PART 2: CLINICAL PRACTICES
Diagnosis and Triage

"From an emotional or psychological standpoint, serious injury is one of the most traumatic things that can happen to an athlete. It can take away an athlete's career at any time. It threatens the feelings of invincibility and immortality that everybody who is young has to some degree. Because athletes are so dependent upon their physical skills and because their identities are so wrapped up in what they do, injury can be tremendously threatening to their self-identity." Geoff Petrie, National Basketball Association All Star and Vice President, Basketball Operations.[65]

Injury is an emotionally disruptive experience for anyone, but perhaps more so for athletes, especially those for whom sport is central to lifestyle and personal identity. As a result, distress is commonplace, even though a diagnosable psychological disorder is not typically seen. The 2 key psychological dynamics of distress are loss and threat, both of which are psychological drivers of the challenge of rehabilitation. Loss reflects change in lifestyle that is imposed by injury, that which the athlete used to do but cannot while recovering. Threat relates to the uncertainty of the future. Loss can potentially evolve into subclinical or full-blown depression, whereas threat can evolve similarly into an anxiety disorder. With injury, recovery is not complete until the athlete is psychologically ready to return to play. Just as athletes must progress through a physical healing process, they must also address the psychological consequences of injury and the challenges of rehabilitation. Efforts to conceptualize the psychological recovery process for athletes began with adaptation of Kubler-Ross'[66] (1969) On Death and Dying. This approach is groundbreaking in that it identifies distress not as a disorder but as a normal consequence of an unfortunate situation; however, it has not withstood either empirical or clinical scrutiny. Research in sport psychology has focused more on the prediction of rehabilitation outcomes (eg, adherence) than on models for clinical intervention. Thus, Heil[65] (1993) proposed the affective cycle of injury (**Fig. 1**) as a clinical model that is sensitive to the medically driven

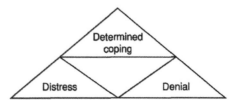

Fig. 1. The affective cycle of injury.

challenges of rehabilitation. It assumes that emotional reactions to injury are cyclical and vary based on daily experiences that create stress or inspiration. The engine of emotion that drives the psychology of rehabilitation has 3 components: (1) distress (eg, loss and threat), (2) denial (unacknowledged distress), and (3) determined coping (vigorous, proactive, goal-driven behavior).

Distress reflects the effects of injury on emotional equilibrium. Denial may be functional when it enables athletes to maintain a positive focus, manage distressing thoughts, or protect themselves from being overwhelmed by negative emotions. Denial is harmful when, for example, failure to recognize the severity of an injury results in poor compliance with a rehabilitation regimen. Determined coping involves moving beyond a resigned sense of acceptance of injury and a passive sense of waiting for the injury to heal. It encompasses exploration, including looking for possibilities, clarifying goals, seeking resources, exploring alternatives, learning new skills, and commitment, such as new focus, vision, teamwork, cooperation, and balance.[67]

The affective cycle of injury assumes that emotional recovery is not a simple linear process, but a cycle that varies over days and weeks, and even within the course of a day. It is useful to envision a macrocycle (which spans the recovery process), minicycles (which are linked to the medical stages of rehabilitation), and microcycles (which reflect the ups and downs of daily life). In the macrocycle of recovery, athletes generally move from distress and denial to determined coping. However, each distinct stage of rehabilitation constitutes a minicycle, which presents new challenges. The microcycle recognizes shifts in emotional response among distress, denial, and determined coping that follow from living with injury. Even as one of the 3 components may predominate in any given stage in rehabilitation, emotional responses typically vary, so that even during periods of determined coping, episodes of denial or distress may appear. Thus, the affective cycle facilitates awareness of and sensitivity to the specific psychological challenges of rehabilitation and how athletes are responding to these challenges.

The Sport Medicine Injury Checklist (**Fig. 2**) is a guide to triage of the injured athlete. The items are not weighted and vary in clinical significance. The checklist simply represents a comprehensive set of factors that offers insight into the psychological status of the athlete and serves as a starting point for triage, diagnosis, and psychological referral, if needed. There is a variety of formal psychological assessment instruments that the psychologist may use in arriving at a diagnostic impression. Inventories such as the Emotional Responses of Athletes to Injury Questionnaire,[27] the aforementioned Reinjury Anxiety Inventory,[27,65,68] and the Coping Responses Inventory[69] may be valuable in gauging athletes' emotions and coping responses during rehabilitation. However, the Sport Medicine Injury Checklist may be particularly germane in a clinical setting, given its easy administration; its provision of visual, direct, and immediate feedback to the sport medicine provider; and the broad range of issues it covers influencing the acute and chronic phases of rehabilitation.

Treatment Intervention

"The more I thought about it, the more cancer seemed like a race to me. Only the destination had changed. They shared grueling physical aspects, as well as a dependence on time, and progress reports every interval, with checkpoints and a slavish reliance on numbers... The idea was oddly restorative: winning my life back would be the biggest victory." Lance Armstrong, World Class Tour Cyclist and Founder, Livestrong Foundation.[70]

A psychologically minded approach to the delivery of medical services is the first line of response to injury and rehabilitation. Facilitating optimal recovery includes

Acute phase

_____ Failure of pain to respond to routine management strategies
_____ Failure of athlete to comply with recommended rehabilitation program
_____ Rehabilitation setbacks
_____ Emotional distress (depression, irritability, confusion, guilt, withdrawal)
_____ Irrational fear or anxiety in specific situations in the otherwise well-adjusted athlete (may be seen as avoidance of feared situation)
_____ Overly optimistic attitude toward injury and recovery
_____ Persistent fatigue
_____ Sleep problems
_____ Gross overestimate or underestimate of rehabilitation progress by athlete

Chronic phase

Current factors
_____ Persistence of pain beyond natural healing
_____ "Odd" descriptions of pain
_____ Inconsistency in "painful" behavior or reports of pain
_____ Failed attempt(s) at return to play
_____ Performance problems following return to play
_____ Inability to identify realistic goals for recovery
_____ Recent stressful changes in sport situation
_____ Stressful life circumstances (within the last year)
_____ Depression (including changes in sleep, appetite, energy, and libido)
_____ Strained relationships with coaches, teammates, or friends
_____ Personality conflicts between treatment providers and athlete
_____ Poor compliance with scheduled visits and medication use
_____ Additional medical treatment sought by athlete without consulting current treatment providers (including emergency room visits)
_____ Iatrogenic problems
_____ Repeated requests for pain (especially psychoactive) medication
_____ Evidence of illicit drug use (recreational or ergogenic)

History
_____ Multiple surgeries at pain site
_____ Chronic pain in the same or another physiological system (may be resolved)
_____ Family members with chronic pain
_____ Problematic psychosocial history (behavior problems in school; vocational, marital, or legal problems; history of physical or sexual abuse)
_____ Problematic psychological history (repeated or prolonged psychological adjustment problems; alcohol/drug problems; eating disorders)

Fig. 2. Sports medicine injury checklist. (_From_ Heil J. Psychology of sport injury. Champaign (IL): Human Kinetics; 1993. p. 133; with permission.)

both being attentive to psychological distress and coaching the athlete on the best path to recovery. Athletes possess a physical intelligence that enables them to be more active agents in the rehabilitation process than general medical patients. As a consequence, they are able to benefit from detailed information about the injury and treatments, and form specific goals and milestones for recovery. As shown in the quote earlier, reframing rehabilitation as an athletic challenge focuses athletes on their strengths and gives them the tools to take control of their rehabilitations. Engaging the athlete in this type of dialogue also builds trust and confidence in the medical provider, which can facilitate adjustment to setbacks and to key transitions in the rehabilitation process, including return to play.

A capsule summary of an intervention plan as might be conducted by a sport psychologist is provided later. The skill-based focus that is unique to sport psychology highlights the expectation that psychological attributes can be cultivated just as physical function can be enhanced. The sport psychologist may be instrumental in addressing the psychological skills listed in the capsule summary, areas in which coaches or teammates may not possess adequate training to address. A detailed discussion of when and where the sport psychologist may be needed during the recovery process is beyond the scope of this article. However, relevant issues may include helping the injured athlete deal with pain and fear (discussed in greater detail later), the reduction of catastrophizing thoughts, reframing negative thoughts and expectations, acting as a source of social support, and liaising between the athlete and various treatment team members. As for the intervention plan, sport psychologists may also provide a range of proactive coping skills that can help injured athletes optimize the likelihood of a safe and successful recovery. A more in-depth review of this plan is available directly from the first and second authors.

Complications

There is an extensive array of psychological factors, positive and negative, that play into the recovery process for better or worse. The psychology of the injured athlete influences both the speed of recovery and the readiness for return to play, or alternatively the transition to a new lifestyle. Because pain and fear are common spoilers in the rehabilitation process, these are discussed in detail. The role of psychological factors in remarkable recovery and as a model for guiding optimal recovery has also been addressed in the literature. Athletes who view the rehabilitation process as a competitive challenge and whose mind-set propels them to new levels of athletic attainment following return to play are said to have achieved a remarkable recovery. For more information see Heil and Podlog[68] (2012).

Pain

"After being injured, I couldn't figure out what pain is good and what is bad. I needed a lot more communication and explanation on the possible types of pains that I might experience. I look back and feel as though there were times where I could have kept training but stopped, and times when I needed to stop, but didn't. Each time it made me feel helpless and lose confidence in my ability in the sport." Iris Zimmermann, Olympic Fencer and Coach.[48]

Pain may emerge as a barrier to rehabilitation: as a potent distractor, as a trigger of anxiety or fear about recovery, or as a question about the efficacy of treatment. In contrast, failure to recognize and accept the limits that pain is signaling can also complicate recovery. Given the complexities of reporting and assessing pain there is the potential for compliance problems to become intertwined with the provider-patient relationship. Failure to respond to pain as a signal of danger or otherwise set reasonable limits on physical activity may also complicate the recovery process. A failure to set limits can indicate a naive enthusiasm but may also reflect a complex set of underlying dynamics, which may manifest as denial[48] or a counterphobic response[71] whereby athletes may push needlessly into pain as a signal of effort or proof of courage.

Pain management in both sport and rehabilitation shares a common skill set: (1) to effectively assess the meaning of pain perceptions, (2) to maintain an appropriate focus in the face of distractions (such as pain perception or catastrophizing cognition), (3) to engage in informed decision making regarding a best course of action, and (4) to regulate the autonomic and other physiologic mechanisms of the pain system.

The pain-sport matrix[65] identifies a four-dimensional strategy that addresses pain assessment, decision making, focusing, and self-regulation. It follows from extensive research with long-distance runners on the psychological strategies of association and dissociation as methods for managing the collective discomfort of pain, fatigue, and exertion during performance.[68,72–74] In this literature, association refers to a focus on relevant performance cues, whereas dissociation implies a specific attempt to detach from the experience of pain.[75]

The pain-sport matrix treats pain and performance as independent dimensions identifying 4 broad classes of pain coping methods, defined by whether the athlete focuses on or focuses away from pain and sport.[68,72] **Fig. 3** provides a visual depiction of the pain-sport matrix. The various types of attentional focus are as follows:

- Associating to both pain and sport can be beneficial when pain signals proper technique. If instead the athlete changes movement patterns to avoid pain, compensatory injury could result.
- Dissociating from both pain and sport during performance is problematic because focus is sacrificed for the sake of pain management. This approach alternatively could be beneficially applied during natural breaks from activity as a way of getting psychological rest from pain or the cognitive demands of sport.
- Dissociating from pain while associating to sports performance is appropriate when pain is understood as routine or benign; otherwise pain becomes a distraction and undermines performance.
- Associating to pain and dissociating from sport is of value in the management of overuse and chronic injury. Because sport performance can fully absorb attention, pain signals may be suppressed to the detriment of athletes' physical well-being. This strategy can be used in breaks between activities to assess pain, or, for example, can be used as a check on muscular guarding.

Fear

"Your mind is racing … you feel your heartbeat pounding in your chest. Your focus is on the heaviness of your breathing and the stream of negative thoughts running through your mind… The image of you falling all the way to the bottom is foremost in your mind." Kathy Kreiner-Phillips, Olympic Alpine Gold Medalist and Sport Psychologist.[64(p114)]

Fear and the risk of injury are integral in sport. As Kreiner-Phillips' comments indicate, fear can take over the moment. In high-risk sports (eg, motor sports, alpine ski racing, X-Games events), the risk of injury and the fear of injury can increase in tandem. However, fear is not necessarily an unhealthy reaction because it can cause athletes to develop a respect for the potential dangers and ensure sensible action. At the same time, fear that consumes athletes puts them at greater risk of injury by creating muscle tension and bracing, tentativeness in execution, and distraction from essential focusing cues. Fear of injury (or reinjury) can range from a routine concern, to a subclinical syndrome, to a diagnosable disorder. The critical task is determining whether fear is benign and simply a distraction, or an indication of a

	Sport	Pain
Association		
Disassociation		

Fig. 3. Pain-sport matrix.

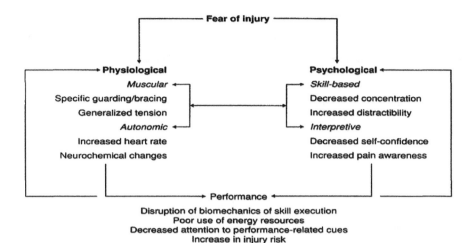

Fig. 4. Fear of injury: a psychophysiologic model of risk.

potential threat. Another test is whether the fear is reasonable and grounded in objective reality or irrational and inappropriate.

The physiologic and psychological elements of the fear response create a complex web of interacting influences. **Fig. 4** shows the ways in which fear can undermine performance and increase injury risk. Fear may elicit a complex set of interacting psychological and physiologic changes. Awareness of autonomic changes or a decrease in concentration may cause athletes to become distracted from their rehabilitation exercises, triggering a downward spiral that results in poor rehabilitation. If fear of reinjury persists as athletes return to sport, they may experience hesitancy, avoidance, poor performance, or muscular guarding (ie, bracing or splinting that either isolates or decreases the mobility of the injured body part), all of which may increase the risk of reinjury. However, if athletes are engaged in a psychologically minded rehabilitation program that both provides detailed information regarding recovery and cultivates confidence, there is a commensurate decrease in fear as they test the formerly injured area in training.

SUMMARY

This article highlights the impact of injury on athletes' psyches. Examination of the research literature revealed the influence of athlete cognitions, emotions, and behaviors on injury rehabilitation processes, as well the impact of the patient-practitioner relationship and social support provisions. Specific performance concerns among returning athletes and tools/inventories for assessing psychological readiness to return to sport are described. The affective cycle of injury as a model for clinical intervention and the Sports Medicine Injury Checklist as a practical guide for assessment and triage are highlighted. A brief overview of the fundamentals of an injury intervention plan (**Box 1**) is provided, and the influence of pain and fear in the rehabilitation process is described. A comprehensive perspective of injury should encompass emotional and cognitive factors as well as physical, functional abilities. The sports medicine professional plays a critical role in psychological assessment and intervention, especially when injury is severe or otherwise complicated.

Box 1
Injury intervention plan

Skill 1: injury education. Providing proactive practical information about injury, healing, and rehabilitation empowers the athlete, cultivates a sense of personal investment in the recovery process, and facilitates compliance with treatment tasks.

Skill 2: rehabilitation and return-to-sport goals. Understanding of rehabilitation goals helps athletes create a sense of personal responsibility and increases their expectations of return to sport by creating a clear path toward recovery.

Skill 3: building the rehabilitation team. Building a team that helps meet the challenges and demands of the new rehabilitation environment helps the athlete overcome feelings of isolation related to separation from the sport/team, and builds confidence in providers, recovery, and return to sport.

Skill 4: managing emotions. Understanding how to identify and cope with the distress inherent in injury helps improve mood and neurovegetative function and modulates the ups and downs of rehabilitation.

Skill 5: visualizing the stages of recovery. Fostering confidence in athletes' ability to cope with injury adversity and endure rehabilitation is driven by depicting a positive future perspective on the recovery process.

Skill 6: focus and distraction control. Facilitating a task focus and providing guidance in distraction control can enable athletes to deal with the uncertainty of rehabilitation and remain appropriately focused on physical, technical, and psychological skills.

Skill 7: working through pain. Managing pain effectively enables the athlete to trust the rehabilitation process, maintain a stable emotional state, and make effective decisions regarding activity and limits.

Skill 8: building confidence in return to play. Accepting fear and treating it as a tool to guide decision making, while cultivating trust in rehabilitation, treatment providers, and self, enables the athlete to transition effectively to sport.

Skill 9: mental toughness and the survival mind-set. Focusing on controlling the controllables (including personal thoughts, feelings, and actions) enable the athlete to gain global skills in coping with adversity and can facilitate remarkable recovery.

Skill 10: becoming a renewed athlete. Assimilating lessons learned from injury and reembracing the aspirations that led to initial participation enable the athlete to return to sport renewed and reinvigorated.

REFERENCES

1. Leddy MH, Lambert MJ, Ogles BM. Psychological consequences of athletic injury among high-level competitors. Res Q Exerc Sport 1994;65(4):347–54.
2. Smith AM, Stuart MJ, Wiese-Bjornstal DM, et al. Competitive athletes: preinjury and postinjury mood state and self-esteem. Mayo Clin Proc 1993;68(10): 939–47.
3. Podlog L, Eklund RC. A longitudinal investigation of competitive athletes' return to sport following serious injury. J Appl Sport Psychol 2006;18(1):44–68.
4. Wadey R, Evans L, Evans K, et al. Perceived benefits following sport injury: a qualitative examination of their antecedents and underlying mechanisms. J Appl Sport Psychol 2011;23(2):142–58.
5. Quinn AM, Fallon BJ. The changes in psychological characteristics and reactions of elite athletes from injury onset until full recovery. J Appl Sport Psychol 1999;11:210–29.

6. Tracey J. The emotional response to the injury and rehabilitation process. J Appl Sport Psychol 2003;15(4):279–93.
7. Podlog L, Eklund RC. Returning to competition after a serious injury: the role of self-determination. J Sports Sci 2010;28(8):819–31.
8. Albinson CB, Petrie T. Cognitive appraisals, stress, and coping: preinjury and postinjury factors influencing psychological adjustment to athletic injury. J Sport Rehabil 2003;12:306–22.
9. Alzate Saez de Heredia R, Ramirez A, Lazaro I. The effect of psychological response on recovery of sport injury. Res Sports Med 2004;12:15–31.
10. Bianco T, Malo S, Orlick T. Sport injury and illness: elite skiers describe their experiences. Res Q Exerc Sport 1999;70(2):157–69.
11. Green SL, Weinberg RS. Relationships among athletic identity, coping skills, social support, and the psychological impact of injury in recreational participants. J Appl Sport Psychol 2001;13:40–59.
12. Manuel JC, Shilt JS, Curl WW, et al. Coping with sports injuries: an examination of the adolescent athlete. J Adolesc Health 2002;31(5):391–3.
13. Smith AM, Scott SG, O'Fallon WM, et al. Emotional responses of athletes to injury. Mayo Clin Proc 1990;65(1):38–50.
14. Brewer BW. Self-identity and specific vulnerability to depressed mood. J Pers 1993;61(3):343–64.
15. Johnston LH, Carroll D. The context of emotional responses to athletic injury: a qualitative analysis. J Sport Rehabil 1998;7:206–20.
16. Sparkes AC. Athletic identity: an Achilles' heel to the survival of self. Qual Health Res 1998;8(5):644–64.
17. Brewer BW. Psychology of injury rehabilitation. In: Tenenbaum G, Eklund RC, editors. Handbook of sport psychology, vol. 3. Hoboken (NJ): John Wiley; 2007.
18. Morrey MA, Stuart MJ, Smith AM, et al. A longitudinal examination of athletes' emotional and cognitive responses to anterior cruciate ligament injury. Clin J Sport Med 1999;9(2):63–9.
19. Fisher AC, Domm MA, Wuest DA. Adherence to sports-injury rehabilitation programs. Phys Sportsmed 1988;16:47–52.
20. Brewer BW, Daly JM, Van Raalte JL, et al. A psychometric evaluation of the rehabilitation adherence questionnaire. J Sport Exerc Psychol 1999;21:167–73.
21. Wittig AF, Schurr KT. Psychological characteristics of women volleyball players: relationships with injuries, rehabilitation, and team success. Pers Soc Psychol Bull 1994;20(3):322–30.
22. Taylor AH, May S. Threat and coping appraisal as determinants of compliance with sports injury rehabilitation: an application of protection motivation theory. J Sports Sci 1996;14(6):471–82.
23. Murphy GC, Foreman PE, Simpson CA, et al. The development of a locus of control measure predictive of injured athletes' adherence to treatment. J Sci Med Sport 1999;2(2):145–52.
24. Milne M, Hall C, Forwell L. Self-efficacy, imagery use, and adherence to rehabilitation by injured athletes. J Sport Rehabil 2005;14:150–67.
25. Daly JM, Brewer BW, Van Raalte JL, et al. Cognitive appraisal, emotional adjustment, and adherence to rehabilitation following knee surgery. J Sport Rehabil 1995;4:23–30.
26. Lampton CC, Lambert ME, Yost R. The effects of psychological factors in sports medicine rehabilitation adherence. J Sports Med Phys Fitness 1993;33(3):292–9.
27. Walker N, Thatcher J, Lavallee D. A preliminary development of the Re-Injury Anxiety Inventory (RIAI). Phys Ther Sport 2010;11(1):23–9.

28. Brewer BW, Cornelius AE, Van Raalte JL, et al. Age-related differences in predictors of adherence to rehabilitation after anterior cruciate ligament reconstruction. J Athl Train 2003;38(2):158–62.

29. Brewer BW, Cornelius AE, van Raalte JL, et al. Comparison of concurrent and retrospective pain ratings during rehabilitation following anterior cruciate ligament reconstruction. J Sport Exerc Psychol 2004;26:610–5.

30. Brewer BW. The role of psychological factors in sport injury rehabilitation outcomes. Int Rev Sport Exerc Psychol 2010;3(1):40–61.

31. Pizzari T, Taylor NF, McBurney H, et al. Adherence to rehabilitation after anterior cruciate ligament reconstructive surgery: implications for outcome. J Sport Rehabil 2005;14:201–14.

32. Feller JA, Webster KE, Taylor NF, et al. Effect of physiotherapy attendance on outcome after anterior cruciate ligament reconstruction: a pilot study. Br J Sports Med 2004;38(1):74–7.

33. Scherzer CB, Brewer BW, Cornelius AE, et al. Psychological skills and adherence to rehabilitation after reconstruction of the anterior cruciate ligament. J Sport Rehabil 2001;10:165–72.

34. Evans L, Hardy L. Injury rehabilitation: a goal-setting intervention study. Res Q Exerc Sport 2002;73(3):310–9.

35. Udry E. Coping and social support among injured athletes following surgery. J Sport Exerc Psychol 1997;19:71–90.

36. Pizzari T, McBurney H, Taylor NF, et al. Adherence to anterior cruciate ligament reconstruction: a qualitative analysis. J Sport Rehabil 2002;11:90–102.

37. Johnston LH, Carroll D. Coping, social support, and injury: changes over time and the effects of level of sports involvement. J Sport Rehabil 2000;9:290–303.

38. Evans L, Hare R, Mullen R. Imagery use during rehabilitation from injury. J Imagery Res Sport Phys Activ 2006;1(1):1.

39. Ross MJ, Berger RS. Effects of stress inoculation training on athletes' postsurgical pain and rehabilitation after orthopedic injury. J Consult Clin Psychol 1996;64(2):406–10.

40. Bianco T, Eklund RC. Conceptual considerations for social support research in sport and exercise settings: the case of sport injury. J Sport Exerc Psychol 2001;23(2):85–107.

41. Brewer BW, Van Raalte JL, Petitpas AJ. Patient-practitioner interactions in sport injury rehabilitation. In: Pargman D, editor. Psychological bases of sport injuries, vol. 3. Morgantown (WV): Fitness Information Technology; 2007. p. 79–94.

42. Larson GA, Starkey CA, Zaichkowsky LD. Psychological aspects of athletic injuries as perceived by athletic trainers. Sport Psychol 1996;10:37–47.

43. Gordon S, Potter M, Ford IW. Toward a psychoeducational curriculum for training sport-injury rehabilitation personnel. J Appl Sport Psychol 1998;10:140–56.

44. Petitpas A, Cornelius A. Practitioner-client relationships: building working alliances. In: Kolt GS, Andersen MB, editors. Psychology in the physical and manual therapies. Edinburgh (Scotland): Churchill Livingstone; 2004. p. 57–70.

45. Wiese-Bjornstal DM, Gardetto DM, Shaffer SM. Effective interaction skills for sports medicine professionals. In: Ray R, Wiese-Bjornstal DM, editors. Counseling in sports medicine. Champaign (IL): Human Kinetics; 1999. p. 55–74.

46. Ray R, Terrell T, Hough D. The role of the sports medicine professional in counseling athletes. In: Ray R, Wiese-Bjornstal D, editors. Counseling in sports medicine. Champaign (IL): Human Kinetics; 1999. p. 3–20.

47. Granquist MD, Podlog L, Engel JR, et al. Certified athletic trainers' perspectives on rehabilitation adherence within collegiate athletic training settings. J Sport Rehabil 2014;23(2):123–33.

48. O'Connor EA, Heil J, Harmer P, et al. Injury. In: Taylor J, Wilson G, editors. Applying sport psychology: four perspectives. Champaign (IL): Human Kinetics; 2005. p. 187–206, 281–283.

49. Lysaght RM, Larmour-Trode S. An exploration of social support as a factor in the return-to-work process. Work 2008;30(3):255–66.

50. Hardy CJ, Burke KL, Crace RK. Social support and injury: a framework for support-based interventions with injured athletes. In: Pargman D, editor. Psychological bases of sport injuries, vol. 2. Morgantown (WV): Fitness Information Technology; 1999. p. 175–98.

51. Mitchell ID, Neil R, Wadey R, et al. Gender differences in athletes' social support during injury rehabilitation. J Sport Exerc Psychol 2009;29(Suppl):S189.

52. Bianco T. Social support and recovery from sport injury: elite skiers share their experiences. Res Q Exerc Sport 2001;72(4):376–88.

53. Gould D, Bridges D, Udry E, et al. Stress sources encountered when rehabilitating from season-ending ski injuries. Sport Psychol 1997;11(4):361–78.

54. Johnston LH, Carroll D. The provision of social support to injured athletes: a qualitative analysis. J Sport Rehabil 1998;7(4):267–84.

55. Robbins JE, Rosenfeld LB. Athletes' perceptions of social support provided by their head coach, assistant coach, and athletic trainer, pre-injury and during rehabilitation. J Sport Behav 2001;24:277–97.

56. Udry E, Gould D, Bridges D, et al. Down but not out: athlete responses to season-ending injuries. J Sport Exerc Psychol 1997;19:229–48.

57. Clement D, Shannon VR. Injured athletes' perceptions about social support. J Sport Rehabil 2011;20(4):457–70.

58. Podlog L, Dionigi R. Coach strategies for addressing psychosocial challenges during the return to sport from injury. J Sports Sci 2010;28(11):1197–208.

59. Taylor J, Stone KR, Mullin MJ, et al. Comprehensive sports injury management: from examination of injury to return to sport. Austin (TX): Pro-Ed; 2003.

60. Andersen MB. Returning to action and the prevention of future injury. In: Crossman J, editor. Coping with sports injuries: psychological strategies for rehabilitation. Melbourne (Australia): Oxford University Press; 2001.

61. Ardern CL, Webster KE, Taylor NF, et al. Return to sport following anterior cruciate ligament reconstruction surgery: a systematic review and meta-analysis of the state of play. Br J Sports Med 2011;45(7):596–606.

62. Podlog L, Eklund RC. The psychosocial aspects of a return to sport following serious injury: a review of the literature from a self-determination perspective. Psychol Sport Exerc 2007;8:535–66.

63. Creighton DW, Shrier I, Shultz R, et al. Return-to-play in sport: a decision-based model. Clin J Sport Med 2010;20(5):379–85.

64. Glazer DD. Development and preliminary validation of the Injury-Psychological Readiness to Return to Sport (I-PRRS) scale. J Athl Train 2009;44(2):185–9.

65. Heil J. Psychology of sport injury. Champaign (IL): Human Kinetics; 1993.

66. Kubler-Ross E. On death and dying: what the dying have to teach doctors, nurses, clergy, and their own families. New York: Macmillan; 1969.

67. Hanin YL. Emotions in Sport. Champaign (IL): Human Kinetics; 2000.

68. Heil J, Podlog L. Injury and performance. In: Murphy S, editor. The Oxford handbook of sport and performance psychology. New York (NY): Oxford University Press; 2012.

69. Billings AG, Moos RH. The role of coping responses and social resources in attenuating the stress of life events. J Behav Med 1981;4(2):139–57.
70. Armstrong L, Jenkins S. It's not about the bike: my journey back to life. New York: Putnam; 2000.
71. Ogilvie BC, Tutko TA. Problem athletes and how to handle them. London: Palham Books; 1966.
72. Heil J. Association-dissociation: clarifying the concept. Paper presented at: Association for the Advancement of Applied Sport Psychology Annual Conference. San Antonio. October 1990.
73. Crust L. Should distance runners concentrate on their bodily sensations, or try to think of something else? Sports Injury Bulletin 2003;30:10–2.
74. Brewer BW, Van Raalte JL, Linder DE. Attentional focus and endurance performance. Applied Research in Coaching and Athletics Annual 1996;11:1–14.
75. Masters KS, Ogles BM. Associative and dissociative cognitive strategies in exercise and running: 20 years later, what do we know? Sport Psychol 1998; 12:253–70.

Index

Note: Page numbers of article titles are in **boldface** type.

Phys Med Rehabil Clin N Am 25 (2014) 931–942
http://dx.doi.org/10.1016/S1047-9651(14)00093-X
1047-9651/14/$ – see front matter © 2014 Elsevier Inc. All rights reserved.

United States Postal Service

Statement of Ownership, Management, and Circulation
(All Periodicals Publications Except Requestor Publications)

1. Publication Title
Physical Medicine and Rehabilitation Clinics of North America

2. Publication Number
0 0 9 - 2 4 3

3. Filing Date
9/14/14

4. Issue Frequency
Feb, May, Aug, Nov

5. Number of Issues Published Annually
4

6. Annual Subscription Price
$275.00

7. Complete Mailing Address of Known Office of Publication (Not printer) (Street, city, county, state, and ZIP+4®)
Elsevier Inc.
360 Park Avenue South
New York, NY 10010-1710

Contact Person
Stephen R. Bushing

Telephone (Include area code)
215-239-3688

8. Complete Mailing Address of Headquarters or General Business Office of Publisher (Not printer)
Elsevier Inc., 360 Park Avenue South, New York, NY 10010-1710

9. Full Names and Complete Mailing Addresses of Publisher, Editor, and Managing Editor (Do not leave blank)

Publisher (Name and complete mailing address)
Linda Belfus, Elsevier Inc., 1600 John F. Kennedy Blvd, Suite 1800, Philadelphia, PA 19103-2899

Editor (Name and complete mailing address)
Jennifer Flynn-Briggs, Elsevier Inc., 1600 John F. Kennedy Blvd., Suite 1800, Philadelphia, PA 19103-2899

Managing Editor (Name and complete mailing address)
Barbara Cohen-Kligerman, Elsevier Inc., 1600 John F. Kennedy Blvd., Suite 1800, Philadelphia, PA 19103-2899

10. Owner (Do not leave blank. If the publication is owned by a corporation, give the name and address of the corporation immediately followed by the names and addresses of all stockholders owning or holding 1 percent or more of the total amount of stock. If not owned by a corporation, give the names and addresses of the individual owners. If owned by a partnership or other unincorporated firm, give its name and address as well as those of each individual owner. If the publication is published by a nonprofit organization, give its name and address.)

Full Name	Complete Mailing Address
Wholly owned subsidiary of	1600 John F. Kennedy Blvd, Ste. 1800
Reed/Elsevier, US holdings	Philadelphia, PA 19103-2899

11. Known Bondholders, Mortgagees, and Other Security Holders Owning or Holding 1 Percent or More of Total Amount of Bonds, Mortgages, or Other Securities. If none, check box   ☐ None

Full Name	Complete Mailing Address
N/A	

12. Tax Status (For completion by nonprofit organizations authorized to mail at nonprofit rates) (Check one)
The purpose, function, and nonprofit status of this organization and the exempt status for federal income tax purposes:
☐ Has Not Changed During Preceding 12 Months
☐ Has Changed During Preceding 12 Months (Publisher must submit explanation of change with this statement)

PS Form 3526, August 2012 (Page 1 of 3 (Instructions Page 3)) PSN 7530-01-000-9931 **PRIVACY NOTICE:** See our Privacy policy in www.usps.com

---

13. Publication Title
Physical Medicine and Rehabilitation Clinics of North America

14. Issue Date for Circulation Data Below
August 2014

15. Extent and Nature of Circulation

			Average No. Copies Each Issue During Preceding 12 Months	No. Copies of Single Issue Published Nearest to Filing Date
a. Total Number of Copies (Net press run)			661	616
b. Paid Circulation (By Mail and Outside the Mail)	(1)	Mailed Outside-County Paid Subscriptions Stated on PS Form 3541. (Include paid distribution above nominal rate, advertiser's proof copies, and exchange copies)	409	377
	(2)	Mailed In-County Paid Subscriptions Stated on PS Form 3541 (Include paid distribution above nominal rate, advertiser's proof copies, and exchange copies)		
	(3)	Paid Distribution Outside the Mails Including Sales Through Dealers and Carriers, Street Vendors, Counter Sales, and Other Paid Distribution Outside USPS®	97	94
	(4)	Paid Distribution by Other Classes Mailed Through the USPS (e.g. First-Class Mail®)		
c. Total Paid Distribution (Sum of 15b (1), (2), (3), and (4))			506	471
d. Free or Nominal Rate Distribution (By Mail and Outside the Mail)	(1)	Free or Nominal Rate Outside-County Copies Included on PS Form 3541	52	65
	(2)	Free or Nominal Rate In-County Copies Included on PS Form 3541		
	(3)	Free or Nominal Rate Copies Mailed at Other Classes Through the USPS (e.g. First-Class Mail)		
	(4)	Free or Nominal Rate Distribution Outside the Mail (Carriers or other means)		
e. Total Free or Nominal Rate Distribution (Sum of 15d (1), (2), (3) and (4))			52	65
f. Total Distribution (Sum of 15c and 15e)			558	536
g. Copies not Distributed (See instructions to publishers #4 (page #3))			103	80
h. Total (Sum of 15f and g)			661	616
i. Percent Paid (15c divided by 15f times 100)			90.68%	87.87%

16 Total circulation includes electronic copies. Report circulation on PS Form 3526-X worksheet.

17. Publication of Statement of Ownership
If the publication is a general publication, publication of this statement is required. Will be printed in the **November 2014** issue of this publication.

18. Signature and Title of Editor, Publisher, Business Manager, or Owner

[signature]

Stephen R. Bushing – Inventory Distribution Coordinator

Date
September 14, 2014

I certify that all information furnished on this form is true and complete. I understand that anyone who furnishes false or misleading information on this form or who omits material or information requested on the form may be subject to criminal sanctions (including fines and imprisonment) and/or civil sanctions (including civil penalties).

PS Form 3526, August 2012 (Page 2 of 3)

Printed and bound by CPI Group (UK) Ltd, Croydon, CR0 4YY

03/10/2024

01040485-0006